Nutrients
and
Epigenetics

Nutrients *and* Epigenetics

Edited by
Sang-Woon Choi
Simonetta Friso

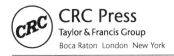

CRC Press
Taylor & Francis Group
Boca Raton London New York

CRC Press is an imprint of the
Taylor & Francis Group, an **informa** business

Cover illustration by Andrea Friso.

CRC Press
Taylor & Francis Group
6000 Broken Sound Parkway NW, Suite 300
Boca Raton, FL 33487-2742

First issued in paperback 2019

ISBN-13: 978-1-4200-6354-7 (hbk)
ISBN-13: 978-0-367-38564-4 (pbk)

Library of Congress Cataloging-in-Publication Data

Nutrients and epigenetics / [edited by] Sang-Woon Choi and Simonetta Friso.
    p. ; cm.
  Includes bibliographical references and index.
  ISBN-13: 978-1-4200-6354-7 (hardcover : alk. paper)
  ISBN-10: 1-4200-6354-5 (hardcover : alk. paper)
  1. Nutrition--Genetic aspects. 2. Nutrient interactions. 3. Genetic regulation. 4. Epigenesis. I. Choi, Sang-Woon. II. Friso, Simonetta.
  [DNLM: 1. Micronutrients--genetics. 2. Chromatin Assembly and Disassembly. 3. DNA Methylation. 4. Epigenesis, Genetic. 5. Histone Code. 6. Nucleosomes--genetics. QU 130.5 N976 2009]

QP144.G45.N876 2009
613.2--dc22
                                                     2008048754

Visit the Taylor & Francis Web site at
http://www.taylorandfrancis.com

and the CRC Press Web site at
http://www.crcpress.com

Contents

Preface

Overt nutritional deficiency diseases, once common worldwide, are difficult to find in developed countries. Some people think nutritional deficiencies are no longer a problem. However, there is evidence indicating that the prevalence of subclinical or marginal deficiencies is higher than expected. These deficiencies are risk factors of chronic diseases such as cancer, neurodegenerative disorders and cardiovascular diseases in the elderly. These deficiencies also pose a problem during development as maternal nutritional insufficiency may increase the risk of an individual developing certain diseases later in life. We expect that current mandatory fortification programs may reduce both the overt and marginal deficiencies of some micronutrients, thus reducing the resulting chronic diseases.

However, recent clinical trials have demonstrated that supplementation with certain nutrients cannot effectively reduce the risk of recurrent cardiovascular diseases or cancers and high levels of supplementation may even be exacerbating the disease process. This evidence highlights the need for further mechanistic research and knowledge regarding nutrients and disease processes. We need to know more about the effects of specific nutrients, especially their function at the molecular level where genes are controlled. Nutrients are not simply food ingredients; they can directly affect the expression of genes that are associated with the development of chronic diseases. In this book we therefore describe how nutrients modulate gene expression through epigenetics, a new mechanism attributed to physiologic and pathologic processes.

Epigenetics refers to the study of heritable changes in gene expression that are not caused by DNA base changes. The epigenetic gene regulatory machinery is responsible for establishing and maintaining diverse patterns of gene expression. Epigenetics is receiving more attention in the field of molecular biology and is regarded as a critical mechanism for embryonic development, aging and carcinogenesis. Throughout life, nutrition influences epigenetic gene regulation and by exploiting this relationship, disease processes associated with epigenetic phenomena can be modulated.

This book has been compiled to update readers about the interrelationships between nutrition and epigenetic phenomena, such as DNA methylation, histone modifications and chromatin remodeling. The book also presents the latest information regarding the role of epigenetics in embryonic development, aging, inflammation and the development of cancer, and it describes how nutrients affect those physiologic and pathologic processes through the modulation of epigenetic phenomena. The importance of fostering future research in this specific field is also emphasized.

We are very grateful to all our authors who enthusiastically dedicated themselves to their respective chapters. We hope our readers gain new knowledge by reading this book and continue to study this exciting field.

The Editors

Sang-Woon Choi is Scientist I at the Jean Mayer United States Department of Agriculture (USDA) Human Nutrition Research Center on Aging at Tufts University and Associate Professor at the Friedman School of Nutrition Science and Policy. He graduated from the College of Medicine, Seoul National University, and received medical training in internal medicine and gastroenterology at the Seoul National University Hospital in Korea. He earned a master's degree in 1988 and a Ph.D. in 1992 from the same university. His research interest during that time was the association between hepatitis B virus infection and the development of primary liver cancer.

To pursue a particular interest in the association between nutrition and cancer, he joined the Jean Mayer USDA Human Nutrition Research Center in 1993. For the past fifteen years, Dr. Choi's research has focused on the question of how one-carbon nutrients, such as folate and vitamin B-12, modulate the process of carcinogenesis. He has focused primarily on epigenetic mechanisms such as DNA methylation and histone modifications, as well as molecular mechanisms underlying nutrient and gene interactions implicated in carcinogenesis, to elucidate the potential chemopreventive properties of one-carbon nutrients. Since age is an important determinant of cancer risk, he has also developed a particular interest in the genetic and epigenetic interactions between aging and nutrients in carcinogenesis.

In 2006 he published, with Dr. Simonetta Friso, a book entitled *Nutrient and Gene Interactions in Cancer* (CRC Press, the Taylor & Francis Publishing Group). He has also authored many outstanding research publications and numerous book chapters and reviews. Owing to his dedication to nutrition research as evidenced through his publications, he received the Director's Scientific Recognition Award in 2006 from the Jean Mayer USDA Human Nutrition Research Center and the Mead Johnson Award in 2008 from the American Society for Nutrition.

Simonetta Friso is Assistant Professor of Internal Medicine at the University of Verona School of Medicine in Italy. She graduated in 1991 from the University of Verona School of Medicine with a thesis on protein function and co-transport systems in red blood cell membrane. In 1996 she obtained the Specialization in Internal Medicine after five years of training at the Verona University Hospital. Her dissertation was on the role of emergent risk factors in thrombophilic status. During that period she dedicated her research work to the study of molecular mechanisms underlying thromboembolic disorders, with particular interest in the identification of novel genetic aberrations affecting coagulation factors, thereby deepening her interest in molecular biology and genetics. The study of gene-nutrient interactions within one-carbon metabolism and their effects on DNA methylation was the topic of her doctoral thesis to obtain the Ph.D. in Experimental Hematology from the National University of Milan in Italy. She then started to focus her research work on the field of gene-nutrient interactions and epigenetics. She developed her interest in the area of nutrition and genetics as a Visiting Scientist at the Jean Mayer USDA Human Nutrition Research Center at Tufts University in Boston between 1998 and 2002. She is the author of several research articles and of a book on nutrient-gene interactions and cancer. She received the 2002 Hamish N. Munro Postdoctoral Fellowship Award for outstanding scientific research on folate metabolism, genetics and DNA methylation, and, in 2006, the Director's Scientific Recognition Award at the Jean Mayer USDA Human Nutrition Research Center at Tufts University for excellence in scientific impact in gene-nutrient interactions and epigenetics.

In recent years she has committed her research work to the identification of molecular mechanisms underlying the interrelationships between nutrients and genes and epigenetics, with her main interest being the effects of B vitamins and polymorphic genes within one-carbon metabolism on DNA methylation, a major epigenetic feature of DNA involved in carcinogenesis and other chronic diseases.

Contributors

Michael J. Boland, Ph.D.
University of Nebraska Medical
  Center
Omaha, Nebraska

Xiaodong Cheng, Ph.D.
Emory University School of
  Medicine
Atlanta, Georgia

Sang-Woon Choi, M.D., Ph.D.
Jean Mayer USDA Human
  Nutrition Research Center on
  Aging at Tufts University
Boston, Massachusetts

Judith K. Christman, Ph.D.
University of Nebraska Medical
  Center
Omaha, Nebraska

Craig A. Cooney, Ph.D.
University of Arkansas for
  Medical Sciences
Little Rock, Arkansas

Roberto Corrocher, M.D.
University of Verona School of
  Medicine
Verona, Italy

Roderick H. Dashwood, Ph.D.
Linus Pauling Institute
Oregon State University
Corvallis, Oregon

Barbara Delage, Ph.D.
Linus Pauling Institute
Oregon State University
Corvallis, Oregon

Dianne Ford, Ph.D.
Human Nutrition Research
  Center
Newcastle University
Newcastle upon Tyne, UK

Simonetta Friso, M.D., Ph.D.
University of Verona School of
  Medicine
Verona, Italy

Da Jia, Ph.D.
Emory University School of
  Medicine
Atlanta, Georgia

John C. Mathers, Ph.D.
Human Nutrition Research Center
Newcastle University
Newcastle upon Tyne, UK

Sharon A. Ross, Ph.D.
National Cancer Institute
National Institutes of Health
Department of Health and
  Human Services
Bethesda, Maryland

Gavin R. Schnitzler, Ph.D.
Tufts University School of
  Medicine
Boston, Massachusetts

chapter one

Introduction

Simonetta Friso and Sang-Woon Choi

Contents

1.1   *Nutrition-epigenetics-phenotype relationship*

A recent study showed that honeybees grow to be either queens or workers depending on whether they are fed royal jelly or beebread.[1] Despite being genetically identical at the larvae level, honeybees fed pure royal jelly are markedly different from worker honeybees. The different honeybee phenotype occurs through epigenetic changes in DNA methylation patterns induced by the type of honey they are fed with, therefore illustrating a strong link between diet-induced epigenetic changes that lead to different development from the same genetic background.[1]

Another paradigmatic example of the nutrient-epigenetic-phenotype relationship is that of the Agouti mouse model where the maternal methyl dietary content affects the coat color of the rodent offspring as well as alters the susceptibility of the animal to certain chronic diseases such as obesity and cancer.[2–4] Additionally, other studies in mammals suggest that environmental *stimuli* such as exposure to different dietary factors can modify DNA methylation and histone acetylation patterns and, therefore, affect gene regulation and the phenotypic expression of a gene.

It is well known that many organisms may respond to different environmental/nutritional factors by exhibiting phenotypic plasticity, meaning that their phenotype may be modified by the nutritional modulations of epigenetic mechanisms.

1.2   The origin of epigenetics

The meaning of *epigenetics* currently refers to genome information that is *super*-imposed on the DNA sequence. The word derives originally from *epigenesis*, a philosophical concept that brings us back to the Greek philosopher Aristotle. Through the theory of *epigenesis*, Aristotle in his book *On the Generation of Animals*, expressed the concept of the progressive differentiation trait of a vital organism, in which its *form*, namely its *being*, emerges to a phenotype from the *unformed*. This conception developed to explain the growth of an organism in contrast to the theory of *preformation*, a different philosophical view sustained by the Greek philosophers Democritus and Leucippus. The idea of preformation implies that the adult organism is already contained in a predetermined status that influences development, as if the embryo is a predelineated miniature of the adult itself. Although quite different from the modern concept of epigenetics, the theory of *epigenesis* expresses the morphogenesis of a vital being through a sequence of progressive steps in which cells and organs differentiate towards the process of development.

When the term *epigenetics* was first proposed by Waddington in the early 1940s it was used to describe "the interactions of genes with their environment, which bring the phenotype into being,"[5] thereby signifying the origin of the phenotype from the genotype, a process that is also influenced by the environment.

It is indeed attractive to pursue scientific research interest toward the interaction between epigenetics and environmental factors, among which a fascinating function is related to the role, at the molecular level, of dietary factors. Advances in this area of research may certainly highlight novel mechanisms of disease pathogenesis and treatment.

1.3   Relationship between genetics
and epigenetics

The maintenance of normal cell homeostasis is regulated by complex mechanisms. Among them is the regulation of gene expression through epigenetic phenomena.[6,7] Epigenetics is now recognized as one of the most important mechanisms in regulating gene function and is responsible for the preservation of patterns of gene expression for different cell types. The way that each cell or organism determines its path through development,[8,9] aging[10,11] or even disease[12,13] is not encoded only in the genome but also in the epigenome code which defines whether, and when, a gene will be programmed to be active or silent despite having the same DNA sequence. One example that implicates epigenetics as a key player is the different disease predisposition, despite identical genomic patrimony, observed in studies of identical monozygotic twins.[14] Epigenetic mechanisms may be considered complementary to genetic functions that modulate gene expression regulation but they can be better defined as the way by which a specific cell or tissue interprets the genome information. It is currently unquestionable that the complete mapping of the genome is just the beginning of the path toward the understanding of gene function, since genetic aberrations alone cannot explain the genesis of many physiological and pathological processes.[15] Due to the convincing implications for possible therapeutic strategies through epigenetics, it is imperative that the interrelationships between genetics, epigenetics and environmental factors are investigated further.[16]

1.4   *Different types of epigenetic phenomena*

DNA methylation and posttranslational modifications of histones have been considered to be the two major epigenetic mechanisms that affect phenotype, but there are many other epigenetic mechanisms, including genomic imprinting, X-chromosome inactivation, small and noncoding RNAs and nucleosome remodeling pattern regulation.[17] The control of gene transcription through DNA methylation and histone modifications are strongly connected to one another in a complex interplay in the nucleosome structure.[18–22] The dynamic functional machinery of chromatin regulation is established by a strict link between DNA methyltransferases, histone tail modifying enzymes and nucleosome-remodeling proteins that eventually decide the chromatin structure and thus regulate gene expression.[21] Nutrients may affect each of the epigenetic steps, providing several possible ways through which nutrients may interfere with the epigenetic machinery.[23]

Epigenetic changes in DNA and chromatin structure are heritable,[24] although they express this characteristic in a dynamic manner. During the division process, the cell remembers the epigenetic mark but, at the same time, such mark can also be modified by environmental factors.[25] Typical epigenetic marks consist of those phenomena that determine the specificity of each tissue and the difference between germ cells and somatic cells as well as between malignant cells and normal cells. Such epigenetic phenomena do not involve alterations in the DNA nucleotide sequence but yet are responsible for the genome function and stability as well as for the prevention of gene disruption and translocations, such as those seen in cancer disease.[26–28] Epigenetic phenomena are also very important for both embryonic development and aging processes where it is known that appropriate nutritional support is a key factor.

1.5   Nutrients, bioactive food components, and epigenetics

Several studies have shown that a number of nutrients and bioactive components affect the pathways involved in gene regulation via epigenetic mechanisms and various modalities were proposed to explain the role of nutrients on DNA methylation.[23] Yet, little is known about the exact mechanisms through which nutrients modulate epigenetics; therefore, it is of great importance to deepen our understanding of the relationship between nutrients and epigenetics on disease pathogenesis with the aim of opening up a novel field for innovative therapeutic strategies. The reversibility of epigenetic phenomena makes them a very intriguing target for altering genome patterns possibly involved in a number of diseases. Most of the studies regard cancer as a disease caused by disordered expression of certain genes that control cell proliferation and differentiation, nudging the cell toward tumorigenesis.[29] A number of trials using epigenetic drugs that modify disordered epigenetic phenomena are already ongoing, with promising results, but a more physiological approach through nutritional modulation also appears to have appealing and fascinating perspectives.

Most of the knowledge regarding the epigenetic modulation of gene expression induced by nutritional factors refers to one-carbon nutrients and metabolites that serve as methyl donors for the universal methyl donor, S-adenosylmethionine whose end product is S-adenosylhomocysteine, an inhibitor of methyltransferases.[10,23,30] To date the role of nutrients in epigenetic mechanisms has been addressed through the function of one-carbon metabolism, donation of methyl groups[31] to DNA and histone tail methylation reactions[32] catalyzed by DNA and histone methyltransferases.[33–35] Most of the knowledge pertains to the function of folate and vitamin B-12 in providing methyl groups for DNA methylation reaction.[36,37] However, other micronutrients or bioactive food components have also implicated in playing a role in epigenetic mechanisms through one-carbon metabolism or by directly affecting the enzymes involved in regulating epigenetic phenomena.

The scope of this book is to focus on the novel attractive roles of nutritional factors in epigenetic mechanisms and their effects on physiologic and pathologic processes. Why is this topic so intriguing? Certainly because epigenetics, although inherited, is reversible; therefore, it is potentially modifiable, also by nutrients. Little is known, however, about nutrition and epigenetic relationships, especially the mechanisms through which nutrients may modulate epigenetics. The growing interest in epigenetics[38] is opening up this fascinating field with captivating insight into the pathogenesis of several diseases, which may lead, hopefully, to therapeutic possibilities.

References

1. Kucharski, R., Maleszka, J., Foret, S., and Maleszka, R. (2008). Nutritional control of reproductive status in honeybees via DNA methylation. *Science* 319, 1827–1830.
2. Wolff, G. L., Kodell, R. L., Moore, S. R., and Cooney, C. A. (1998). Maternal epigenetics and methyl supplements affect agouti gene expression in Avy/a mice. *FASEB J* 12, 949–957.
3. Cooney, C. A., Dave, A. A., and Wolff, G. L. (2002). Maternal methyl supplements in mice affect epigenetic variation and DNA methylation of offspring. *J Nutr* 132, 2393S–2400S.
4. Cropley, J. E., Suter, C. M., Beckman, K. B., and Martin, D. I. (2006). Germ-line epigenetic modification of the murine A vy allele by nutritional supplementation. *Proc Natl Acad Sci USA* 103, 17308–17312.
5. Waddington, C. H. (1942). The epigenotype. *Endeavour* 1, 18–20.
6. Bird, A. (2007). Perceptions of epigenetics. *Nature* 447, 396–398.
7. Jaenisch, R., and Bird, A. (2003). Epigenetic regulation of gene expression: How the genome integrates intrinsic and environmental signals. *Nat Genet* 33 Suppl, 245–254.
8. Lunyak, V. V., and Rosenfeld, M. G. (2008). Epigenetic regulation of stem cell fate. *Hum Mol Genet* 17, R28–R36.
9. Chen, L., and Daley, G. Q. (2008). Molecular basis of pluripotency. *Hum Mol Genet* 17, R23–R27.
10. Choi, S. W., Friso, S., Keyes, M. K., and Mason, J. B. (2005). Folate supplementation increases genomic DNA methylation in the liver of elder rats. *Br J Nutr* 93, 31–35.
11. Fraga, M. F., and Esteller, M. (2007). Epigenetics and aging: The targets and the marks. *Trends Genet* 23, 413–418.
12. Jones, P. A., and Baylin, S. B. (2002). The fundamental role of epigenetic events in cancer. *Nat Rev Genet* 3, 415–428.
13. Laird, P. W. (2003). The power and the promise of DNA methylation markers. *Nat Rev Cancer* 3, 253–266.
14. Fraga, M. F., Ballestar, E., Paz, M. F., Ropero, S., Setien, F., Ballestar, M. L., Heine-Suner, D., Cigudosa, J. C., Urioste, M., Benitez, J., Boix-Chornet, M., Sanchez-Aguilera, A., Ling, C., Carlsson, E., Poulsen, P., Vaag, A., Stephan, Z., Spector, T. D., Wu, Y. Z., Plass, C., and Esteller, M. (2005). Epigenetic differences arise during the lifetime of monozygotic twins. *Proc Natl Acad Sci USA* 102, 10604–10609.
15. Robertson, K. D., and Wolffe, A. P. (2000). DNA methylation in health and disease. *Nat Rev Genet* 1, 11–19.
16. Egger, G., Liang, G., Aparicio, A., and Jones, P. A. (2004). Epigenetics in human disease and prospects for epigenetic therapy. *Nature* 429, 457–463.
17. Turner, B. M. (2007). Defining an epigenetic code. *Nat Cell Biol* 9, 2–6.
18. Kouzarides, T. (2007). Chromatin modifications and their function. *Cell* 128, 693–705.
19. Goldberg, A. D., Allis, C. D., and Bernstein, E. (2007). Epigenetics: A landscape takes shape. *Cell* 128, 635–638.
20. Bernstein, B. E., Meissner, A., and Lander, E. S. (2007). The mammalian epigenome. *Cell* 128, 669–681.

21. Tong, J. K., Hassig, C. A., Schnitzler, G. R., Kingston, R. E., and Schreiber, S. L. (1998). Chromatin deacetylation by an ATP-dependent nucleosome remodelling complex. *Nature* 395, 917–921.
22. Ulyanova, N. P., and Schnitzler, G. R. (2005). Human SWI/SNF generates abundant, structurally altered dinucleosomes on polynucleosomal templates. *Mol Cell Biol* 25, 11156–11170.
23. Ross, S. A. (2003). Diet and DNA methylation interactions in cancer prevention. *Ann NY Acad Sci* 983, 197–207.
24. Wolffe, A. P. (1994). Inheritance of chromatin states. *Dev Genet* 15, 463–470.
25. Wolffe, A. P., and Matzke, M. A. (1999). Epigenetics: Regulation through repression. *Science* 286, 481–486.
26. Baylin, S. B., Esteller, M., Rountree, M. R., Bachman, K. E., Schuebel, K., and Herman, J. G. (2001). Aberrant patterns of DNA methylation, chromatin formation and gene expression in cancer. *Hum Mol Genet* 10, 687–692.
27. Esteller, M. (2008). Epigenetics in cancer. *N Engl J Med* 358, 1148–1159.
28. Jones, P. A., and Baylin, S. B. (2007). The epigenomics of cancer. *Cell* 128, 683–692.
29. Wiseman, M. (2008). The second World Cancer Research Fund/American Institute for Cancer Research expert report. Food, nutrition, physical activity, and the prevention of cancer: A global perspective. *Proc Nutr Soc* 67, 253–256.
30. Balaghi, M., and Wagner, C. (1993). DNA methylation in folate deficiency: Use of CpG methylase. *Biochem Biophys Res Commun* 193, 1184–1190.
31. Wainfan, E., Dizik, M., Stender, M., and Christman, J. K. (1989). Rapid appearance of hypomethylated DNA in livers of rats fed cancer-promoting, methyl-deficient diets. *Cancer Res* 49, 4094–4097.
32. Friso, S., and Choi, S. W. (2002). Gene-nutrient interactions and DNA methylation. *J Nutr* 132, 2382S–2387S.
33. O'Gara, M., Zhang, X., Roberts, R. J., and Cheng, X. (1999). Structure of a binary complex of HhaI methyltransferase with S-adenosyl-L-methionine formed in the presence of a short non-specific DNA oligonucleotide. *J Mol Biol* 287, 201–209.
34. Ooi, S. K., Qiu, C., Bernstein, E., Li, K., Jia, D., Yang, Z., Erdjument-Bromage, H., Tempst, P., Lin, S. P., Allis, C. D., Cheng, X., and Bestor, T. H. (2007). DNMT3L connects unmethylated lysine 4 of histone H3 to de novo methylation of DNA. *Nature* 448, 714–717.
35. Zhang, X., Yang, Z., Khan, S. I., Horton, J. R., Tamaru, H., Selker, E. U., and Cheng, X. (2003). Structural basis for the product specificity of histone lysine methyltransferases. *Mol Cell* 12, 177–185.
36. Choi, S. W., Friso, S., Ghandour, H., Bagley, P. J., Selhub, J., and Mason, J. B. (2004). Vitamin B-12 deficiency induces anomalies of base substitution and methylation in the DNA of rat colonic epithelium. *J Nutr* 134, 750–755.
37. Brunaud, L., Alberto, J. M., Ayav, A., Gerard, P., Namour, F., Antunes, L., Braun, M., Bronowicki, J. P., Bresler, L., and Gueant, J. L. (2003). Vitamin B12 is a strong determinant of low methionine synthase activity and DNA hypomethylation in gastrectomized rats. *Digestion* 68, 133–140.
38. American Association for Cancer Research Human Epigenome Task Force; European Union, Network of Excellence, Scientific Advisory Board. (2008). Moving AHEAD with an international human epigenome project. *Nature* 454, 711–715.

chapter two

Methylation on the nucleosome
From DNA to histone

Da Jia and Xiaodong Cheng

Contents

2.1   Introduction

With the completion of the human genome sequence and the genomes of other model organisms used in basic and translational research, the future focuses on understanding functional roles for gene products (proteins) in cellular physiology and pathology, in particular oncogenesis, metastasis, and biomarkers. Proteomics, epigenetics, and transcriptional regulation dominate biomedical research headlines today and will continue to do so in coming decades.

Nucleosomes—the fundamental building blocks of all eukaryotic chromatin—consist of ~146 base pairs of DNA wrapped twice around a histone octamer[1] (Figure 2.1a). Chromatin, rather than being a passive platform to store genetic information, can regulate transcriptional processes based on its modifications on both components: DNA and histones. In mammals, DNA methylation occurs at the C5 position of cytosine mostly within the context of a CpG dinucleotide (Figure 2.1b).

Histones are posttranslationally modified by various enzymatic reactions, including methylation, primarily at their flexible N-termini. These modifications play an important role in modulating chromatin structure, and thus regulate gene expression, DNA repair, DNA recombination, and many other chromatin-dependent processes.[2] Histone methylation can occur in lysine or arginine residues (Figures 2.1c and 2.1d). Both DNA and histone methylation are *S*-adenosyl-L-methionine dependent. AdoMet (also called SAdoMet, SAM, or SAMe) is the second most used enzymatic cofactor after ATP and is one of the hottest (and expensive) food supplements currently on the market. However, the real benefits and risks of AdoMet as a nutrient are still unclear.

DNA methylation, together with histone modifications, defines epigenetic programs. Epigenetic mechanisms are responsible for maintaining the patterns of gene expression for different cell types.[3] Many biological phenomena, including genomic imprinting, gene silencing, X chromosome inactivation, position effect, reprogramming, and the progress of carcinogenesis, are epigenetic processes. DNA methylation and histone modifications are intricately connected with each other. For example, mouse ES cells that lack the H3 lysine 9 (H3K9) methyltransferases Suv39h1 and Suv39h2 show slight demethylation of satellite DNA.[4] Methylation of histone H3 lysine 4 (H3K4) has been suggested to protect gene promoters from de novo DNA methylation in somatic cells.[5,6] The mammalian de novo DNA methylation machinery, the Dnmt3L-Dnmt3a complex—required for the de novo methylation of imprinting control regions in female germ cells and for the de novo methylation of dispersed repeated sequences in male germ cells—could convert patterns of histone H3 lysine 4 methylation, which are not known to be transmitted by mitotic inheritance, into patterns of DNA methylation that mediate the heritable transcriptional silencing of the affected sequences.[7]

There are many recent reviews in the field of histone lysine methylation and demethylation, DNA methylation and epigenetics.[8–13] Here, we summarize the most recent structural and biochemical advances in the field. In particular, we focus on the structural features that contribute to the specificity of the enzymes, which are responsible for generation and recognition of chromatin modifications.

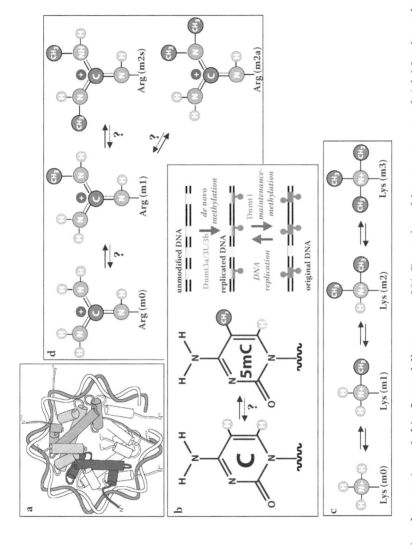

Figure 2.1 (A color version of this figure follows page 20.) Examples of known targets of AdoMet-dependent methylation. (a) A model of nucleosome. (b) DNA cytosine methylation at ring carbon C5 position. (c) Protein lysine methylation, and (d) protein arginine methylation. Note: only the deprotonated amino group (NH₂) has a free lone pair of electrons capable of nucleophilic attack on the AdoMet methyl group.

2.2   DNA methylation

2.2.1   Mammalian DNA methyltransferases

In mammals, DNA methyltransferases (Dnmts) consist of four members that form two distinguished families: Dnmt1 and Dnmt3 (Figure 2.2a). Although Dnmt3 is responsible for establishing the initial de novo methylation pattern, Dnmt1 maintains this pattern during the cell cycle[14] (Figure 2.1b).

The Dnmt3 family consists of two active de novo Dnmts, Dnmt3a and Dnmt3b, and one regulatory factor, Dnmt3-like protein (Dnmt3L)[15] (Figure 2.2a). Dnmt3a and Dnmt3b have a similar domain arrangement: both contain a variable region at the N-terminus followed by a PWWP domain, a Cys-rich 3-zinc binding domain (six CXXC motifs), and a C-terminal catalytic domain. Dnmt3L shares a high degree of sequence similarity with Dnmt3a and Dnmt3b in the Cys-rich 3-zinc binding domain but lacks the conserved residues required for DNA methyltransferase activity in the C-terminal domain. DNMT2, a protein annotated historically based on its high sequence and structure similarity to known DNA methyltransferases,[16] methylates cytosine 38 in the anticodon loop of tRNA^{Asp} (Figure 2.2b).[17]

At the time of this writing (October 2007), no structural information is available for any part of Dnmt1, while structures are available for the PWWP domain of Dnmt3b[18] (Figure 2.2c), the full-length Dnmt3L in complex with histone H3 peptide[7] (Figure 2.2d), and a complex between the C-terminal domains of Dnmt3a and Dnmt3L[19] (Figure 2.3).

2.2.2   Dnmt3L is a regulatory factor for de novo DNA methylation

The phenotype of Dnmt3L knockout mice is indistinguishable from that of Dnmt3a conditional knockout with altered sex-specific de novo methylation of DNA sequences in male and female germ cells.[20–22] These results indicate that Dnmt3a and Dnmt3L are both required for the methylation of the most imprinted loci in germ cells. Dnmt3L that co-localizes and co-immunoprecipitates with Dnmt3a and Dnmt3b[23] enhances de novo methylation by Dnmt3a and Dnmt3b.[24–28] The minimum domains required for interaction between Dnmt3L and Dnmt3a (or Dnmt3b) and stimulated activity are mapped to the C-terminal domains of both proteins,[25–29] as

Figure 2.2 **(Opposite)** (*A color version of this figure follows page 20.*) Members of the DNMT family. (a) Schematic representation of Dnmt1 and Dnmt3. (b) Dnmt2 is a tRNA^{Asp} methyltransferase.[17] (c) The PWWP domain structure of Dnmt3b, rich in basic residues.[18] (d) Structure of DNMT3L with a bound histone H3 N-terminal tail (orange).[7]

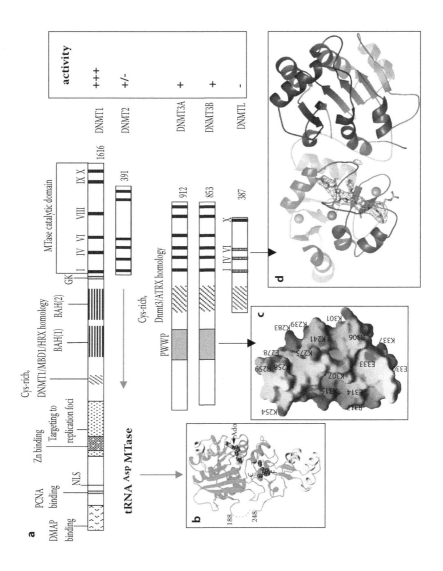

Figure 2.2.

illustrated by the complex structure between the C-terminal domains of Dnmt3a and Dnmt3L[19] (Figure 2.3a).

Both Dnmt3a-C and Dnmt3L-C have the classical fold characteristic for AdoMet-dependent methyltransferases,[30] but the reaction product S-adenosyl-L-homocysteine was found only in Dnmt3a-C and not in Dnmt3L-C. This is consistent with Dnmt3a-C being the catalytic component of the complex, while Dnmt3L is inactive and unable to bind cofactor.[27] The overall complex is elongated, with a butterfly shape (Figure 2.3a). The complex contains two monomers of Dnmt3a-C and two of Dnmt3L-C, forming a tetramer (3L-3a-3a-3L) with two 3L-3a interfaces and one 3a-3a interface. Substitution of key noncatalytic residues in the Dnmt3a-3L interface or Dnmt3a-3a interface eliminated enzymatic activity, indicating that both interfaces (3a-3L and 3a-3a) are essential for catalysis. Dnmt3L might stabilize the conformation of the active-site loop of Dnmt3a (containing the key nucleophile Cys706), via interactions with the C-terminal portion of the active-site loop. These stabilizing interactions could explain the stimulation of Dnmt3a2 activity by Dnmt3L (Figure 2.3b).[24–28]

2.2.3 The dimeric Dnmt3a suggests a model for de novo DNA methylation involving detection of CpG spacing

Among the known active DNA methyltransferases, Dnmt3a and Dnmt3b have the smallest DNA binding domain (absent in Dnmt3L). This domain includes ~50 residues in Dnmt3a/b compared to, for example, ~85 residues in the bacterial GCGC methyltransferase M.HhaI.[31] However, dimerization via the 3a-3a interface brings two active sites together and effectively doubles the DNA-binding surface. Superimposing the Dnmt3a structure onto that of M.HhaI complexed with a short oligonucleotide[31] yielded a model of Dnmt3a-DNA complex with a short DNA duplex bound to each active site (Figure 2.3a, top panel). The two DNA segments can be connected

Figure 2.3 (**Opposite**) (*A color version of this figure follows page 20.*) A model of Dnmt3a-Dnmt3L tetramer with bound DNA substrate. (a) Top panel: a surface representation of Dnmt3a-3L tetramer, with two short DNA molecules adopted by superimposition of the HhaI-DNA complex structure[31] onto individual Dnmt3a-C. Middle panel: the Dnmt3a-3L tetramer with one contiguous curved DNA molecule covering two active sites. Bottom panel: the Dnmt3a dimer could methylate two CpGs separated by one helical turn in one binding event. (b) Top panel: schematic representation of the primary structures of Dnmt3a2 and Dnmt3L. Mouse Dnmt3a2 lacks 219 amino acids that are part of full-length Dnmt3a. Middle panel: SDS-PAGE gels of the purified recombinant proteins. Bottom panel: the methyl transfer activities of Dnmt3a2 proteins (lane 1), Dnmt3a2/Dnmt3L complex (lane 2), and Dnmt3a-C/Dnmt3L-C complex (lane 3).

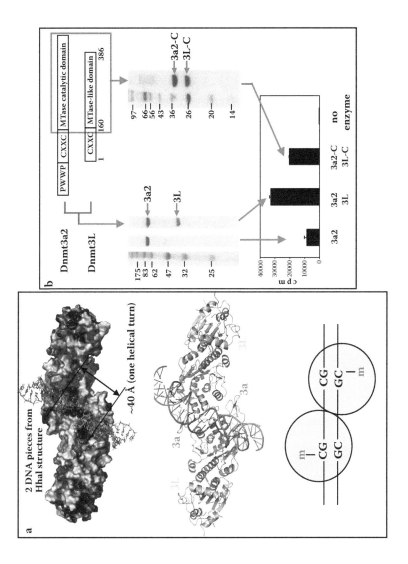

Figure 2.3.

easily to form a contiguous DNA, such that the two active sites are located in the major groove about 40 Å apart (Figure 2.3a, middle panel). This model suggests that dimeric Dnmt3a could methylate two CpGs separated by one helical turn in one binding event (Figure 2.3a, lower panel). A periodicity in the activity of Dnmt3a on long DNA revealed a correlation of methylated CpG sites at distances of 8 to 10 base pairs, suggesting that oligomerization leads Dnmt3a to methylate DNA in a periodic pattern.[19] A similar periodicity is observed for the frequency of CpG sites in the differentially methylated regions of 12 maternally imprinted mouse genes.[19] These results suggest a basis for the recognition and methylation of differentially methylated regions in imprinted genes, involving detection of both CpG spacing and nucleosome modification (see below).

The catalytic domain of Dnmt3b is about 80% identical to that of Dnmt3a with no gaps or insertions between the two sequences. Point mutations in human DNMT3B are responsible for a human disorder called ICF (immunodeficiency, centromere instability, and facial anomalies) syndrome that results in death before adulthood.[32,33] Most ICF mutations cluster in the C-terminal catalytic domain of DNMT3B. If assuming the DNMT3B monomer will have a similar structure to that of Dnmt3a, ICF mutations reduce the enzymatic activity of DNMT3B in several alternative ways: affecting overall stability (V699G, V726G, and A766P), altering conformation of the active-site loop (G663S, L664T), impairing interaction with the methyl donor AdoMet (A585V, V606A, and A603T), affecting the proposed 3b-3b interface (analogous to the 3a-3a interface; V818M, D817G, and H814R), or impairing its proposed interaction with DNA (R823G). Interestingly, no ICF mutation is located in the proposed interface between Dnmt3b and Dnmt3L, suggesting that such mutations are lethal or, more likely, that Dnmt3b and Dnmt3L have nonoverlapping functions. The latter possibility is consistent with the in vivo phenotypes of the respective knockouts,[22] and the lack of an effect on target methylation when DNMT3L and DNMT3B are co-expressed in human cells.[24]

2.2.4   *Dnmt3L connects unmethylated lysine 4 of histone H3 to de novo DNA methylation*

Dnmt3a2 (Figure 2.3b)—a germ cell specific isoform of Dnmt3a that is also required for genomic imprinting[34]—and Dnmt3b and the four core histones were identified as the main proteins that interact in vivo with the product of an epitope-tagged allele of the endogenous *Dnmt3L* gene.[7] Peptide interaction assays showed that Dnmt3L specifically interacts with the extreme amino-terminal of histone H3; this interaction was strongly inhibited by methylation at lysine 4 of histone H3 but was insensitive to modifications at other positions.[7] Cocrystallization of Dnmt3L with the tail of H3 revealed that the H3 tail bound to the Cys-rich 3-zinc binding domain of Dnmt3L (Figure 2.2d), and substitution of key residues in the binding site eliminated the H3-Dnmt3L interaction. These data indicate that Dnmt3L recognizes histone H3 tails that are unmethylated at lysine 4 and induces de novo DNA methylation by activation of Dnmt3a2. There have been reports of an inverse relationship between H3K4 methylation and allele-specific DNA methylation at differentially methylated regions, that is, the lack of H3K4 methylation at the methylated allele and the presence of H3K4 methylation at the unmethylated allele.[35–38] The Dnmt3L-Dnmt3a complex suggests a novel mechanism wherein absence of H3K4 methylation is recognized by the Cys-rich 3-zinc binding domain of Dnmt3L,[7] while its C-terminal methyltransferase-like domain interacts with the active DNA methyltransferase Dnmt3a to establish a heritable DNA methylation pattern. Hence, H3K4 methylation could protect unmethylated differentially methylated regions from DNA methylation by the Dnmt3a-Dnmt3L complex.

2.3 Histone lysine methylation, recognition, and demethylation

2.3.1 SET domain-containing histone lysine methyltransferases (HKMTs)

The SET domain-containing proteins (reviewed in Reference 10) catalyze histone lysine methylation, except Dot1p which methylates histone H3 lysine 79[39,40] without SET domain. The SET domain, comprising about 130 amino acids, can be found in many proteins in eukaryotes—at least 132 SET domains are encoded in the human genome by searching Pfam. The SET domain was initially identified in three epigenetic modifiers in *Drosophila*: Suppressor of variegation 3-9, Enhancer of Zeste, and Trithorax.[41] Based on the sequences flanking the conserved core of the SET domain, SET domain proteins have been grouped into several families: SUV, SET1, SET2, EZ, and RIZ families (reviewed in Reference 10). A few enzymes, such as SET7/9 and SET8, do not fall within any given family. Interestingly, such a classification has a very good correlation with grouping based on the substrate specificity except for a few examples. For instance, many members within the SUV family, the largest family of HKMTs, have been shown to methylate H3K9.

The SET domain is rich in short β-sheets and has a pseudo-knot structure (Figure 2.4), where a C-terminal sequence passes through a loop formed by the preceding sequence. Such a unique knot structure brings together the active site, the methyl-donor and the substrate binding pockets. Complex structures between the SET domain and substrate demonstrate the substrate lysine is inserted in a narrow hydrophobic channel, where the methylene part of the lysine residue makes van der Waals contacts with

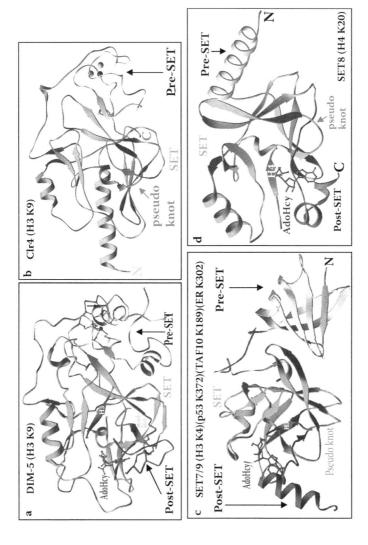

Figure 2.4 (A color version of this figure follows page 20.) SET domain protein (histone) lysine methyltransferase (HKMT) structures. (a) Ribbon diagram of DIM-5 protein (one of the smallest members of the SUV family) contains four segments: a weakly conserved N-terminal region (cyan), a pre-SET domain containing nine invariant cysteines (yellow), the SET region containing four signature motifs (green and magenta), and the post-SET domain containing three invariant cysteines (gray). (b) *S. pombe* Clr4. (c) Human SET7/9, and (d) Human SET8 (or PR-SET7).

the aromatic residues from enzymes. The channel terminates in a narrow pore, where the target nitrogen lies in close proximity to the methyl-donor AdoMet, allowing for the transfer of methyl groups.

In addition to substrate sequence specificity (which lysine to methylates), HKMTs also differ in the number of methyl groups (one, two or three) they transfer, referred to as product specificity.[42] SET7/9 protein generates exclusively H3K4me1;[42,43] DIM-5, on the other hand, generates primarily H3K9me3.[42,44] This product specificity is determined by a single amino acid in the active site pocket:[42] F281 of DIM-5 and Y305 of SET7/9, which occupy a structurally similar position in both enzymes. Swapping the two residues can invert the methylation product specificity without affecting the overall reaction rate. Sequence alignment suggests that the tyrosine/phenylalanine switch rule may be generalized for many HKMTs with known product specificity.[45]

2.3.2   Protein domains (chromo, tudor, PHD, and ankyrin repeats) that recognize lysine in four different methylation states

Lysine residue can exist in four different methylation states: unmodified (me0), mono- (me1), di- (me2), or trimethylated (me3) at the side chain amine group (Figure 2.1c). A defined methylation state can result in differing functional consequences and its significance is highlighted by a variety of genomic-scale analyses of histone modification.[46,47] The histone side chain lysine in different states are recognized by a variety of protein domains: chromo domain, tudor domain, PHD, and ankyrin-repeat domain.

The founding member of the methyl-lysine binding domain is heterochromatin protein 1 (HP1) chromo domain that recognizes H3K9me3 via a cage consisting of three hydrophobic residues (Figure 2.5a).[48,49] The chromo domain of Polycomb recognizes H3K27me3.[50,51]

PHD (plant homeodomain) is comprised of 60 to 80 amino acids and found in every eukaryotic organism. All structurally characterized PHD (and RING fingers) adopt a "cross-braced" topology of two-metal Zn^{2+}-coordinating residues.[52] A subset of PHD binds the methyl lysine of histone peptides.[53–56] The molecular recognition of methyl lysine is primarily through the caging of methyl lysine by aromatic residues, such as those of BPTF (bromodomain PHD finger transcription factor)[57] and ING2 (inhibitor of growth family 2)[58] (Figures 2.5b and 2.5c). The BPTF PHD features a full aromatic cage (Figure 2.5b), reminiscent of the binding of the HP1 or Polycomb chromo domain to trimethyl lysine,[48–51] whereas ING2 has only half a hydrophobic cage (Figure 2.5c), with a serine and a methionine finishing the H3K4 binding pocket, similar to recognition of H3K4me3 by the CHD1 (chromo-ATPase/helicase-DNA-binding) double

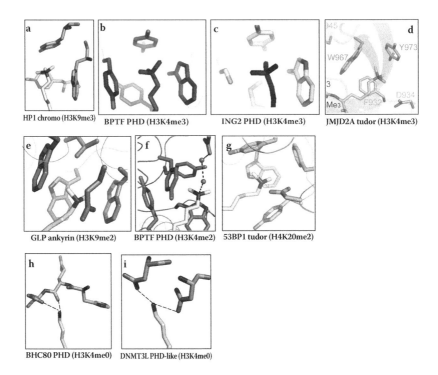

Figure 2.5 (*A color version of this figure follows page 20.*) Protein domains recognizing histone lysine side chains in methylated and unmethylated states. (a) Recognition of H3K9me3 by HP1 chromo domain. Recognition of H3K4me3 by (b) BPTF PHD, (c) ING2 PHD, and (d) IMJD2A double tudor domain. (e) Recognition of H3K9me2 by GLP ankyrin repeats, (f) H3K4me2 by BPTF PHD, and (g) H4K20me2 by 53BP1 double tudor domain. Despite having a different fold, 53bp1 double tudor domain and GLP ankyrin repeats form a strikingly similar cage. Both form a cage using three hydrophobic residues and one acidic residue. 53bp1 has reduced binding to H4K20me1 and excludes H4K20me3.[69] BPTF PHD has preference for H3K4me3, but binds H3K4me2 with only slightly decreased affinity. BPTF also utilizes a hydrophobic cage with an acidic residue, whose contacts are mediated through a water-mediated network of hydrogen bonds.[57] (h) BHC80 PHD and (i) DNMT3L PHD-like domains recognize H3K4me0.

chromo domain[59,60] and JMJD2A (a demethylase, see below) double tudor domain[61] (Figure 2.5d).

In contrast to the PHD of BPTF and ING2,[53,54] which binds H3K4me3, the PHD of BHC80, a component of the LSD1 demethylase complex, binds unmethylated H3K4 (H3K4me0), and this interaction is specifically abrogated by methylation of H3K4.[62] The PHD of BHC80 adopts a fold highly similar to that of BPTF and ING2. All engage the H3 peptide as an antiparallel β-sheet, with recognition of the H3 *N*-amine and the H3A1 side chain. H3R2 is buried in a pocket in BPTF and ING2, but is not contacted by BHC80. Only BHC80 contacts H3R8, whereas in BPTF and ING2, the H3 peptide meanders off the face of the PHD before R8. The aromatic cage is absent from BHC80. The molecular recognition of unmodified lysine is primarily through bonds (electrostatic bridges and hydrogen bonds) to the unmodified epsilon amino group, and steric exclusion of methyl groups (Figure 2.5h).

As a family, PHD shows flexibility in peptide binding, making it difficult to predict whether an individual PHD is a histone-binding module and whether it binds lysine or methyl lysine on the basis of its primary sequence. Indeed, the robustness of the PHD scaffold, and its plasticity as a binding module have been noted.[63] The array of PHD in chromatin-interacting and -modifying proteins, many of which lack the consensus binding sequence for H3K4me3 that is found in the BPTF and ING PHDs, might have histone binding activities of unknown specificity. In this regard, the DNA methyltransferase 3-like protein, Dnmt3L (see above), binds H3K4me0 through its Cys-rich 3-zinc binding domain[7] (Figure 2.5i). Structural comparison reveals the similarity in their common mode of interaction with histone H3K4me0, which raises the question of whether de novo DNA methylation (by Dnmt3L) is linked to the action of H3K4 LSD1 demethylase and its associated complex components. In this regard, conditional gene deletion of LSD1 established that LSD1 is essential for mouse development.[64]

A more recent example of a protein module capable of binding methyl-lysine histone tails is the ankyrin repeats of G9a and GLP (G9a-like protein) HKMTs.[65] G9a and GLP are the major euchromatin-associated H3K9 methyltransferases that repress transcription by mono- and dimethylating H3K9.[66–68] Interestingly, G9a and GLP ankyrin repeats bind with strong preference to histone H3 N-terminal tail peptides mono- or dimethylated at K9—the histone mark generated by their associated methyltransferase activity in the same polypeptide. The crystal structure of the GLP ankyrin repeats bound to a H3K9me2 peptide revealed the basis for recognition of the methylated lysine by a partial hydrophobic cage with three tryptophans and one acidic residue (Figure 2.5e). A nearly identical hydrophobic cage with one acidic residue is also present in the structure of 53bp1, a H4K20me2 binding double tudor domain[69] (Figure 2.5g), and to a lesser extent, JMJD2A, a H3K4me3 binding double tudor domain (Figure 2.5d).

2.3.3   *Histone lysine demethylation by oxidation or hydroxylation*

Methylation can function as a reversible signal, as in the case of O(xygen)-methylation, in which the side chain carboxyl groups of glutamate residues or the C-terminal carboxyl groups are reversibly methylated.[70,71] There are many examples of N(itrogen)-methylations (of arginine, lysine, glutamine, asparagine, histidine residues, and the amino group at the N terminus) in the cell. While it is not certain that all N-methylations are reversible, recent discoveries showed a human nuclear amine oxidase, LSD1, functions as a protein di/mono-methyl-lysine demethylase via an oxidation reaction;[72–74] and JmjC-domain-containing hydroxylase-like proteins are able to demethylate mono-, di-, or tri-methylated lysines.[75,76]

LSD1 (also known as BHC110), named after protein lysine-specific-demethylase 1,[72] is found in histone modification complexes that control cell-specific gene expression. Within these complexes, REST (RE1-silencing transcription factor) corepressor CoREST enables LSD1 to demethylate nucleosomes,[73,74] while BHC80 (BRAF–HDAC complex) inhibits LSD1 activity.[73] The LSD1 polypeptide chain can be divided into several structural/functional regions (Figure 2.6a): the N-terminal putative nuclear localization signal, followed by a SWIRM (Swi3p, Rsc8p, and Moira) domain

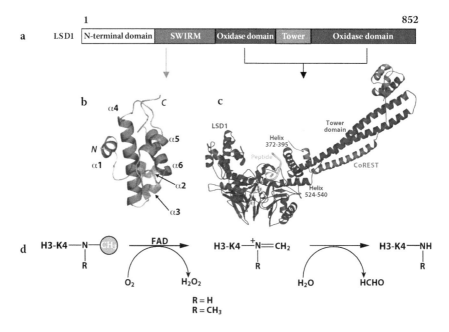

Figure 2.6 (A color version of this figure follows page 20.) Demethylation by oxidation. (a) Schematic representation of human LSD1 domain organization. The oxidase domain contains an atypical insertion of Tower domain not found in other oxidases. (b) The solution NMR structure of the SIWRM domain of LSD1.[77] (c) Crystal structure of LSD1 (residues 171–836)-CoREST (residues 308–440) in complex with pLys4Met H3 peptide (residues 1–16). LSD1 is in blue, CoREST in red, and the peptide in green. The FAD cofactor is shown as a yellow ball-and-stick.[86] (d) Scheme of the demethylation reaction catalyzed by LSD1.

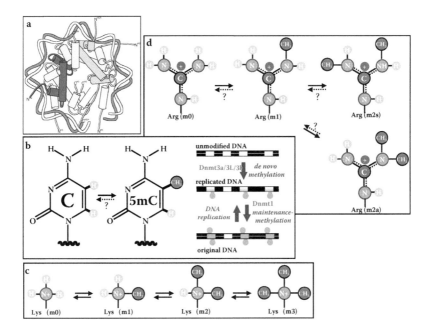

Color Figure 2.1 Examples of known targets of AdoMet-dependent methylation. (a) A model of nucleosome. (b) DNA cytosine methylation at ring carbon C5 position. (c) Protein lysine methylation, and (d) protein arginine methylation. Note: only the deprotonated amino group (NH_2) has a free lone pair of electrons capable of nucleophilic attack on the AdoMet methyl group.

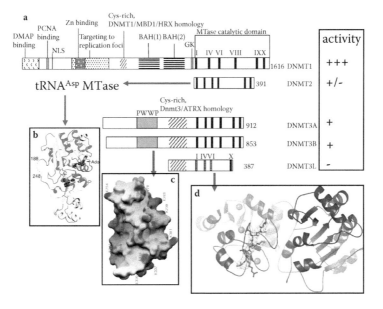

Color Figure 2.2 Members of the DNMT family. (a) Schematic representation of Dnmt1 and Dnmt3. (b) Dnmt2 is a tRNA[Asp] methyltransferase.[17] (c) The PWWP domain structure of Dnmt3b, rich in basic residues.[18] (d) Structure of DNMT3L with a bound histone H3 N-terminal tail (orange).[7]

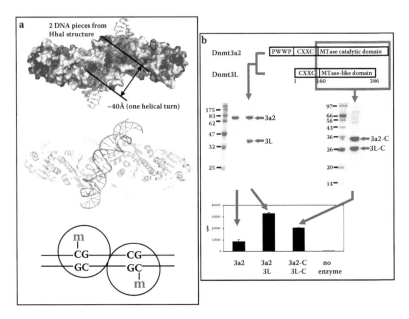

Color Figure 2.3 A model of Dnmt3a-Dnmt3L tetramer with bound DNA substrate. (*See text for full caption.*)

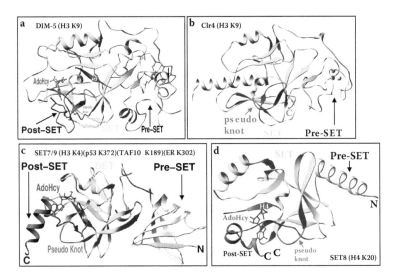

Color Figure 2.4 SET domain protein (histone) lysine methyltransferase (HKMT) structures. (*See text for full caption.*)

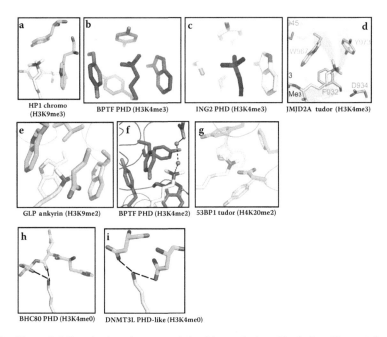

a
| | | | | |
|HP1 chromo (H3K9me3)|BPTF PHD (H3K4me3)|ING2 PHD (H3K4me3)|JMJD2A tudor (H3K4me3)|

GLP ankyrin (H3K9me2) BPTF PHD (H3K4me2) 53BP1 tudor (H4K20me2)

BHC80 PHD (H3K4me0) DNMT3L PHD-like (H3K4me0)

Color Figure 2.5 Protein domains recognizing histone lysine side chains. (*See text for full caption.*)

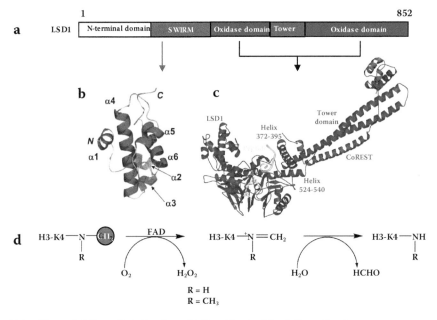

Color Figure 2.6 Demethylation by oxidation. (*See text for full caption.*)

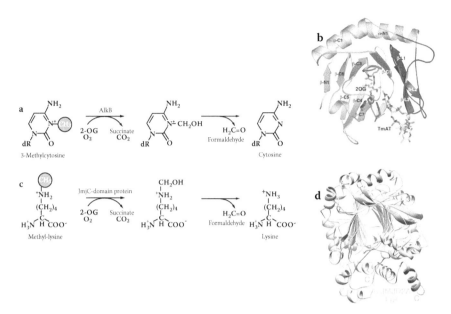

Color Figure 2.7 Demethylation by hydroxylation. (*See text for full caption.*)

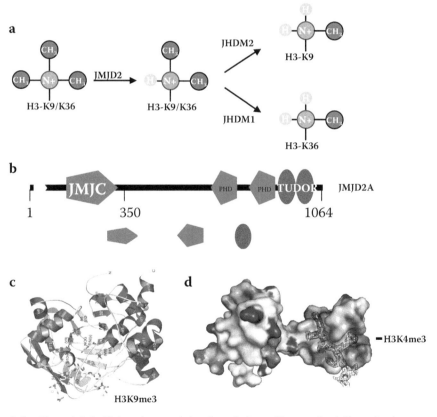

Color Figure 2.8 JmjC-domain-containing demethylases. (*See text for full caption.*)

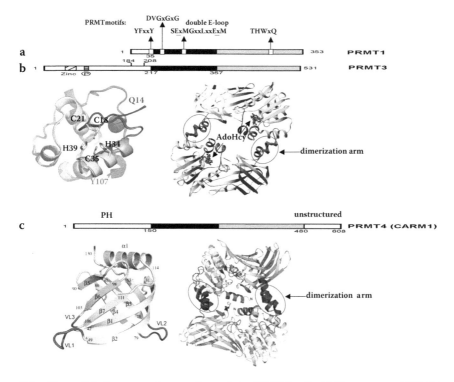

Color Figure 2.9 Representative members of the PRMT family. (a) The conserved PRMT core domain is in black and the unique β-barrel domain to the PRMT family is in gray. The four invariant sequence motifs are labeled. (b) PRMT3: N-terminal C2H2 zinc-finger (PDB code 1WIR) and the ring-like core domain.[118] (c) PRMT4/CARM1: N-terminal PH domain and the ring-like core domain.[117]

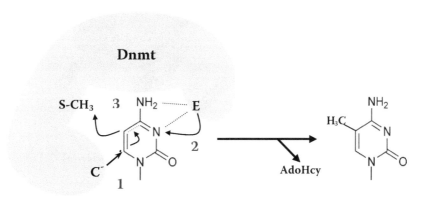

Color Figure 3.1 DNA (cytosine-C5) methyltransferase catalyzed methyl transfer. Blue Dnmt ovals represent different regions of the same Dnmt protein. S-CH₃ symbolizes the *S*-methyl moiety of *S*-adenosyl methionine. Refer to the text for other details.

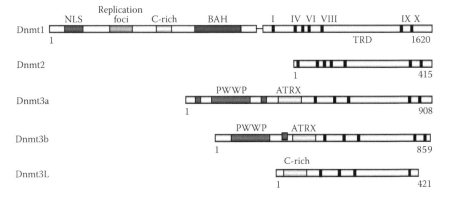

Color Figure 3.2 Mammalian DNA methyltransferases. Shaded regions indicate protein binding domains. Black bars indicate conserved sequences in the catalytic domains.

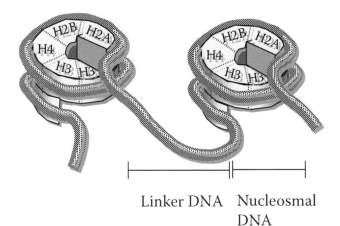

Linker DNA   Nucleosmal DNA

Color Figure 4.1 Basic chromatin structure. Two nucleosomes are shown, with histone octamer proteins in blue and genomic double-stranded DNA in green. Each nucleosome wraps ~146 bp of DNA, and nucleosomes are separated by linker DNA.

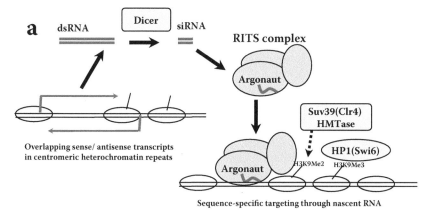

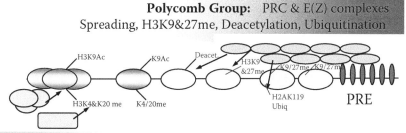

Color Figure 4.2 Model for HP1-mediated heterochromatin. (a) Model for the mechanism by which double-stranded DNA from pericentromeric repeats results in formation of HP1-containing silent heterochromatin over these same repeats. (b) Model for the spread of heterochromatin to variably cover or uncover nearby loci, resulting in position effect variegation.

Polycomb Group: PRC & E(Z) complexes
Spreading, H3K9&27me, Deacetylation, Ubiquitination

Trithorax Group: ALL/Trithorax, Ash1 & SWI/SNF
Activating methylation, remodeled chromatin

Color Figure 4.3 Model for functional antagonism of Polycomb and Thrithorax complexes. Polycomb group complexes nucleated at PREs may spread by deacetylating H3K9 and H3K27 and then methylating these residues. Methyl H3K9 and H3K27 is a signal that is then bound by other Polycomb group proteins. Polycomb-mediated heterochromatin also requires enzymes that ubiquitinate H2A at K119. Trithorax group proteins may counter this repressive effect by rearranging nucleosome positions with SWI/SNF (nucleosome on the right), and by laying down activating histone methylation marks (H3K4me and H3K20me).

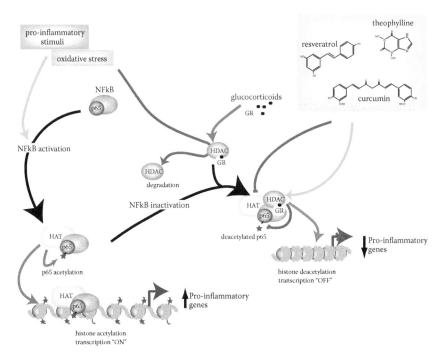

Color Figure 6.1 Histone acetylation and pro-inflammatory genes. (*See text for full caption.*)

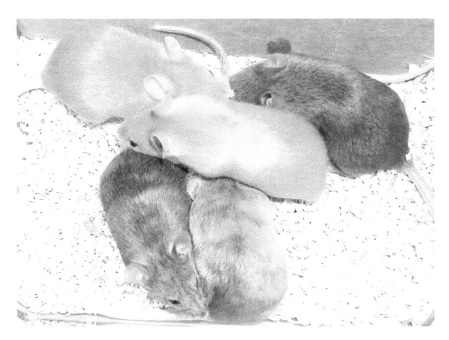

Color Figure 7.3 Examples of mice from the yellow agouti mouse model. Strain VY mice showing A^{vy}/a mice, top left, a clear yellow, Y5 mouse; top right, a pseudoagouti, Y0 mouse; middle, a slightly mottled, Y4 mouse; bottom left, a heavily mottled, Y2, mouse; and bottom right, a mottled, Y3 mouse. These five mice are genetically identical. Coat color patterns are due to the degree of A^{vy} expression.

(Figure 2.6b)[77]—found in several nucleosome-interacting proteins—and a monoamine oxidase domain (Figure 2.6c), capable of demethylating lysines in a flavin-dependent manner.[78] From a sequence conservation standpoint, LSD1 belongs to the class of flavin-dependent monoamine oxidases (such as human monoamino oxidase B), which typically catalyze the oxidation of an amine-containing substrate using molecular oxygen as the electron acceptor.[79] The amino group of the methylated Lys is oxidized, presumably to generate the corresponding imine compound, which is subsequently hydrolyzed to produce formaldehyde (Figure 2.6d). Substrate oxidation leads to the two-electron reduction of the protein-bound FAD cofactor, which is regenerated to its oxidized form by molecular oxygen to produce hydrogen peroxide. Biochemically, LSD1 demethylates H3K4me1 or H3K4me2 equally well, but does not demethylate H3K4me3.[78] LSD1 also demethylates nonhistone substrates, such as p53.[80] In vitro, LSD1 removes both monomethylation (K370me1) and dimethylation (K370me2) at p53 K370, a Smyd2-dependent monomethylation site.[81] However, in vivo, LSD1 shows a strong preference to reverse K370me2, which is performed by a distinct, but unknown, methyltransferase.

Thus far, crystal structures of LSD1 alone,[82,83] LSD1 in complex with CoREST,[84] and LSD1-CoREST in complex with H3 peptide[85,86] have been determined. Using a 21-residue peptide bearing a methionine in place of target methyl-K4 showed a 30-fold increase in binding affinity making the mutant peptide a strong inhibitor and an ideal candidate for structural work. Forneris et al.[86] were able to resolve the first 16 residues of the H3 peptide, in perfect agreement with their previous biochemical data that LSD1 is active on peptide substrates longer than 16 amino acids.[78] This study is the first in which a long, structured histone tail has been visualized in histone-modifying enzymes and protein domains that recognize (decode) methyl-lysine signals. In comparison, a similar study of LSD1-histone peptide, using the approach of covalent tethering of peptide substrate to cofactor FAD, observed the first 7 residues (out of 21 residues used) of H3 peptide,[85] while the tandem tudor domains of 53BP1 in complex with a 10- or 14-residue H4 peptide observed only two structured residues, H4R19 and H4K20me2.[69]

Studies of DNA repair in *Escherichia coli* demonstrated that methyl groups of 1-methyladenine (1-meA) and 3-methylcytosine (3-meC) in DNA can be removed by the AlkB family of enzymes through oxidative demethylation[87–89] (Figures 2.7a and 2.7b). The similarity between the chemistry of removing a methyl group from 1-meA and 3-meC and methyl-lysine (Figure 2.7c) prompted the proposal that the fission yeast protein Epe1 is a putative histone demethylase that could act by oxidative demethylation.[90] Epe1 modulates the stability of silent chromatin and contains a JmjC domain.[91] The Epe1 protein can be modeled onto the structure of the 2-oxoglutarate-Fe(II)-dependent dioxygenase, factor

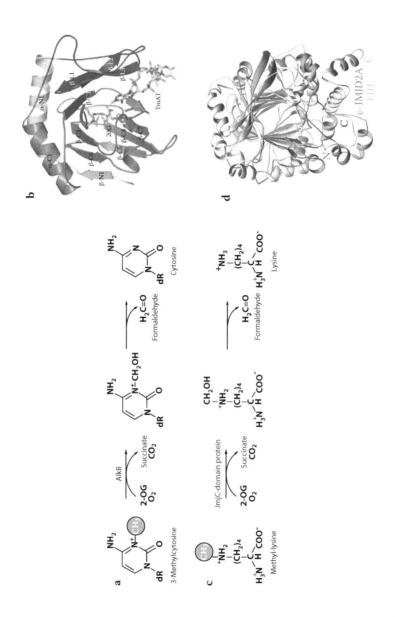

Figure 2.7.

inhibiting hypoxia inducible factor (FIH), which is a protein hydroxylase that also contains a JmjC domain.[92] JmjC domain-containing proteins are predicted to be metalloenzymes that regulate chromatin function.[93] Using a biochemical assay based on the detection of formaldehyde, one of the predicted release products, coupled with chromatography, JHDM1 (JmjC domain-containing histone demethylase 1) and JHDM2A were found to demethylate mono- and dimethylated H3K36[94] and H3K9,[75] respectively. Another JmjC domain-containing protein, JMJD2A, is found to reverse trimethylated H3K9/K36 to di- but not mono- or unmethylated products[76] (Figure 2.8a). Indeed, the structure of the N-terminal catalytic core JmjC-containing domain of JMJD2A is a close relative of FIH but with apparent differences outside of the jellyroll region (Figure 2.7d).[95] Structural studies reveal that JMJD2A predominately recognizes the backbone of peptides, allowing the enzyme to recognize both H3K9me3 and H3K36me3.[96–98]

The human genome encodes at least 50 JmjC proteins.[13] Analogous to the SET domain, the JmjC domain is flanked by a variety of domains. Based on the domain architecture and multiple sequence alignment, JmjC proteins are classified into seven different groups and each group has specific activity toward specific lysine residues[99] (Table 2.1). Thus, chromatin-associated JmjC-domain proteins may generally be protein N(itrogen)-demethylases that can remove methyl group(s) from many protein substrates containing a variety of modified residues.

2.4   Histone arginine methylation

Protein arginine methylation is a common posttranslational modification in eukaryotes. There are two major types of protein arginine (R) methyltransferases (PRMTs). Both catalyze the formation of monomethyl (me1)-arginine, but type I PRMTs also form asymmetric dimethyl (me2a)-arginine and type II PRMTs form symmetric dimethyl (me2s)-arginine[100] (Figure 2.1d). Nine very similar paralogous mammalian PRMT genes have been reported so far.[101] Among them, PRMT1, PRMT4/CARM1, and PRMT6 methylate histones H3,[102–104] H3R17,[105] H3R2,[106] H4R3,[107,108] and H2B,[109] in addition to many other substrates.

Figure 2.7 **(Opposite)** (*A color version of this figure follows page 20.*) Demethylation by hydroxylation. (a) Mechanism of demethylation of 3-methylcytosine by AlkB. (b) Structure of *E. coli* AlkB with Fe(II), 2-oxoglutarate (2OG), and a methylated trinucleotide.[89] The sphere representing the Fe cofactor is colored in orange, whereas atoms in 2OG, and dT-(1-me-dA)-dT are colored according to atomic identity (carbon, white; oxygen, red; nitrogen, blue; and phosphorous, orange). (c) Mechanism of demethylation of histones by JmjC-domain proteins. (d) The superposition of N-terminal catalytic core of JMJD2A (colored green) and FIH (colored yellow).[95] The double-stranded helix (jellyroll region) is well conserved.

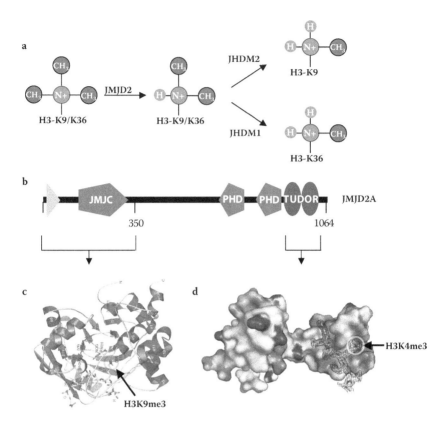

Figure 2.8 (A color version of this figure follows page 20.) JmjC-domain-containing demethylases. (a) JMJD2A demethylates trimethylated H3-K9/K36 to dimethyl lysine,[76] while JHDM2A and JHDM1A demethylate, respectively, dimethylated H3K9[94] and H3K36.[75] (b) Domain organization of JMJD2A. (c) The H3K9me3 peptide bound to the N-terminal catalytic domain of JMJD2A–Ni(ii)–Zn(ii)–NOG.[96] (d) The H3K4me3 peptide bound to the C-terminal double tudor domain.[61]

Histone arginine methylation is a component of the "histone code" that directs a variety of processes involving chromatin.[110,111] For example, methylation of histone H4 arginine 3 (H4R3) by PRMT1 facilitates H4 acetylation and enhances transcriptional activation by nuclear hormone receptors synergistically with CARM1,[107,108,112,113] in that CARM1 prefers acetylated histone tails in generating H3R17 methylation.[108,114] In vitro, p53-mediated transcription was stimulated the greatest when all three coactivators (PRMT1, CARM1, and p300) were present, whether added sequentially or at the same time.[109] Preincubation of a chromatin template with p53 and PRMT1 significantly stimulated the histone acetyltransferase activity of p300 and, similarly, preincubation of the template with p53 and p300 stimulated H3 arginine methylation by CARM1. More recently, methylation of histone

Table 2.1 Demethylases that remove protein (histone) lysine methylation

Enzyme	Specificity	References
LSD1	H3K4me1,2	72
	p53K370me2	80
JHDM1A	H3K36me1,2	75
JHDM1B		
JHDM2A	H3K9me1,2	94
JHDM2B		
JHDM2C		
HR		
JMJD2A/JHDM3A	H3K9me2,3	76
JMJD2B	H3K36me2,3	
JMJD2C/GASC1		
JMJD2D		
JARID1A/RBP2	H3K4me2,3	55
JARID1B/PLU1		
JARID1C/SMCX		
JARID1D/SMCY		
UTX	H3K27me2,3	124
JMJD3		125
		126
		127

H3R2 by PRMT6 and H3K4 was shown to be mutually exclusive.[106,115] H3R2 methylation by PRMT6 was prevented by the presence of H3K4me3 and, conversely, the H3R2me2a mark prevented methylation of H3K4 by the SET1 complex in yeast[115] and an MLL complex in mammalian cells.[106]

The PRMT proteins all contain a conserved core region of approximately 310 amino acids (Figure 2.9a). The sequences beyond the conserved PRMT core region are all N-terminal additions; however, CARM1 also has a C-terminal addition. The size of the N-terminal addition varies (~20 amino acids in PRMT1 to ~200 in PRMT3). The varied N-terminals could subject each PRMT to a different regulation. For example, PRMT2 includes an SH3 domain that mediates protein-protein interaction in the Src family signaling pathways. However, the recombinant PRMT2 with or without the N-terminal SH3 domain is inactive.[116] PRMT3 contains a C2H2 zinc finger (Figure 2.9b) and tyrosine phosphorylation site, suggesting a link to other signaling pathways. PRMT4/CARM1, recruited by several transcription factors, methylates a large variety of proteins and plays a critical role in gene expression, and it contains an N-terminal PH domain,[117]

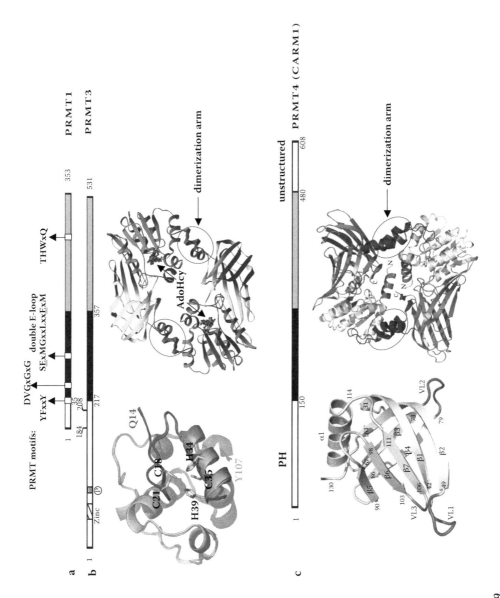

Figure 2.9.

a scaffold frequently found to regulate protein-protein interactions in a large variety of biological processes.

Structural studies reveal a striking structural conservation of the PRMT catalytic core[117–121] forming a ring-like dimer (Figure 2.9). It is conceivable that binding of the protein substrate within this ring-like structure could facilitate the processive dimethylation of Arg residues by allowing the product of the first methylation reaction, monomethyl-arginine, to enter the active site of the second molecule of the dimer without releasing the substrate from the ring. In support of this possibility there is the fact that mutants of rat PRMT1, yeast RMT1/Hmt1, and PRMT4/CARM1 in which the dimerization arm is either deleted (residues 188–222),[120] replaced with alanines,[119] or mutated[122] exist as monomers in solution and lack methylation activity.

2.5 Summary

With the increasing interest in protein (histone) methylation as a mechanism for gene regulation, we will undoubtedly discover other exciting roles for methyltransferases, methyl-reading modules, and demethylases and the cellular processes that they direct. One interesting observation is that several histone-(de)methylating complexes contain components of both synthesis and binding to a specific histone mark, such as Suv39h-HP1 (for H3K9me3) (reviewed in Reference 123) and LSD1-BHC80 (for H3K4me0),[62] where the components that make (or remove) and recognize a specific histone mark are separate proteins. G9a and GLP histone methylating proteins contain modules, within the same polypeptide, for both making (via the SET domain) and recognizing (via the ankyrin repeats) a given methyl mark. Both activities are critical to the function of the protein as a corepressor,[65] and the requirement of both methyltransferase and product binding activities to establish global methylation patterns indicates that both activities are critical for the repression of many cellular genes. On the other hand, JMJD2A, a histone lysine demethylase, contains modules, within the same peptide, for both removing (H3K9/K36me3 via the JmjC domain) and recognizing (H3K4me3 or H4K20me3 via the double tudor domain) different marks (see Figure 2.8). Furthermore, sequential rounds of methylation and methyl mark binding may provide a processive mechanism to effectively spread silent/activation marks over many kilobases.

Figure 2.9 **(Opposite)** (*A color version of this figure follows page 20.*) Representative members of the PRMT family. (a) The conserved PRMT core domain is in black and the unique β-barrel domain to the PRMT family is in gray. The four invariant sequence motifs are labeled. (b) PRMT3: N-terminal C2H2 zinc-finger (PDB code 1WIR) and the ring-like core domain.[118] (c) PRMT4/CARM1: N-terminal PH domain and the ring-like core domain.[117]

References

1. Luger, K., Mader, A. W., Richmond, R. K., Sargent, D. F., and Richmond, T. J. (1997). Crystal structure of the nucleosome core particle at 2.8 A resolution. *Nature* 389, 251–260.
2. Kouzarides, T. (2007). Chromatin modifications and their function. *Cell* 128, 693–705.
3. Turner, B. M. (2007). Defining an epigenetic code. *Nature Cell Biol* 9, 2–6.
4. Lehnertz, B. (2003). Suv39h-mediated histone H3 lysine 9 methylation directs DNA methylation to major satellite repeats at pericentric heterochromatin. *Curr Biol* 13, 1192–1200.
5. Weber, M. (2007). Distribution, silencing potential and evolutionary impact of promoter DNA methylation in the human genome. *Nature Genet* 39, 457–466.
6. Appanah, R., Dickerson, D. R., Goyal, P., Groudine, M., and Lorincz, M. C. (2007). An unmethylated 3[prime] promoter-proximal region is required for efficient transcription initiation. *PLoS Genet* 3, e27.
7. Ooi, S. K. T., Qiu, C., Bernstein, E., Li, K., Jia, D., Yang, Z., Erdjument-Bromage, H., Tempst, P., Lin, S.-P., Allis, C. D., Cheng, X., and Bestor, T. H. (2007). DNMT3L connects unmethylated lysine 4 of histone H3 to de novo methylation of DNA. *Nature* 448, 714–717.
8. Anand, R., and Marmorstein, R. (2007). Structure and mechanism of lysine specific demethylase enzymes. *J Biol Chem* 282, 35425–35429.
9. Berger, S. L. (2007). The complex language of chromatin regulation during transcription. *Nature* 447, 407–412.
10. Cheng, X., Collins, R. E., and Zhang, X. (2005). Structural and sequence motifs of protein (histone) methylation enzymes. *Annu Rev Biophys Biomol Structure* 34, 267–294.
11. Cheng, X., and Zhang, X. (2007). Structural dynamics of protein lysine methylation and demethylation. *Mut Research* 618, 102–115.
12. Goll, M. G., and Bestor, T. H. (2005). Eukaryotic cytosine methyltransferases. *Annu Rev Biochem* 74, 481–514.
13. Klose, R. J., and Zhang, Y. (2007). Regulation of histone methylation by demethylimination and demethylation. *Nat Rev* 8, 307–318.
14. Chen, T., and Li, E. (2006). Establishment and maintenance of DNA methylation patterns in mammals. *Current Topics Microbiol Immunol* 301, 179–201.
15. Bestor, T. H. (2000). The DNA methyltransferases of mammals. *Human Mol Genet* 9, 2395–2402.
16. Dong, A., Yoder, J. A., Zhang, X., Zhou, L., Bestor, T. H., and Cheng, X. (2001). Structure of human DNMT2, an enigmatic DNA methyltransferase homolog that displays denaturant-resistant binding to DNA. *Nucleic Acids Res* 29, 439–448.
17. Goll, M. G., Kirpekar, F., Maggert, K. A., Yoder, J. A., Hsieh, C. L., Zhang, X., Golic, K. G., Jacobsen, S. E., and Bestor, T. H. (2006). Methylation of tRNAAsp by the DNA methyltransferase homolog Dnmt2. *Science* 311, 395–398.
18. Qiu, C., Sawada, K., Zhang, X., and Cheng, X. (2002). The PWWP domain of mammalian DNA methyltransferase Dnmt3b defines a new family of DNA-binding folds. *Nat Struc Biol* 9, 217–224.
19. Jia, D., Jurkowska, R. Z., Zhang, X., Jeltsch, A., and Cheng, X. (2007). Structure of Dnmt3a bound to Dnmt3L suggests a model for de novo DNA methylation. *Nature* 449, 248–251.

20. Bourc'his, D., Xu, G. L., Lin, C. S., Bollman, B., and Bestor, T. H. (2001). Dnmt3L and the establishment of maternal genomic imprints. *Science* 294, 2536–2539.
21. Bourc'his, D., and Bestor, T. H. (2004). Meiotic catastrophe and retrotransposon reactivation in male germ cells lacking Dnmt3L. *Nature* 431, 96–99.
22. Kaneda, M. (2004). Essential role for de novo DNA methyltransferase Dnmt3a in paternal and maternal imprinting. *Nature* 429, 900–903.
23. Hata, K., Okano, M., Lei, H., and Li, E. (2002). Dnmt3L cooperates with the Dnmt3 family of de novo DNA methyltransferases to establish maternal imprints in mice. *Development* 129, 1983–1993.
24. Chedin, F., Lieber, M. R., and Hsieh, C. L. (2002). The DNA methyltransferase-like protein DNMT3L stimulates de novo methylation by Dnmt3a. *Proc Natl Acad Sci USA* 99, 16916–16921.
25. Suetake, I., Shinozaki, F., Miyagawa, J., Takeshima, H., and Tajima, S. (2004). DNMT3L stimulates the DNA methylation activity of Dnmt3a and Dnmt3b through a direct interaction. *J Biol Chem* 279, 27816–27823.
26. Chen, Z. X., Mann, J. R., Hsieh, C. L., Riggs, A. D., and Chedin, F. (2005). Physical and functional interactions between the human DNMT3L protein and members of the de novo methyltransferase family. *J Cell Biochem* 95, 902–917.
27. Gowher, H., Liebert, K., Hermann, A., Xu, G., and Jeltsch, A. (2005). Mechanism of stimulation of catalytic activity of Dnmt3A and Dnmt3B DNA-(cytosine-C5)-methyltransferases by Dnmt3L. *J Biol Chem* 280, 13341–13348.
28. Kareta, M. S., Botello, Z. M., Ennis, J. J., Chou, C., and Chedin, F. (2006). Reconstitution and mechanism of the stimulation of de novo methylation by human DNMT3L. *J Biol Chem* 281, 25893–25902.
29. Margot, J. B., Ehrenhofer-Murray, A. E., and Leonhardt, H. (2003). Interactions within the mammalian DNA methyltransferase family. *BMC Mol Biol* 4, 7.
30. Schubert, H. L., Blumenthal, R. M., and Cheng, X. (2003). Many paths to methyltransfer: a chronicle of convergence. *Trends Biochem Sci* 28, 329–335.
31. Klimasauskas, S., Kumar, S., Roberts, R. J., and Cheng, X. (1994). HhaI methyltransferase flips its target base out of the DNA helix. *Cell* 76, 357–369.
32. Okano, M., Bell, D. W., Haber, D. A., and Li, E. (1999). DNA methyltransferases Dnmt3a and Dnmt3b are essential for de novo methylation and mammalian development. *Cell* 99, 247–257.
33. Xu, G. L., Bestor, T. H., Bourc'his, D., Hsieh, C. L., Tommerup, N., Bugge, M., Hulten, M., Qu, X., Russo, J. J., and Viegas-Pequignot, E. (1999). Chromosome instability and immunodeficiency syndrome caused by mutations in a DNA methyltransferase gene. *Nature* 402, 187–191.
34. Chen, T., Ueda, Y., Xie, S., and Li, E. (2002). A novel Dnmt3a isoform produced from an alternative promoter localizes to euchromatin and its expression correlates with active de novo methylation. *J Biol Chem* 277, 38746–38754.
35. Fournier, C. (2002). Allele-specific histone lysine methylation marks regulatory regions at imprinted mouse genes. *EMBO J* 21, 6560–6570.
36. Vu, T. H., Li, T., and Hoffman, A. R. (2004). Promoter-restricted histone code, not the differentially methylated DNA regions or antisense transcripts, marks the imprinting status of IGF2R in human and mouse. *Hum Mol Genet* 13, 2233–2245.
37. Yamasaki, Y. (2005). Neuron-specific relaxation of Igf2r imprinting is associated with neuron-specific histone modifications and lack of its antisense transcript Air. *Hum Mol Genet* 14, 2511–2520.

38. Delaval, K. (2007). Differential histone modifications mark mouse imprinting control regions during spermatogenesis. *EMBO J.* 26, 720–729.

39. Min, J., Feng, Q., Li, Z., Zhang, Y., and Xu, R. M. (2003). Structure of the catalytic domain of human DOT1L, a non-SET domain nucleosomal histone methyltransferase. *Cell* 112, 711–723.

40. Sawada, K., Yang, Z., Horton, J. R., Collins, R. E., Zhang, X., and Cheng, X. (2004). Structure of the conserved core of the yeast Dot1p, a nucleosomal histone H3 lysine79 methyltransferase. *J Biol Chem* 279, 43296–43306.

41. Jenuwein, T., Laible, G., Dorn, R., and Reuter, G. (1998). SET domain proteins modulate chromatin domains in eu- and heterochromatin. *Cell Mol Life Sci* 54, 80–93.

42. Zhang, X., Yang, Z., Khan, S. I., Horton, J. R., and Tamaru, H. (2003). Structural basis for the product specificity of histone lysine methyltransferases. *Mol Cell* 12, 177–185.

43. Xiao, B., Jing, C., Wilson, J. R., Walker, P. A., and Vasisht, N. (2003). Structure and catalytic mechanism of the human histone methyltransferase SET7/9. *Nature* 421, 652–656.

44. Tamaru, H., Zhang, X., McMillen, D., Singh, P. B., and Nakayama, J. (2003). Trimethylated lysine 9 of histone H3 is a mark for DNA methylation in *Neurospora crassa*. *Nat Genet* 34, 75–79.

45. Collins, R. E., Tachibana, M., Tamaru, H., Smith, K. M., Jia, D., Zhang, X., Selker, E. U., Shinkai, Y., and Cheng, X. (2005). In vitro and in vivo analyses of a Phe/Tyr switch controlling product specificity of histone lysine methyltransferases. *J Biol Chem* 280, 5563–5570.

46. Pokholok, D. K., Harbison, C. T., Levine, S., Cole, M., Hannett, N. M., Lee, T. I., Bell, G. W., Walker, K., Rolfe, P. A., Herbolsheimer, E., Zeitlinger, J., Lewitter, F., Gifford, D. K., and Young, R. A. (2005). Genome-wide map of nucleosome acetylation and methylation in yeast. *Cell* 122, 517–527.

47. Ruthenburg, A. J., Allis, C. D., and Wysocka, J. (2007). Methylation of lysine 4 on histone H3: Intricacy of writing and reading a single epigenetic mark. *Mol Cell* 25, 15–30.

48. Jacobs, S. A., and Khorasanizadeh, S. (2002). Structure of HP1 chromodomain bound to a lysine 9-methylated histone H3 tail. *Science* 295, 2080–2083.

49. Nielsen, P. R., Nietlispach, D., Mott, H. R., Callaghan, J., Bannister, A., Kouzarides, T., Murzin, A. G., Murzina, N. V., and Laue, E. D. (2002). Structure of the HP1 chromodomain bound to histone H3 methylated at lysine 9. *Nature* 416, 103–107.

50. Min, J., Zhang, Y., and Xu, R. M. (2003). Structural basis for specific binding of Polycomb chromodomain to histone H3 methylated at Lys 27. *Genes Dev* 17, 1823–1828.

51. Fischle, W., Wang, Y., Jacobs, S. A., Kim, Y., Allis, C. D., and Khorasanizadeh, S. (2003). Molecular basis for the discrimination of repressive methyl-lysine marks in histone H3 by Polycomb and HP1 chromodomains. *Genes Dev* 17, 1870–1881.

52. Bienz, M. (2006). The PHD finger, a nuclear protein-interaction domain. *Trends Biochem Sci* 31, 35–40.

53. Shi, X., Hong, T., Walter, K. L., Ewalt, M., Michishita, E., Hung, T., Carney, D., Pena, P., Lan, F., Kaadige, M. R., Lacoste, N., Cayrou, C., Davrazou, F., Saha, A., Cairns, B. R., Ayer, D. E., Kutateladze, T. G., Shi, Y., Cote, J., Chua, K. F., and Gozani, O. (2006). ING2 PHD domain links histone H3 lysine 4 methylation to active gene repression. *Nature* 442, 96–99.

54. Wysocka, J., Swigut, T., Xiao, H., Milne, T. A., Kwon, S. Y., Landry, J., Kauer, M., Tackett, A. J., Chait, B. T., Badenhorst, P., Wu, C., and Allis, C. D. (2006). A PHD finger of NURF couples histone H3 lysine 4 trimethylation with chromatin remodelling. *Nature* 442, 86–90.

55. Iwase, S., Lan, F., Bayliss, P., de la Torre-Ubieta, L., Huarte, M., Qi, H. H., Whetstine, J. R., Bonni, A., Roberts, T. M., and Shi, Y. (2007). The X-linked mental retardation gene SMCX/JARID1C defines a family of histone H3 lysine 4 demethylases. *Cell* 128, 1077–1088.

56. Shi, X., Kachirskaia, I., Walter, K. L., Kuo, J. H., Lake, A., Davrazou, F., Chan, S. M., Martin, D. G., Fingerman, I. M., Briggs, S. D., Howe, L., Utz, P. J., Kutateladze, T. G., Lugovskoy, A. A., Bedford, M. T., and Gozani, O. (2007). Proteome-wide analysis in *Saccharomyces cerevisiae* identifies several PHD fingers as novel direct and selective binding modules of histone H3 methylated at either lysine 4 or lysine 36. *J Biol Chem* 282, 2450–2455.

57. Li, H., Ilin, S., Wang, W., Duncan, E. M., Wysocka, J., Allis, C. D., and Patel, D. J. (2006). Molecular basis for site-specific read-out of histone H3K4me3 by the BPTF PHD finger of NURF. *Nature* 442, 91–95.

58. Pena, P. V., Davrazou, F., Shi, X., Walter, K. L., Verkhusha, V. V., Gozani, O., Zhao, R., and Kutateladze, T. G. (2006). Molecular mechanism of histone H3K4me3 recognition by plant homeodomain of ING2. *Nature* 442, 100–103.

59. Flanagan, J. F., Mi, L. Z., Chruszcz, M., Cymborowski, M., Clines, K. L., Kim, Y., Minor, W., Rastinejad, F., and Khorasanizadeh, S. (2005). Double chromodomains cooperate to recognize the methylated histone H3 tail. *Nature* 438, 1181–1185.

60. Sims, R. J. III, Chen, C. F., Santos-Rosa, H., Kouzarides, T., Patel, S. S., and Reinberg, D. (2005). Human but not yeast CHD1 binds directly and selectively to histone H3 methylated at lysine 4 via its tandem chromodomains. *J Biol Chem* 280, 41789–41792.

61. Huang, Y., Fang, J., Bedford, M. T., Zhang, Y., and Xu, R. M. (2006). Recognition of histone H3 lysine-4 methylation by the double tudor domain of JMJD2A. *Science* 312, 748–751.

62. Lan, F., Collins, R. E., De Cegli, R., Alpatov, R., Horton, J. R., Shi, X., Gozani, O., Cheng, X., and Shi, Y. (2007). Recognition of unmethylated histone H3 lysine 4 links BHC80 to LSD1-mediated gene repression. *Nature* 448, 718–722.

63. Kwan, A. H., Gell, D. A., Verger, A., Crossley, M., Matthews, J. M., and Mackay, J. P. (2003). Engineering a protein scaffold from a PHD finger. *Structure* 11, 803–813.

64. Wang, J., Scully, K., Zhu, X., Cai, L., Zhang, J., Prefontaine, G. G., Krones, A., Ohgi, K. A., Zhu, P., Garcia-Bassets, I., Liu, F., Taylor, H., Lozach, J., Jayes, F. L., Korach, K. S., Glass, C. K., Fu, X. D., and Rosenfeld, M. G. (2007). Opposing LSD1 complexes function in developmental gene activation and repression programmes. *Nature* 446, 882–887.

65. Collins, R. E., Northrop, J. P., Horton, J. R., Lee, D. Y., Zhang, X., Stallcup, M. R., and Cheng, X. (2008). The ankyrin repeats of G9a and GLP histone methyltransferases are mono- and dimethyllysine binding modules. *Nat Struct Mol Biol* 15, 245–250.

66. Tachibana, M., Sugimoto, K., Nozaki, M., Ueda, J., and Ohta, T. (2002). G9a histone methyltransferase plays a dominant role in euchromatic histone H3 lysine 9 methylation and is essential for early embryogenesis. *Genes Dev* 16, 1779–1791.

67. Rice, J. C., Briggs, S. D., Ueberheide, B., Barber, C. M., and Shabanowitz, J. (2003). Histone methyltransferases direct different degrees of methylation to define distinct chromatin domains. *Mol Cell* 12, 1591–1598.

68. Tachibana, M., Ueda, J., Fukuda, M., Takeda, N., Ohta, T., Iwanari, H., Sakihama, T., Kodama, T., Hamakubo, T., and Shinkai, Y. (2005). Histone methyltransferases G9a and GLP form heteromeric complexes and are both crucial for methylation of euchromatin at H3-K9. *Genes Dev* 19, 815–826.

69. Botuyan, M. V., Lee, J., Ward, I. M., Kim, J. E., Thompson, J. R., Chen, J., and Mer, G. (2006). Structural basis for the methylation state-specific recognition of histone H4-K20 by 53BP1 and Crb2 in DNA repair. *Cell* 127, 1361–1373.

70. Longin, S., and Goris, J. (2006). Reversible methylation of protein phosphatase 2A. *Enzymes* 24, 303–324.

71. Antomattei, F. M., and Weis, R. M. (2006). Reversible methylation of glutamate residues in the receptor proteins of bacterial sensory systems. *Enzymes* 24, 325–382.

72. Shi, Y., Lan, F., Matson, C., Mulligan, P., and Whetstine, J. R. (2004). Histone demethylation mediated by the nuclear amine oxidase homolog LSD1. *Cell* 119, 941–953.

73. Shi, Y. J., Matson, C., Lan, F., Iwase, S., Baba, T., and Shi, Y. (2005). Regulation of LSD1 histone demethylase activity by its associated factors. *Mol Cell* 19, 857–864.

74. Lee, M. G., Wynder, C., Cooch, N., and Shiekhattar, R. (2005). An essential role for CoREST in nucleosomal histone 3 lysine 4 demethylation. *Nature* 437, 432–435.

75. Tsukada, Y., Fang, J., Erdjument-Bromage, H., Warren, M. E., Borchers, C. H., Tempst, P., and Zhang, Y. (2006). Histone demethylation by a family of JmjC domain-containing proteins. *Nature* 439, 811–816.

76. Whetstine, J. R., Nottke, A., Lan, F., Huarte, M., Smolikov, S., Chen, Z., Spooner, E., Li, E., Zhang, G., Colaiacovo, M., and Shi, Y. (2006). Reversal of histone lysine trimethylation by the JMJD2 family of histone demethylases. *Cell* 125, 467–481.

77. Tochio, N., Umehara, T., Koshiba, S., Inoue, M., Yabuki, T., Aoki, M., Seki, E., Watanabe, S., Tomo, Y., Hanada, M., Ikari, M., Sato, M., Terada, T., Nagase, T., Ohara, O., Shirouzu, M., Tanaka, A., Kigawa, T., and Yokoyama, S. (2006). Solution structure of the SWIRM domain of human histone demethylase LSD1. *Structure* 14, 457–468.

78. Forneris, F., Binda, C., Vanoni, M. A., Battaglioli, E., and Mattevi, A. (2005). Human histone demethylase LSD1 reads the histone code. *J Biol Chem* 280, 41360–41365.

79. Binda, C., Mattevi, A., and Edmondson, D. E. (2002). Structure-function relationships in flavoenzyme-dependent amine oxidations: A comparison of polyamine oxidase and monoamine oxidase. *J Biol Chem* 277, 23973–23976.

80. Huang, J., Sengupta, R., Espejo, A. B., Lee, M. G., Dorsey, J. A., Richter, M., Opravil, S., Shiekhattar, R., Bedford, M. T., Jenuwein, T., and Berger, S. L. (2007). p53 is regulated by the lysine demethylase LSD1. *Nature* 449, 105–108.

81. Huang, J., Perez-Burgos, L., Placek, B. J., Sengupta, R., Richter, M., Dorsey, J. A., Kubicek, S., Opravil, S., Jenuwein, T., and Berger, S. L. (2006). Repression of p53 activity by Smyd2-mediated methylation. *Nature* 444, 629–632.

82. Chen, Y., Yang, Y., Wang, F., Wan, K., Yamane, K., Zhang, Y., and Lei, M. (2006). Crystal structure of human histone lysine-specific demethylase 1 (LSD1). *Proc Natl Acad Sci USA* 103, 13956–13961.

83. Stavropoulos, P., Blobel, G., and Hoelz, A. (2006). Crystal structure and mechanism of human lysine-specific demethylase-1. *Nat Struct Mol Biol* 13, 626–632.

84. Yang, M., Gocke, C. B., Luo, X., Borek, D., Tomchick, D. R., Machius, M., Otwinowski, Z., and Yu, H. (2006). Structural basis for CoREST-dependent demethylation of nucleosomes by the human LSD1 histone demethylase. *Mol Cell* 23, 377–387.

85. Yang, M., Culhane, J. C., Szewczuk, L. M., Gocke, C. B., Brautigam, C. A., Tomchick, D. R., Machius, M., Cole, P. A., and Yu, H. (2007). Structural basis of histone demethylation by LSD1 revealed by suicide inactivation. *Nat Struct Mol Biol* 14, 535–539.

86. Forneris, F., Binda, C., Adamo, A., Battaglioli, E., and Mattevi, A. (2007). Structural basis of LSD1-CoREST selectivity in histone H3 recognition. *J Biol Chem* 282, 20070–20074.

87. Falnes, P. O., Johansen, R. F., and Seeberg, E. (2002). AlkB-mediated oxidative demethylation reverses DNA damage in *Escherichia coli*. *Nature* 419, 178–182.

88. Trewick, S. C., Henshaw, T. F., Hausinger, R. P., Lindahl, T., and Sedgwick, B. (2002). Oxidative demethylation by *Escherichia coli* AlkB directly reverts DNA base damage. *Nature* 419, 174–178.

89. Yu, B., Edstrom, W. C., Benach, J., Hamuro, Y., Weber, P. C., Gibney, B. R., and Hunt, J. F. (2006). Crystal structures of catalytic complexes of the oxidative DNA/RNA repair enzyme AlkB. *Nature* 439, 879–884.

90. Trewick, S. C., McLaughlin, P. J., and Allshire, R. C. (2005). Methylation: Lost in hydroxylation? *EMBO Rep* 6, 315–320.

91. Ayoub, N., Noma, K., Isaac, S., Kahan, T., Grewal, S. I., and Cohen, A. (2003). A novel jmjC domain protein modulates heterochromatization in fission yeast. *Mol Cell Biol* 23, 4356–4370.

92. Elkins, J. M., Hewitson, K. S., McNeill, L. A., Seibel, J. F., Schlemminger, I., Pugh, C. W., Ratcliffe, P. J., and Schofield, C. J. (2003). Structure of factor-inhibiting hypoxia-inducible factor (HIF) reveals mechanism of oxidative modification of HIF-1 alpha. *J Biol Chem* 278, 1802–1806.

93. Clissold, P. M., and Ponting, C. P. (2001). JmjC: Cupin metalloenzyme-like domains in jumonji, hairless and phospholipase A2beta. *Trends Biochem Sci* 26, 7–9.

94. Yamane, K., Toumazou, C., Tsukada, Y., Erdjument-Bromage, H., Tempst, P., Wong, J., and Zhang, Y. (2006). JHDM2A, a JmjC-containing H3K9 demethylase, facilitates transcription activation by androgen receptor. *Cell* 125, 483–495.

95. Chen, Z., Zang, J., Whetstine, J., Hong, X., Davrazou, F., Kutateladze, T. G., Simpson, M., Mao, Q., Pan, C. H., Dai, S., Hagman, J., Hansen, K., Shi, Y., and Zhang, G. (2006). Structural insights into histone demethylation by JMJD2 family members. *Cell* 125, 691–702.

96. Ng, S. S., Kavanagh, K. L., McDonough, M. A., Butler, D., Pilka, E. S., Lienard, B. M., Bray, J. E., Savitsky, P., Gileadi, O., von Delft, F., Rose, N. R., Offer, J., Scheinost, J. C., Borowski, T., Sundstrom, M., Schofield, C. J., and Oppermann, U. (2007). Crystal structures of histone demethylase JMJD2A reveal basis for substrate specificity. *Nature* 448, 87–91.

97. Chen, Z., Zang, J., Kappler, J., Hong, X., Crawford, F., Wang, Q., Lan, F., Jiang, C., Whetstine, J., Dai, S., Hansen, K., Shi, Y., and Zhang, G. (2007). Structural basis of the recognition of a methylated histone tail by JMJD2A. *Proc Natl Acad Sci USA* 104, 10818–10823.

98. Couture, J. F., Collazo, E., Ortiz-Tello, P. A., Brunzelle, J. S., and Trievel, R. C. (2007). Specificity and mechanism of JMJD2A, a trimethyllysine-specific histone demethylase. *Nat Struct Mol Biol* 14, 689–695.

99. Klose, R. J., Kallin, E. M., and Zhang, Y. (2006). JmjC-domain-containing proteins and histone demethylation. *Nat Rev Genet* 7, 715–727.

100. Branscombe, T. L., Frankel, A., Lee, J. H., Cook, J. R., and Yang, Z. (2001). PRMT5 (Janus kinase-binding protein 1) catalyzes the formation of symmetric dimethylarginine residues in proteins. *J Biol Chem* 276, 32971–32976.

101. Bedford, M. T., and Richard, S. (2005). Arginine methylation an emerging regulator of protein function. *Mol Cell* 18, 263–272.

102. Chen, D., Ma, H., Hong, H., Koh, S. S., and Huang, S. M. (1999). Regulation of transcription by a protein methyltransferase. *Science* 284, 2174–2177.

103. Schurter, B. T., Koh, S. S., Chen, D., Bunick, G. J., and Harp, J. M. (2001). Methylation of histone H3 by coactivator-associated arginine methyltransferase 1. *Biochemistry* 40, 5747–5756.

104. Ma, H., Baumann, C. T., Li, H., Strahl, B. D., and Rice, R. (2001). Hormone-dependent, CARM1-directed, arginine-specific methylation of histone H3 on a steroid-regulated promoter. *Curr Biol* 11, 1981–1985.

105. Bauer, U. M., Daujat, S., Nielsen, S. J., Nightingale, K., and Kouzarides, T. (2002). Methylation at arginine 17 of histone H3 is linked to gene activation. *EMBO Rep* 3, 39–44.

106. Guccione, E., Bassi, C., Casadio, F., Martinato, F., Cesaroni, M., Schuchlautz, H., Luscher, B., and Amati, B. (2007). Methylation of histone H3R2 by PRMT6 and H3K4 by an MLL complex are mutually exclusive. *Nature* 49, 933–937.

107. Strahl, B. D., Briggs, S. D., Brame, C. J., Caldwell, J. A., and Koh, S. S. (2001). Methylation of histone H4 at arginine 3 occurs in vivo and is mediated by the nuclear receptor coactivator PRMT1. *Curr Biol* 11, 996–1000.

108. Wang, H., Huang, Z. Q., Xia, L., Feng, Q., and Erdjument-Bromage, H. (2001). Methylation of histone H4 at arginine 3 facilitating transcriptional activation by nuclear hormone receptor. *Science* 293, 853–857.

109. An, W., Kim, J., and Roeder, R. G. (2004). Ordered cooperative functions of PRMT1, p300, and CARM1 in transcriptional activation by p53. *Cell* 117, 735.

110. Strahl, B. D., and Allis, C. D. (2000). The language of covalent histone modifications. *Nature* 403, 41–45.

111. Kouzarides, T. (2002). Histone methylation in transcriptional control. *Curr Opin Genet Dev* 12, 198–209.

112. Xu, W., Chen, H., Du, K., Asahara, H., and Tini, M. (2001). A transcriptional switch mediated by cofactor methylation. *Science* 294, 2507–2517.

113. Lee, Y. H., Koh, S. S., Zhang, X., Cheng, X., and Stallcup, M. R. (2002). Synergy among nuclear receptor coactivators: Selective requirement for protein methyltransferase and acetyltransferase activities. *Mol Cell Biol* 22, 3621–3632.

114. Daujat, S., Bauer, U. M., Shah, V., Turner, B., Berger, S., and Kouzarides, T. (2002). Crosstalk between CARM1 methylation and CBP acetylation on histone H3. *Curr Biol* 12, 2090–2097.

115. Kirmizis, A., Santos-Rosa, H., Penkett, C. J., Singer, M. A., Vermeulen, M., Mann, M., Bahler, J., Green, R. D., and Kouzarides, T. (2007). Arginine methylation at histone H3R2 controls deposition of H3K4 trimethylation. *Nature* 449, 928–932.

116. Scott, H. S., Antonarakis, S. E., Lalioti, M. D., Rossier, C., Silver, P. A., and Henry, M. F. (1998). Identification and characterization of two putative human arginine methyltransferases (HRMT1L1 and HRMT1L2). *Genomics* 48, 330–340.

117. Troffer-Charlier, N., Cura, V., Hassenboehler, P., Moras, D., and Cavarelli, J. (2007). Functional insights from structures of coactivator-associated arginine methyltransferase 1 domains. *EMBO J* 26, 4391–4401.

118. Zhang, X., Zhou, L., and Cheng, X. (2000). Crystal structure of the conserved core of protein arginine methyltransferase PRMT3. *EMBO J* 19, 3509–3519.

119. Weiss, V. H., McBride, A. E., Soriano, M. A., Filman, D. J., Silver, P. A., and Hogle, J. M. (2000). The structure and oligomerization of the yeast arginine methyltransferase, Hmt1. *Nat Struct Biol* 7, 1165–1171.

120. Zhang, X., and Cheng, X. (2003). Structure of the predominant protein arginine methyltransferase PRMT1 and analysis of its binding to substrate peptides. *Structure* 11, 509–520.

121. Yue, W. W., Hassler, M., Roe, S. M., Thompson-Vale, V., and Pearl, L. H. (2007). Insights into histone code syntax from structural and biochemical studies of CARM1 methyltransferase. *EMBO J* 26, 4402–4412.

122. Higashimoto, K., Kuhn, P., Desai, D., Cheng, X., and Xu, W. (2007). Phosphorylation-mediated inactivation of coactivator-associated arginine methyltransferase 1. *Proc Natl Acad Sci USA* 104, 12318–12323.

123. Grewal, S. I., and Jia, S. (2007). Heterochromatin revisited. *Nat Rev Genet* 8, 35–46.

124. Lee, M. G., Villa, R., Trojer, P., Norman, J., Yan, K. P., Reinberg, D., Di Croce, L., and Shiekhattar, R. (2007). Demethylation of H3K27 regulates Polycomb recruitment and H2A ubiquitination. *Science* 318, 447–450.

125. Lan, F., Bayliss, P. E., Rinn, J. L., Whetstine, J. R., Wang, J. K., Chen, S., Iwase, S., Alpatov, R., Issaeva, I., Canaani, E., Roberts, T. M., Chang, H. Y., and Shi, Y. (2007). A histone H3 lysine 27 demethylase regulates animal posterior development. *Nature* 449, 689–694.

126. De Santa, F., Totaro, M. G., Prosperini, E., Notarbartolo, S., Testa, G., and Natoli, G. (2007). The histone H3 lysine-27 demethylase Jmjd3 links inflammation to inhibition of Polycomb-mediated gene silencing. *Cell* 130, 1083–1094.

127. Agger, K., Cloos, P. A., Christensen, J., Pasini, D., Rose, S., Rappsilber, J., Issaeva, I., Canaani, E., Salcini, A. E., and Helin, K. (2007). UTX and JMJD3 are histone H3K27 demethylases involved in HOX gene regulation and development. *Nature* 449, 731–734.

chapter three

Mammalian DNA methyltransferases
Catalytic mechanism, structure, and functions

Michael J. Boland and Judith K. Christman

Contents

3.1   Introduction

5-Methylcytosine (5mC) was first detected in mammalian DNA 60 years ago[1] and within six years, it was demonstrated that the only dinucleotide with significant 5mC content was 5mC,G.[2,3] It took almost another decade to determine that cytosine residues were enzymatically methylated after incorporation into DNA, establishing the basis for epigenetic modulation of gene expression.[4,5] The first demonstrations that inhibition of DNA methylation could induce differentiation of cultured cells were published in the late 1970s.[6–8] Since then, it has become increasingly clear that DNA methylation plays a number of important roles in cellular homeostasis and regulation of normal mammalian development. Methylation of DNA promotes genomic stability through repression of mitotic recombination and transposition, assuring proper chromatid segregation and maintenance of higher-order heterochromatin structure.[9–11] Genomic methylation patterns also play a crucial role during embryogenesis, leading to temporal transcriptional repression of critical developmental programs during cellular differentiation through its ability to regulate chromatin structure.[12–14] Additionally, DNA methylation is integral to the processes of genomic imprinting and gene dosage compensation in females through inactivation of one X chromosome.[15,16] A variety of tumors exhibit aberrant DNA methylation patterns. The most common change is an early global loss or reduction in DNA methylation, that is hypomethylation.[17–20] This is followed by localized promoter hypermethylation of tumor-suppressor genes (see Reference 21 for a comprehensive review of epigenetic events associated with cancer).

Methylation of bases in mammalian DNA only occurs at position 5 of the cytosine pyrimidine ring, with the majority of DNA methylation occurring in CpG dideoxynucleotides (5′-CG-3′). In normal somatic cells, approximately 1% to 4 % of all cytosine residues are methylated depending on cell/tissue type. This reflects the methylation of 70% to 80% of all CpG sites in the genome.[22] Although CpG sites are underrepresented in the mammalian genome, it is hypothesized that during evolution there has been selection for regions of high CpG density that are located in repeated satellite DNA and gene promoter-associated CpG islands.[23] The majority of methylated cytosines are located in LINE/SINE transposons, long-terminal repeats of endogenous retroviruses and short, tandemly repeated satellite DNA that is present in centromeres and pericentromeric regions juxtaposed to centromeres (reviewed in Reference 24).

In contrast, CpG sites in CpG islands associated with the promoters of ~70% of mammalian genes[25,26] generally remain unmethylated during normal tissue differentiation. The exception is imprinted genes and a subgroup of genes repressed in a tissue specific manner.[24,25,27] Recent examination of

DNA methylation patterns in a variety of human tissues indicated that ~85% of CpG islands in somatic cells remain unmethylated.[28-30] It was also found that the CpG islands of many transcriptionally inactive genes possess low levels of DNA methylation, suggesting that additional epigenetic mechanisms are in place to regulate gene expression in a coordinate and combinatorial manner.[30] This supports earlier observations that transcriptional silencing precedes DNA methylation of retroviral elements, proviral sequences and genes silenced during X chromatin inactivation (reviewed in Reference 24).

3.2 Mechanism of DNA methylation

Mammalian DNA methyltransferases (Dnmts) were first purified in the late 1960s and shown to catalyze the transfer of a methyl group from *S*-adenosyl-L-methionine (AdoMet, SAM) to carbon 5 of the cytosine pyrimidine ring, resulting in 5-methylcytosine.[31-33] The mechanistic basis of this transfer was established in a prokaryotic Dnmt, M.HhaI.[34] Biochemical and structural studies of Dnmts have complemented each other in providing a mechanistic view of DNA methylation (Figure 3.1). Mechanistic and structural studies suggest that both bacterial and mammalian Dnmts exist in a relaxed or open conformation when not associated with DNA.[6,35,36] Binding of Dnmts to their recognition sites in DNA induces a conformational change in the enzyme resulting in a closed conformation that is primed for methyl-transfer and the methylation reaction is initiated after extrahelical flipping of the target cytosine into the Dnmt active site.[37] Nucleophilic attack on target cytosine carbon 6 (C6) by the thiolate anion of the conserved Dnmt active site cysteine forms a covalent

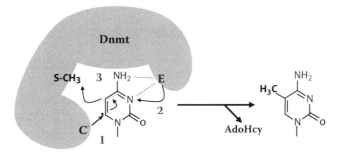

Figure 3.1 (*A color version of this figure follows page 20.*) DNA (cytosine-C5) methyltransferase catalyzed methyl transfer. Blue Dnmt ovals represent different regions of the same Dnmt protein. S-CH$_3$ symbolizes the *S*-methyl moiety of *S*-adenosyl methionine. Refer to the text for other details.

intermediate between enzyme and substrate resulting in saturation of the double bond between C5 and C6 (Figure 3.1, step 1). Electron rearrangement across C4 and C5 (dashed red line) in concert with enzymatic protonation of C3 (step 2) creates a temporary electrophilic center at C5, thereby priming it for methyl acceptance by nucleophilic attack on the methylsulfonium moiety of AdoMet (step 3). Following methyl transfer, an activated water molecule abstracts a proton from C5 allowing β-elimination to occur followed by release of the enzyme and *S*-adenosyl-L-homocysteine (AdoHcy, SAH).

3.3   *Mammalian DNA methyltransferases*

There are three families of mammalian Dnmts: Dnmt1, Dnmt2 and the Dnmt3 family, which consists of three members, 3a, 3b and 3L (Figure 3.2). The C-terminal catalytic domain of mammalian methyltransferases is homologous to that of bacterial methyltransferases. Each Dnmt possesses characteristic and highly conserved DNA (cytosine-C5) methyltransferase motifs within their catalytic domains that are necessary for transmethylation.[38] The conserved Dnmt motifs (I, IV, VI, VIII, IX, X) are indicated by black bars. Together, motifs I and X form the AdoMet binding pocket; the phylogenetically conserved active site ProCys dipeptide resides in motif IV. A glutamyl residue located in the conserved GluAsnVal tripeptide of motif VI is responsible for protonating position 3 of the target cytosine and motif IX organizes the structure of the target recognition domain (TRD) located between motifs VIII and IX. The N-terminus of each of the mammalian Dnmts contains regulatory domains/motifs specific to that enzyme. These motifs are responsible

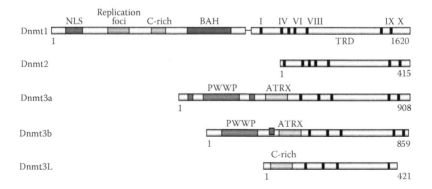

Figure 3.2 (A color version of this figure follows page 20.) Mammalian DNA methyltransferases. Shaded regions indicate protein binding domains. Black bars indicate conserved sequences in the catalytic domains.

for the interactions of Dnmts with other proteins, nuclear/subnuclear localization and genomic targeting.

3.4   DNA methyltransferase 1

DNA methyltransferase 1 (Dnmt1) was the first Dnmt to be identified and cloned.[39] It possesses a 5- to 30-fold preference for hemimethylated substrates[40–43] and is targeted to replication foci through an N-terminal interaction with PCNA.[44–48] Because of these characteristics, Dnmt1 is considered to be the major maintenance methyltransferase in mammalian cells and to be responsible for restoring the fully methylated status of CpG sites on the newly synthesized daughter strand following replication.

Dnmt1 is ubiquitously expressed during postimplantation and post-natal development. However, it is regulated by alternative splicing events during gametogenesis. These lead to production of an oocyte-specific Dnmt1 that is actively sequestered in the cytoplasm and a spermatocyte-specific form that is translationally repressed during meiosis.[49,50]

Embryonic stem (ES) cells that lack Dnmt1 (*Dnmt1-/-*) proliferate normally and do not display any morphologic abnormalities even though the absence of Dnmt1 leads to a 70% reduction in overall 5mC content of DNA.[51] Gene-targeting of *Dnmt1* in the mouse results in embryonic lethality,[51] with a number of abnormal phenotypes that are now known to be a consequence of severe global hypomethylation. These include altered gene expression, reduced cell proliferation and increased incidence of apoptosis coincident with aberrant chromosomal recombination. Rhee and colleagues reported that the 5mC level in *DNMT1-/-* HCT116 colorectal cells did not cause more than a 20% reduction in global methylation.[52] This led them to conclude that DNMT3B cooperates with DNMT1 to maintain genomic methylation levels.[53] However, the homologous recombination technique used by Rhee et al. to generate the *DNMT1-/-* and *DNMT1-/-/ DNMT3B-/-* HCT116 cell lines was found to produce a hypomorphic allele resulting in low-level expression of a truncated DNMT1 protein that retained methyltransferase activity.[54] In contrast, RNAi depletion of the truncated DNMT1 protein resulted in dramatically decreased methylation levels and cell survival. This suggests that DNMT1 is essential for normal cell proliferation and/or survival.[54] Chen et al.[55] provided support for this suggestion by generating a conditional *DNMT1* knockout in HCT116 cells that results in a complete loss of DNMT1 activity and activation of the G_2/M checkpoint, leading to arrest in the G_2 phase of the cell cycle. The small fraction of DNMT1 null HCT116 cells that escaped arrest displayed severe mitotic abnormalities, such as tetraploidy, uncongressed and misaligned chromosomes, chromosome fragments and anaphase bridges. Eventually the cells succumbed to the mitotic defects and either died during the following mitosis or arrested in a tetraploid state.[55]

3.5   DNA methyltransferase 2

Dnmt2 was the second mammalian DNA methyltransferase to be discovered.[56] Although Dnmt2 contains all of the necessary motifs required for methylation, it has very little activity when tested with DNA substrates.[56,57] Thus, the in vivo function of Dnmt2 remained elusive until recently, when Lyco and colleagues demonstrated that the *Drosophila melanogaster* Dnmt2 homolog has DNA methyltransferase activity that is restricted to a narrow window of early development (see Kunert et al.[58]). Two reports have presented evidence that Dnmt2 also functions as an RNA methyltransferase, specifically methylating the anticodon loop of tRNA[(Asp)].[59] In zebrafish, Dnmt2-cataylzed tRNA[(Asp)] methylation activity occurs in the cytoplasm and is essential for proper organ development.[60] There are other examples of RNA methyltransferases that can methylate DNA substrates in vitro,[61] suggesting that the duality of enzymes that carry out DNA and RNA methylation may be a more general phenomenon than is currently appreciated.

3.6   The Dnmt3 family: de novo methyltransferases

Two strong lines of evidence suggested the existence of enzymes that could methylate DNA de novo (i.e., methylate a fully unmethylated CpG site) long before they were identified in 1998. First, there was evidence for a genome-wide event that resulted in significant loss of methylation of bulk genomic DNA in mouse embryos during the postfertilization, preimplantation stage that was completed at the blastula stage.[62,63] This loss of DNA methylation within the cells of the inner cell mass was reversed by de novo methylation during the period from blastocyst implantation at mouse embryonic day 3.5 (E3.5) to a time shortly before gastrulation (E7.0).[63–65] Second, ES cells nullizygous for Dnmt1, the only DNA methyltransferase that had been identified at that time, were viable and contained reduced but stable levels of 5-methylcytosine.[51] However, when *Dnmt1[-/-]* ES cells were forced to differentiate, the levels of 5-methylcytosine were further reduced, indicating downregulation of a DNA methyltransferase(s) during the differentiation process.[51] In addition, *Dnmt1[-/-]* ES cells were found to retain the ability to de novo methylate integrated proviral DNA.[66]

   The de novo methyltransferases, Dnmt3a and Dnmt3b, were discovered by a BLAST (Basic Logical Alignment Search Tool) search of the EST (Expressed Sequence Tag) database using a full-length bacterial methyltransferase sequence as bait.[67] Structurally, Dnmt3a and Dnmt3b share little homology to either Dnmt1 or Dnmt2. The exceptions are the conserved methyltransferase catalytic motifs. Both Dnmt3a and 3b are highly expressed in ES cells but their expression decreases dramatically as the cells differentiate into embryoid bodies.[67] Northern blotting revealed the presence of *Dnmt3a* transcripts in adult heart, brain and lungs and reduced expression in the liver, kidney and testis adult tissues. In contrast, *Dnmt3b* was found to be strongly expressed in the testes but barely detectable in other tissues examined. Weak, but reproducible expression of *Dnmt3b*, was observed in liver, lung, spleen and heart tissue. These results provided the first indication that Dnmt3a and 3b are temporally regulated during development.[67]

3.7   *Dnmt3a and Dnmt3b possess distinct functions during embryogenesis*

Dnmt3a and 3b share a certain degree of target redundancy (e.g., pericentromeric satellite repeats[68]). However, evidence suggests that they perform nonoverlapping functions at different stages of embryogenesis. Recent studies demonstrate that Dnmt3a and Dnmt3b have different expression profiles during cellular differentiation. For example, Dnmt3b is strongly expressed in totipotent cells of the inner cell mass, epiblast and embryonic ectoderm during early embryogenesis (E 4.5–E7.5) but Dnmt3a is not expressed in appreciable amounts during the same time period.[69] It should be noted that this is the period during mouse development when genome-wide remethylation of DNA occurs.[63] One study showed that during olfactory receptor neuron development, Dnmt3b expression is restricted to primitive mitotic progenitors, whereas Dnmt3a is found in more differentiated postmitotic neurons.[70] The same study also demonstrated sequential expression of Dnmt3b and Dnmt3a in the retina, taste buds and central nervous system (CNS), suggesting conservation of differential de novo methyltransferase expression during embryogenesis. These findings have been bolstered by those of Feng et al.,[71] who found that Dnmt3b expression in the developing CNS is restricted to early neurogenesis and declines rapidly as development proceeds. In contrast, Dnmt3a is primarily expressed in post-mitotic CNS neurons from the newborn stage to adulthood.[71] Additionally, *Dnmt3a*[-/-] and *Dnmt3b*[-/-] mice die at different stages of development. *Dnmt3a*[-/-] mice develop to term but become runted and die at ~4 weeks of age, while *Dnmt3b*[-/-] embryos develop normally until E9.0 and then die from a myriad of developmental defects, including growth impairment and neural tube defects.[72]

The de novo methyltransferases also display distinct target preferences and modes of activity.[73] Dnmt3a has been demonstrated to possess a CpG site-selectivity that differs from that of Dnmt3b.[74] Dnmt3a also exhibits a preference for methylating naked DNA or the naked part of nucleosomal DNA (i.e., the linker region)[75] while Dnmt3b is capable of methylating DNA within the nucleosome core and displays reduced activity to naked DNA when compared to Dnmt3a. In contrast to Dnmt1, which is expressed during the S phase of the cell cycle,[76] neither Dnmt3a nor 3b is localized to replication foci.[77] They are targeted to and methylate pericentromeric satellite DNA.[72,78] However, Dnmt3b, but not 3a, is responsible for methylation of the centromeric satellite repeats in ES cells and mouse embryos.[72]

3.8   Alternate isoforms of Dnmt3a and Dnmt3b

The *Dnmt3a* locus produces two main transcripts: full-length Dnmt3a and Dnmt3a2, which lacks 249 N-terminal amino acids. Dnmt3a2 is the predominant isoform expressed in ES and EC (embryonal carcinoma) cells.[79] The N-terminus of both proteins contains a PWWP and an ATRX-like domain that serve to regulate the nuclear localization, genomic targeting and protein interactions of each protein. For example, Dnmt3a primarily localizes to heterochromatin[80] while Dnmt3a2 can be found throughout the nucleus suggesting that it may also localize to euchromatin.[79]

The *Dnmt3b* locus produces five major splice variants of Dnmt3b, 3b2–6, which are highly conserved between human and mouse.[72,81] The full-length transcript/protein is referred to as Dnmt3b1 whereas Dnmt3b2 is encoded by an mRNA generated by an alternative splicing event that removes the N-terminal exons 10 and 11 (amino acids 362–383). Dnmt3b3 is produced by splicing at exons 10/11 and exons 21/22 (amino acids 750–814) in the catalytic domain while 3b4 is a C-terminal truncated protein that lacks exons 10/11 and 21–23. Dnmt3b5 lacks exons 10/11 and 22 (amino acids 773–814) and the C-terminal 45 amino acids are out of frame. Dnmt3b6 is missing exons 21 and 22 (amino acids 750–814). Each of the variants has a separate expression profile and some have been implicated in development of cancer but the precise nature of their biological role has yet to be elucidated. With the exception of Dnmt 3b2, all of the alternate isoforms are predicted to be catalytically inactive due to lack of specific methyltransferase motifs. The major transcripts produced in ES and EC cells are those of Dnmt3b1 and 3b6,[79] although two additional isoforms (3b7, 3b8) specific to mouse ES cells have also been described.[82] Despite its lack of catalytic activity, Dnmt3b4 has been implicated in the negative regulation of methylation in hepatocellular carcinoma.[83] Dnmt3b3 may also play a role in the regulation of methylation.[82] All of the alternative isoforms possess the PWWP and ATRX-like domains which are the primary mediators of Dnmt3b-protein interactions. Thus, all of the alternative Dnmt3b isoforms would be expected to interact with those proteins that interact with Dnmt3b1 through these domains.

Genomic targeting of DNA methyltransferases has begun to be elucidated. Specific domains/motifs within the N-terminal domains of each of the Dnmts are responsible for their subnuclear and genomic localization. Dnmt1 is targeted to replication foci through a targeting motif[45] and retained at replication foci through a PCNA-binding motif.[44,46] The PWWP domains of Dnmt3a and 3b are responsible for targeting them to pericentromeric heterochromatin.[68,84] One mechanism for targeting Dnmts to a particular promoter to mediate transcriptional repression is through interactions between the Dnmt and a sequence-specific transcription factor or a corepressor. For example, a ternary complex is formed between Dnmt3a and Myc and Miz1. Miz recruits the Dnmt3a:Myc complex to the *Cdkn1a* promoter. Myc selectively targets Dnmt3a to the *Cdkn1a* promoter where it induces DNA methylation and gene silencing.[85] In addition, Dnmt3a but not Dnmt3b localizes to the *Il18r1* promoter as well as the promoters of many Stat4-dependent genes during helper T cell differentiation.[86] Together, these experiments demonstrate that DNA methyltransferases possess distinct genomic targets.

3.9   Dnmt3L

DNA methyltransferase 3-like (Dnmt3L) shares some degree of homology to Dnmt3a/3b but lacks the conserved PC and ENV motifs necessary for catalysis, as well as the C-terminal half of motif IX and all of motif X.[87,88] Therefore, it possesses no inherent catalytic activity. A number of studies have provided evidence for the role of Dnmt3L as part of the DNA methylation machinery. Physical interaction of Dnmt3L with Dnmt3a and Dnmt3b stimulates their activity as well as that of their alternate isoforms.[89–94] Original studies identified a role for Dnmt3L in the establishment of maternal imprints in the oocyte.[87] These findings were confirmed when Li and colleagues generated and characterized Dnmt3L-deficient mouse embryos (Hata et al.[88]). Female *Dnmt3L*[-/-] mice failed to establish maternal imprints in the oocyte and male *Dnmt3L* homozygous null mice were sterile, suggesting a role for Dnmt3L in maternal imprinting and spermatogenesis. The same study identified an interaction between Dnmt3L and Dnmt3a/3b. In the absence of Dnmt3a or 3b, Dnmt3L is localized in the cytoplasm. However, co-expression of either Dnmt3a or Dnmt3b with Dnmt3L leads to co-localization of Dnmt3L with Dnmt3a or 3b in the nucleus.[88] Consistent with the ability of Dnmt3L to stimulate the activity of Dnmt3a or 3b, specific *DNMT3B* mutations found in ICF (immunodeficiency, centromeric instability and facial anomalies) syndrome patients that reduce the catalytic activity do so by affecting the ability of Dnmt3L to interact with Dnmt3b.[95]

3.10   Methylated-DNA binding proteins

The Bird laboratory originally identified a protein that could bind methylated DNA and, in so doing, repress transcription.[96] Since then a number of methyl-CpG binding proteins have been identified[97] and collectively they can be regarded as the "effector" molecules of DNA methylation-mediated transcriptional repression. Each of the five members (MeCP2 and MBD1–4) possesses a domain that binds methylated DNA and their mode of action is to exclude binding of the transcriptional machinery. The MBD proteins are also thought to tether other epigenetic regulators (i.e., histone deacetylases [HDACs] and histone methyltransferases [HMTases]) to chromatin in order to establish and maintain transcription repression. Evidence suggests that they have nonoverlapping functions within the cell. For example, MBD2 resides in a complex that includes HDAC1 and HDAC2 among other proteins,[98] whereas MBD3 is a component of the ubiquitous NuRD/Mi2 chromatin remodeling complex.[99,100] MBD1 has been shown to interact with the histone methyltransferase Suv39h and the chromodomain protein HP1,[101] as well as a subunit of chromatin assembly factor 1 (CAF-1)[102] to mediate transcriptional repression. In addition to its role in transcriptional repression,[103] MBD4 possesses thymine-DNA glycosylase activity,[104] although the in vivo relevance of this activity has yet to be demonstrated. Each of the MBD proteins possesses a characteristic binding affinity for DNA that is determined in part by density and spacing of methylated CpG sites, as well as neighboring sequence contexts.[105]

3.11 DNA methylation and chromatin structure

Based on structure, chromatin can be divided into two classes: euchromatin and heterochromatin.[10] Euchromatin is the fraction of the genome that is transcriptionally active and exits in a relaxed, decondensed state during interphase. Heterochromatin remains condensed throughout the cell cycle and is generally considered transcriptionally inactive. Centromeres and pericentromeric regions are the best examples of heterochromatin. These regions are late replicating and can be distinguished cytologically during interphase because they form highly condensed chromatin regions that are densely stained with 4′,6-diamidino-2-phenylindole (DAPI). Heterochromatin can also be found at and around the promoters of transcriptionally inactive genes.

The structural basis of heterochromatin formation is beginning to be elucidated, primarily through intensive study of the mouse and yeast (Schizosaccharomyces pombe) genomes.[106,107] Pericentromeric heterochromatin is composed of highly repetitive satellite DNA sequences that are known as the major satellite repeats in murine cells. These repeats consist of 234 bp monomers that are tandemly arranged into higher-order nucleosomal arrays over regions spanning 240 to 2,000 kb in length. Pericentromeric nucleosomes (and those of heterochromatin in general) contain a variety of epigenetic modifications that are stably inherited through mitosis and cell division. Generally, the N-terminal histone tails are hypoacetylated;

histone 3 (H3) exhibits the repressive marks of methylation at lysine 9 (H3K9me) and lysine 27 (H3K27me)[108] and CpG sites in DNA are heavily methylated. Heterochromatic DNA methylation and H3K9me/H3K27me signals are "read" by effector molecules such as the methyl-CpG binding proteins (e.g., MeCP2) and heterochromatin protein 1 (HP1)/polycomb group proteins (PcG), respectively.[109,110] Through intermolecular interactions, these molecules form large proteinaceous complexes that preserve the higher-order structure of heterochromatin during interphase and also propagate transcriptional repression across cell generations.[111–113]

A significant in vivo function of Dnmt3b is the establishment and maintenance of DNA methylation at the centromeric and pericentromeric satellite repeats,[68,72] chromosomal regions that are normally dense in CpG methylation. Reduction or loss of DNA methylation (hypomethylation) in pericentromeric heterochromatin has been linked to genomic instability in the rare autosomal recessive disease, ICF (immunodeficiency, centromeric instability and facial anomalies) syndrome.[114,115] ICF syndrome is usually diagnosed in infants or children and these patients often die in infancy or early childhood. Mortality is typically attributed to infection resulting from agammaglobulinemia (primarily of IgG and IgA). However, with age many patients exhibit combined immunodeficiency due to lymphocyte depletion or low stimulation indices of B or T cells. ICF patients also have mild facial abnormalities that include but are not limited to hypertelorism, low-set ears, epicanthic folds and macroglossia.[116]

Except for a few documented cases,[117] patients with ICF syndrome possess biallelic mutations in *DNMT3B* that ablate or drastically reduce the catalytic function of DNMT3B. This leads to hypomethylation of the satellite repeats in pericentromeric heterochromatin.[118,119] Hypomethylation of these repeats results in chromatin decondensation and enhanced chromosomal rearrangements leading to chromosomal arm deletions and/or multiradiate chromosomes.[120] Human chromosomes 1, 9 and 16 contain the largest regions of pericentromeric satellite DNA. Therefore, aberrant recombination occurs most frequently between the qh regions of chromosomes 1 and 16 (and to a lesser extent with chromosome 9) in mitogen-activated lymphocytes. The cytogenetic phenotypes of ICF patients reinforce the concept that maintaining proper DNA methylation patterns is crucial not only for regulation of gene expression but also for regulation of chromatin structure and suppression of abnormal recombination.

In addition to the constitutive heterochromatin found at centromeres and juxtacentromeric regions, the constitutive heterochromatin in subtelomeric regions is also regulated by DNA methylation. Loss of *Dnmt* expression induces hypomethylation of subtelomeric chromatin that contributes to telomere elongation and enhanced illegitimate recombination among the telomeres of sister chromatids.[121]

3.12 Crosstalk between DNA methylation and other epigenetic systems

There are three main categories of epigenetic regulatory processes: (1) ATP-dependent chromatin remodeling, (2) DNA methylation and (3) posttranslational modifications of histones and Polycomb group (PcG) proteins (i.e., methylation, acetylation, phosphorylation, SUMOylation, ubiquitination and biotinylation). PcG proteins function in large multi-protein complexes termed Polycomb Repressive Complexes (PRCs) that consist of chromatin remodeling proteins and enzymes that posttrans-lationally modify specific histone residues (e.g., trimethylation of H3K27 [H3K27me3]) to establish and maintain the heritable repression of tran-scriptional programs involved in cellular identity/memory. Exciting and intensive current research has implicated RNA molecules and the RNAi machinery in the regulation of epigenetic modifications such as DNA and histone methylation. The extremely complex interplay between the different epigenetic regulatory systems is just beginning to be appreci-ated. Some of the seminal studies that demonstrate a link between DNA methylation and other epigenetic systems are addressed in the next section.

3.13 DNA methylation and chromatin remodeling

One of the inherent problems associated with modifying the components of condensed heterochromatin is enzymatic access to the cognate DNA or histone substrate. A mammalian cell contains a number of proteins that utilize ATP-hydrolysis to remodel nucleosomes via disruption of histone-DNA interactions resulting in nucleosome sliding and chromatin "opening."[122] It is still somewhat unclear how these remodeling machines affect epigenetic modification of DNA and histones. However, they clearly have definitive roles in the regulation of DNA methylation. For instance, mutation of the α-thalassemia/mental-retardation, X-linked (ATRX) pro-tein, a member of the SNF2 family, alters the DNA methylation pattern at ribosomal (r) DNA repeats as well as the subtelomeric heterochromatin repeats.[123] Interestingly, the helicase domain of ATRX interacts with the methylated-DNA binding domain of MeCP2 and ATRX can be recruited to heterochromatin in a manner that depends on DNA methylation.[124] Furthermore, mutations of MeCP2 that occur in patients with X-linked mental retardation disrupt its interaction with ATRX.[124] Although ATRX is known to influence DNA methylation patterns, the mechanisms it uti-lizes to do so remain uncharacterized.

The prototypic ATP-dependent chromatin remodeling protein, hSNF2, and its homolog, lymphoid-specific helicase (Lsh) interact with

DNMT3B.[125,126] Interestingly, Lsh plays a direct role in the regulation of DNA methylation patterns established by Dnmt3a and Dnmt3b.[126,127] Lsh homozygous null mice survive to birth but exhibit a ≈50% reduction in global DNA methylation in all tissues, particularly at repetitive regions of the genome.[126,128] Recently it has been shown that Lsh acts to coordinate various epigenetic systems (i.e., de novo DNA methylation and Polycomb-mediated histone methylation) to regulate spatiotemporal transcriptional repression during development.[129]

3.14 DNA methylation and posttranslational modifications (PTMs) of histones

The relationship between histone deacetylation and acetylation with transcriptional repression and derepression, respectively, has been known for many years.[130] Indication of a functional link between histone deacetylation and DNA methylation was identified when treatment of Friend erythroleukemia cells with sodium butyrate, a general inhibitor of histone deacetylases (HDACs),[131] was found to result in decreased global DNA methylation during differentiation.[132] In the last several years, a functional synergism between Dnmts and HDACs in transcriptional repression has been established. Each of the Dnmts (except Dnmt2) binds and recruits HDACs to induce transcriptional silencing.[80,133–136] Further functional association between DNA methylation and histone deacetylation in transcriptional repression was established by the demonstration that genes silenced by DNA methylation could be reexpressed by inhibiting both DNA methylation and histone deacetylation.[137–139]

A link between DNA methylation and two separate epigenetic systems that regulate histone methylation to mediate heritable transcriptional repression and the establishment of constitutive heterochromatin have been described. These systems involve PcG and Su(var) (suppressor of variegation) HMTases (histone methyltransferases). As mentioned above, PcG proteins function in multiprotein complexes; three of which (PRC1, PRC2 and PRC3), have been characterized to date. It is generally thought that PRC2 (containing PcG proteins EED, EZH2, Suz12 and YY1) is involved in the initiation of silencing, whereas PRC1 (consisting of BMI1, HPC, HPH and RING1) plays a role in the stable maintenance of repression. The particular EED isoform of PRC3 has been demonstrated to target EZH2-directed methylation to specific lysine residues of H1 or H3.[140] Schlesinger et al.[141] have presented evidence that preexisting trimethylation of histone 3 lysine 27 (H3K27me3) mediated by PRC2 HMTase, EZH2, may serve as the basis for targeted de novo DNA methylation in colon cancer cells. Consistent with this idea that PRC1 functions to maintain repression is the fact that Dnmt1 and PRC2 are required to recruit PRC1 to pericentromeric PcG bodies.[142]

Direct communication between the DNA methylation machinery and the Polycomb system was discovered when Vire et al. demonstrated that EZH2 interacted with DNMTs and could direct de novo DNA methylation to promoters regulated by PRC2/3 complexes.[143] Another report indicates that regulation of transcription via H3K27me3 and DNA methylation may be more complex as knockdown of EZH2 does not affect preexisting DNA methylation but does increase basal-level transcription from genes that are not regulated by DNA methylation.[144]

Recently, structural studies have provided clues to the nature and regulation of de novo methylation by PcG-mediated histone methylation. Jia et al. solved the crystal structure of Dnmt3a bound to Dnmt3L.[145] They observed what appeared to be an 8 to 10 bp periodicity of methylation based on the physical characteristics of the Dnmt3a:Dnmt3L configuration, a finding that is in agreement with biochemical studies that indicate Dnmt3a functions in a distributive manner.[146] Another study discovered that Dnmt3L could bind histones lacking methylation of H3K4 and recruit Dnmt3a2 to induce DNA methylation.[147] Moreover, Dnmt3L did not bind histones possessing H3K4me3 but still bound histones with trimethylation of H3K9 and H3K27.[147] This suggests that histone modifications associated with active transcription (H3K4me3) but not those associated with transcriptional repression indirectly inhibit DNA methylation by interfering with Dnmt3L binding to chromatin. Taken together, these studies portray a mode of action for Dnmt3a-catalyzed de novo methylation and a means by which certain regions of the genome are protected from de novo DNA methylation as had been previously suggested.[30,148]

Interactions between Dnmt3b and the H3K9 methyltransferase, Suv39h, demonstrated a link between DNA and H3K9 methylation.[149] Utilizing ES cells nullizygous for both isoforms of Suv39h in addition to *Dnmt1* single and *Dnmt3a/Dnmt3b* double knockout ES cells, these authors demonstrated a dependence on preexisting H3K9me3 to direct DNA methylation to pericentromeric satellite repeats. However, DNA methylation at centromeric satellite repeats was found to be independent of H3K9 methylation.[149] Because Dnmt3b is responsible for methylation of centromeric and pericentromeric satellite DNA,[72,78] this implies tight regulation of DNA methylation based on genomic location. Additionally, methylation of H3K9 by G9a leads to HP1 binding followed by recruitment and stimulation of DNMT1 to mediate local DNA methylation both in vitro and in vivo.[150]

3.15   *DNA methylation and siRNA-mediated transcriptional gene silencing (TGS)*

One of the more exciting and currently controversial fields of epigenetic regulation involves the hypothesis that small interfering RNAs (siRNAs) direct TGS and influence chromatin structure by targeting enzymes involved in DNA methylation and histone modifications to certain genomic regions. Numerous reports have established a definitive role for RNA-directed DNA methylation (RdDM) and TGS in plants.[151–154] RdDM in *Arabidopsis thaliana* involves the processing of dsRNAs into siRNAs by the endonuclease, Dicer; a member of the RNAi machinery. Once assembled into the RNA-induced transcriptional silencing (RITS) multiprotein complex, these siRNAs that are complementary to promoter regions then become guide molecules for MET1(*A. thaliana* Dnmt1 homolog)-catalyzed CpG or CMT3-catalyzed non-CpG methylation leading to TGS. In addition, mechanisms involving the RNAi pathway are responsible for establishing constitutive heterochromatin in organisms from *S. pombe* and *Tetrahymena* to *Arabidopsis* and *Drosophila*; see References 155 and 156 for review. It is generally assumed that mammals possess a similar mechanism but application of the principles established in plants, yeast and flies to mammals is in its infancy. Early studies identified an unusually high concentration of chromatin-associated RNA in heterochromatin relative to euchromatin in a number of cell types.[157] Recently, an RNA component has been implicated in the formation of pericentromeric heterochromatin in mammals.[108] It has long been known that Dnmts bind and are inhibited by RNA[158] and Dnmt3a and 3b (but not Dnmt1) bind chemically synthesized RNAs designed to mimic siRNAs in vitro.[159] Studies using Dicer null mouse ES cells implicate Dicer in the regulation of DNA methylation and repressive histone modifications at the centromeric repeats.[160] A contradictory second study came to the conclusion that Dicer is dispensable for maintenance of DNA methylation and H3K9 methylation at pericentromeric heterochromatin in ES cells.[161] Additional work is needed to determine the precise role of Dicer and the RNAi pathway in the establishment and maintenance of mammalian centromeric and pericentromeric heterochromatin.

3.16   RNA-directed DNA methylation in mammals?

It is well established that small, noncoding RNA molecules can function to induce targeted DNA methylation in plants.[162,163] These RNA "guide" molecules are processed by the RNAi machinery from larger molecules that arise from many sources, including transposons and transgenes. A component of RNA-directed DNA methylation is a seemingly plant-specific RNA-dependent RNA polymerase (RNA Pol IV). No such polymerase has been identified in mammals to date but there are examples of RNA-directed DNA methylation in mammals nonetheless. For example, genomic imprinting via DNA methylation has been associated with antisense RNA.[164,165] Furthermore, aberrant antisense RNA transcription has been shown to direct de novo methylation of a nonimprinted CpG island implicated in the development of α-thalassemia.[166]

The first indication that siRNAs can direct de novo DNA methylation to an endogenous promoter to induce TGS in human cells was demonstrated independently by Morris et al.[167] and Kawasaki and Taira,[168] although the latter publication has since been retracted.[169] Morris et al. transfected 293T cells with an siRNA that was complementary to a promoter region of a stably integrated EF1A transgene that is essential for transcription of the transgene. They found that transcriptional repression of the EF1A transgene was dependent on the complementary siRNA and derepression could be achieved by treatment with the HDAC and Dnmt inhibitors trichostatin A and 5-azacytidine, respectively.[167] In addition, they determined that siRNA-induced repression partially resulted from de novo DNA methylation of the transgene promoter. Induction of repressive histone modifications together with DNA methylation at multiple promoters via siRNA-directed TGS has been reported and characterized in human cells and includes the Polycomb H3K27 methyltransferase, EZH2, as well as DNMT3A and the RNAi-associated protein, Argonaute-1.[170,171] It will be interesting to determine the extent of the role that siRNA-directed TGS plays in endogenous Polycomb-mediated transcriptional repression.

There are other examples of RNA-directed, PcG-mediated methylation of H3K27. The long noncoding RNA (ncRNA) termed HOTAIR was found to associate with PRC2, where it acted to mediate H3K27 methylation and transcriptional silencing in *trans* at the *HOXD* locus.[172] Unfortunately, the DNA methylation status of this locus was not examined. However, based on the fact that Polycomb complexes can directly stimulate DNA methylation[143] and RNA molecules can mediate localized H3K27 methylation as well as DNA methylation,[167,170,171] one can speculate that DNA methylation is involved in this process as well. An emerging model is that the combination of ncRNAs, chromatin modeling, Polycomb-mediated gene silencing and DNA methylation function together to provide a general mechanism for self-reinforcing, mitotically heritable transcriptional repression during differentiation.

3.17   *DNA methyltransferases and DNA repair*

The underrepresentation of CpG dinucleotides in DNA from humans and many other eukaryotes is thought to result from unrepaired deamination of cytosine (C) and 5-methylcytosine (5mC), resulting in U·G and T·G mismatches.[173] Failure to repair these lesions prior to DNA replication leads to C·G-to-T·A transitions. It has been estimated that C·G-to-T·A transitions account for approximately 30% of all germline and somatic point mutations.[174] Two thymine glycosylases, thymine-DNA glycosylase (Tdg) and methyl-CpG binding domain 4 (Mbd4) are believed to be responsible for excising T·G and-U·G mismatches.[175–177] However, while Mbd4 knockout has a modest effect on T·G mismatch repair,[178] T·G mismatches in a CpG dinucleotide are the preferred substrates for TdG.[178–181] Recently, two groups have reported that interactions between Dnmt3a and Dnmt 3b and Tdg play an important role in postreplicative repair of T:G mismatches.[182,183] While Dnmt3a and 3b are localized differently in the nucleus, the overall mechanism of the repair appears to be identical, that is, after the complexed Tdg removes T, the mismatched base excision repair (BER) is initiated and a C is inserted, restoring the CpG site by a replication independent process.[184] The results of these studies suggest that Dnmt3b and Dnmt3a may serve to recruit or target Tdg to defined regions of heterochromatin and to stimulate its activity once bound to the T·G mismatch. It remains to be determined what factors regulate the remethylation of the hemimethylated site that is created during the repair process and the precise role of small RNAs in regulating BER.

3.18   What next?

The studies reviewed in this chapter highlight the many roles played by DNA methyltransferases that are completely or at least partially independent of their ability to transfer methyl groups to cytosine residues. Two recently published studies suggest that DNMT3a and DNMT3b may also be involved in a cyclical deamination of 5mC to T in the promoter of an actively transcribed gene. Deamination leads to creation of a T·G mismatch that is repaired within a few hours, presumably through repair by BER, restoring a hemimethylated site.[185,186] As recently reviewed, there has been a long history of reported "demethylating" enzymes that, even if active, have turned out to be much more inefficient than passive loss of methylation during replication.[187] However, if the observation that Dnmt3a and Dnmt3b can be converted to highly active deaminators of 5-mC in DNA can be replicated in other laboratories, these findings may lead to new insights into the effects of environmental factors on DNA methylation and gene expression.

References

1. Hotchkiss, R. D. (1948). The quantitative separation of purines, pyrimidines and nucleosides by paper chromatography. *J Biol Chem* 168, 315–332.
2. Chargaff, E., and Crampton, C. F. (1953). Separation of calf thymus deoxyribonucleic acid into fractions of different composition. *Nature* 172, 289–282.
3. Sinsheimer, R. L. (1954). The action of pancreatic desoxyribonuclease. I. Isolation of mono- and dinucleotides. *J Biol Chem* 208, 445–459.

4. Gold, M., and Hurwitz, J. (1963). The enzymatic methylation of the nucleic acids. *Cold Spring Harbor Symp Quant Biol* 28, 149–156.

5. Srinivasan, P. R., and Borek, E. (1964). Enzymatic alteration of nucleic acid structure. *Science* 145, 548–553.

6. Christman, J. K. (2002). 5-Azacytidine and 5-aza-2'-deoxycytidine as inhibitors of DNA methylation: Mechanistic studies and their implications for cancer therapy. *Oncogene* 21, 5483–5495.

7. Christman, J. K. (1977). Correlation between hypomethylation of DNA and expression of globin genes in Friend erythroleukemia cells. *Eur J Biochem* 81, 53–61.

8. Constantinides, P. G., Taylor, S. M., and Jones, P. A. (1978). Phenotypic conversion of cultured mouse embryo cells by aza pyrimidine nucleosides. *Dev Biol* 66, 57–71.

9. Chen, R. Z., Pettersson, U., Beard, C., Jackson-Grusby, L., and Jaenisch, R. (1998). DNA hypomethylation leads to elevated mutation rates. *Nature* 395, 89–93.

10. Li, E. (2002). Chromatin modification and epigenetic reprogramming in mammalian development. *Nat Rev Genet* 3, 662–673.

11. Rizwana, R., and Hahn, P. J. (1999). CpG methylation reduces genomic instability. *J Cell Sci* 112 (Pt 24), 4513–4519.

12. Hashimshony, T., Zhang, J., Keshet, I., Bustin, M., and Cedar, H. (2003). The role of DNA methylation in setting up chromatin structure during development. *Nat Genet* 34, 187–192.

13. Siegfried, Z., Eden, S., Mendelsohn, M., Feng, X., Tsuberi, B. Z., and Cedar, H. (1999). DNA methylation represses transcription in vivo. *Nat Genet* 22, 203–206.

14. Oda, M., Yamagiwa, A., Yamamoto, S., Nakayama, T., Tsumura, A., Sasaki, H., Nakao, K., Li, E., and Okano, M. (2006). DNA methylation regulates long-range gene silencing of an X-linked homeobox gene cluster in a lineage-specific manner. *Genes Dev* 20, 3382–3394.

15. Heard, E. (2004). Recent advances in X-chromosome inactivation. *Curr Opin Cell Biol* 16, 247–255.

16. Reik, W., Kelsey, G., and Walter, J. (1999). Dissecting de novo methylation. *Nat Genet* 23, 380–382.

17. Narayan, A., Ji, W., Zhang, X. Y., Marrogi, A., Graff, J. R., Baylin, S. B., and Ehrlich, M. (1998). Hypomethylation of pericentromeric DNA in breast adenocarcinomas. *Int J Cancer* 77, 833–838.

18. Qu, G., Dubeau, L., Narayan, A., Yu, M. C., and Ehrlich, M. (1999). Satellite DNA hypomethylation vs. overall genomic hypomethylation in ovarian epithelial tumors of different malignant potential. *Mutat Res* 423, 91–101.

19. Qu, G. Z., Grundy, P. E., Narayan, A., and Ehrlich, M. (1999). Frequent hypomethylation in Wilms tumors of pericentromeric DNA in chromosomes 1 and 16. *Cancer Genet Cytogenet* 109, 34–39.

20. Jackson, K., Yu, M. C., Arakawa, K., Fiala, E., Youn, B., Fiegl, H., Muller-Holzner, E., Widschwendter, M., and Ehrlich, M. (2004). DNA hypomethylation is prevalent even in low-grade breast cancers. *Cancer Biol Ther* 3, 1225–1231.

21. Jones, P. A., and Baylin, S. B. (2002). The fundamental role of epigenetic events in cancer. *Nat Rev Genet* 3, 415–428.

22. Ehrlich, M. (1982). Amount and distribution of 5-methylcytosine in human DNA from different types of tissues or cell. *Nucleic Acids Res* 10, 2709–2721.

23. Gardiner-Garden, M., and Frommer, M. (1987). CpG islands in vertebrate genomes. *J Mol Biol* 196, 261–282.

24. Bird, A. (2002). DNA methylation patterns and epigenetic memory. *Genes Dev* 16, 6–21.

25. Ioshikhes, I. P., and Zhang, M. Q. (2000). Large-scale human promoter mapping using CpG islands. *Nat Genet* 26, 61–63.

26. Saxonov, S., Berg, P., and Brutlag, D. L. (2006). A genome-wide analysis of CpG dinucleotides in the human genome distinguishes two distinct classes of promoters. *Proc Natl Acad Sci USA* 103, 1412–1417.

27. Grunau, C., Hindermann, W., and Rosenthal, A. (2000). Large-scale methylation analysis of human genomic DNA reveals tissue-specific differences between the methylation profiles of genes and pseudogenes. *Hum Mol Genet* 9, 2651–2663.

28. Eckhardt, F., Lewin, J., Cortese, R., Rakyan, V. K., Attwood, J., Burger, M., Burton, J., Cox, T. V., Davies, R., Down, T. A., Haefliger, C., Horton, R., Howe, K., Jackson, D. K., Kunde, J., Koenig, C., Liddle, J., Niblett, D., Otto, T., Pettett, R., Seemann, S., Thompson, C., West, T., Rogers, J., Olek, A., Berlin, K., and Beck, S. (2006). DNA methylation profiling of human chromosomes 6, 20 and 22. *Nat Genet* 38, 1378–1385.

29. Rollins, R. A., Haghighi, F., Edwards, J. R., Das, R., Zhang, M. Q., Ju, J., and Bestor, T. H. (2006). Large-scale structure of genomic methylation patterns. *Genome Res* 16, 157–163.

30. Weber, M., Hellmann, I., Stadler, M. B., Ramos, L., Paabo, S., Rebhan, M., and Schubeler, D. (2007). Distribution, silencing potential and evolutionary impact of promoter DNA methylation in the human genome. *Nat Genet* 39, 457–466.

31. Kalousek, F., and Morris, N. (1969). The purification and properties of deoxyribonucleic acid methylase from rat spleen. *J Biol Chem* 244, 1157–1163.

32. Sheid, B., and Bilik, E. (1969). Studies on DNA methylase activity in mammalian tissue. *Experentia* 25, 361–362.

33. Sheid, B., Srinivasan, P. R., and Borek, E. (1968). Deoxyribonucleic acid methylase of mammalian cells. *Biochemistry (Moscow)* 7, 280–285.

34. Wu, J. C., and Santi, D. V. (1987). Kinetic and catalytic mechanism of HhaI methyltransferase. *J Biol Chem* 262, 4778–4786.

35. Brank, A. S., Eritja, R., Garcia, R. G., Marquez, V. E., and Christman, J. K. (2002). Inhibition of HhaI DNA (cytosine-C5) methyltransferase by oligodeoxyribonucleotides containing 5-aza-2'-deoxycytidine: Examination of the intertwined roles of co-factor, target, transition state structure and enzyme conformation. *J Mol Biol* 323, 53–67.

36. Cheng, X., Kumar, S., Posfai, J., Pflugrath, J. W., and Roberts, R. J. (1993). Crystal structure of the HhaI DNA methyltransferase complexed with S-adenosyl-L-methionine. *Cell* 74, 299–307.

37. Klimasauskas, S., Kumar, S., Roberts, R. J., and Cheng, X. (1994). HhaI methyltransferase flips its target base out of the DNA helix. *Cell* 76, 357–369.

38. Posfai, J., Bhagwat, A. S., Posfai, G., and Roberts, R. J. (1989). Predictive motifs derived from cytosine methyltransferases. *Nucleic Acids Res* 17, 2421–2435.

39. Bestor, T., Laudano, A., Mattaliano, R., and Ingram, V. (1988). Cloning and sequencing of a cDNA encoding DNA methyltransferase of mouse cells. The carboxyl-terminal domain of the mammalian enzymes is related to bacterial restriction methyltransferases. *J Mol Biol* 203, 971–983.

40. Pradhan, S., Bacolla, A., Wells, R. D., and Roberts, R. J. (1999). Recombinant human DNA (cytosine-5) methyltransferase. I. Expression, purification, and comparison of de novo and maintenance methylation. *J Biol Chem* 274, 33002–33010.

41. Pradhan, S., Talbot, D., Sha, M., Benner, J., Hornstra, L., Li, E., Jaenisch, R., and Roberts, R. J. (1997). Baculovirus-mediated expression and characterization of the full-length murine DNA methyltransferase. *Nucleic Acids Res* 25, 4666–4673.

42. Yoder, J. A., Soman, N. S., Verdine, G. L., and Bestor, T. H. (1997). DNA (cytosine-5)-methyltransferases in mouse cells and tissues. Studies with a mechanism-based probe. *J Mol Biol* 270, 385–395.

43. Brank, A. S., Van Bemmel, D. M., and Christman, J. K. (2002). Optimization of Baculovirus mediated expression and purification of hexahistidine-tagged murine (Cytosine-C5) methyltransferase in *Spodoptera frugiperda* 9 cells. *Protein Expr Purif* 25, 31–34.

44. Iida, T., Suetake, I., Tajima, S., Morioka, H., Ohta, S., Obuse, C., and Tsurimoto, T. (2002). PCNA clamp facilitates action of DNA cytosine methyltransferase 1 on hemimethylated DNA. *Genes Cells* 7, 997–1007.

45. Leonhardt, H., Page, A. W., Weier, H. U., and Bestor, T. H. (1992). A targeting sequence directs DNA methyltransferase to sites of DNA replication in mammalian nuclei. *Cell* 71, 865–873.

46. Chuang, L. S. H., Ian, H.-I., Koh, T.-W., Ng, H.-H., Xu, G., and Li, B. F. L. (1997). Human DNA-(cytosine-5) methyltransferase-PCNA complex as a target for p21WAF1. *Science* 277, 1996–2000.

47. Schermelleh, L., Haemmer, A., Spada, F., Rosing, N., Melinger, D., Rothbauer, U., Cardoso, M. C., and Leonhardt, H. (2007). Dynamics of Dnmt1 interaction with the replication machinery and its role in postreplicative maintenance of DNA methylation. *Nucleic Acids Res* 35, 4301–4312.

48. Sporbert, A., Domaing, P., Leonhardt, H., and Cardoso, M. C. (2005). PCNA acts as a stationary loading platform for transiently interacting Okazaki fragment maturation proteins. *Nucleic Acids Res* 33, 3521–3528.

49. Mertineit, C., Yoder, J. A., Taketo, T., Laird, D. W., Trasler, J. M., and Bestor, T. H. (1998). Sex-specific exons control DNA methyltransferase in mammalian germ cells. *Development* 125, 889–897.

50. Doherty, A. S., Bartolomei, M. S., and Schultz, R. M. (2002). Regulation of stage-specific nuclear translocation of Dnmt1o during preimplantation mouse development. *Dev Biol* 242, 255–266.

51. Li, E., Bestor, T. H., and Jaenisch, R. (1992). Targeted mutation of the DNA methyltransferase gene results in embryonic lethality. *Cell* 69, 915–926.

52. Rhee, I., Jair, K.-W., Yen, R.-W. C., Lengauer, C., Herman, J. G., Kinzler, K. W., Vogelstein, B., Baylin, S. B., and Schuebel, K. E. (2000). CpG methylation is maintained in human cancer cells lacking DNMT1. *Nature* 404, 1003–1007.

53. Rhee, I., Bachman, K. E., Park, B. H., Jair, K. W., Yen, R. W., Schuebel, K. E., Cui, H., Feinberg, A. P., Lengauer, C., Kinzler, K. W., Baylin, S. B., and Vogelstein, B. (2002). DNMT1 and DNMT3b cooperate to silence genes in human cancer cells. *Nature* 416, 552–556.

54. Egger, G., Jeong, S., Escobar, S. G., Cortez, C. C., Li, T. W., Saito, Y., Yoo, C. B., Jones, P. A., and Liang, G. (2006). Identification of DNMT1 (DNA methyltransferase 1) hypomorphs in somatic knockouts suggests an essential role for DNMT1 in cell survival. *Proc Natl Acad Sci USA* 103, 14080–14085.

55. Chen, T., Hevi, S., Gay, F., Tsujimoto, N., He, T., Zhang, B., Ueda, Y., and Li, E. (2007). Complete inactivation of DNMT1 leads to mitotic catastrophe in human cancer cells. *Nat Genet* 39, 391–396.

56. Okano, M., Xie, S., and Li, E. (1998). Dnmt2 is not required for de novo and maintenance methylation of viral DNA in embryonic stem cells. *Nucleic Acids Res* 26, 2536–2540.

57. Hermann, A., Schmitt, S., and Jeltsch, A. (2003). The human Dnmt2 has residual DNA-(cytosine-C5) methyltransferase activity. *J Biol Chem* 278, 31717–31721.

58. Kunert, N., Marhold, J., Stanke, J., Stach, D., and Lyko, F. (2003). A Dnmt2-like protein mediates DNA methylation in Drosophila. *Development* 130, 5083–5090.

59. Goll, M. G., Kirpekar, F., Maggert, K. A., Yoder, J. A., Hsieh, C.-L., Zhang, X., Golic, K. G., Jacobsen, S. E., and Bestor, T. H. (2006). Methylation of tRNAAsp by the DNA methyltransferase homolog Dnmt2. *Science* 311, 395–398.

60. Rai, K., Chidester, S., Zavala, C. V., Manos, E. J., James, S. R., Karpf, A. R., Jones, D. A., and Cairns, B. R. (2007). Dnmt2 functions in the cytoplasm to promote liver, brain, and retina development in zebrafish. *Genes Dev* 21, 261–266.

61. Sakita-Suto, S., Kanda, A., Suzuki, F., Sato, S., Takata, T., and Tatsuka, M. (2007). Aurora-B regulates RNA methyltransferase NSUN2. *Mol Biol Cell* 18, 1107–1117.

62. Kafri, T., Gao, X., and Razin, A. (1993). Mechanistic aspects of genome-wide demethylation in the preimplantation mouse embryo. *Proc Natl Acad Sci USA* 90, 10558–10562.

63. Monk, M., Boubelik, M., and Lehnert, S. (1987). Temporal and regional changes in DNA methylation in the embryonic, extraembryonic and germ cell lineages during mouse embryo development. *Development* 99, 371–382.

64. Jahner, D., Stuhlmann, H., Stewart, C. L., Harbers, K., Lohler, J., Simon, I., and Jaenisch, R. (1982). De novo methylation and expression of retroviral genomes during mouse embryogenesis. *Nature* 298, 623–628.

65. Kafri, T., Ariel, M., Brandeis, M., Shemer, R., Urven, L., McCarrey, J., Cedar, H., and Razin, A. (1992). Developmental pattern of gene-specific DNA methylation in the mouse embryo and germ line. *Genes Dev* 6, 705–714.

66. Lei, H., Oh, S. P., Okano, M., Juttermann, R., Goss, K. A., Jaenisch, R., and Li, E. (1996). De novo DNA cytosine methyltransferase activities in mouse embryonic stem cells. *Development* 122, 3195–3205.

67. Okano, M., Xie, S., and Li, E. (1998). Cloning and characterization of a family of novel mammalian DNA (cytosine-5) methyltransferases. *Nat Genet* 19, 219–220.

68. Chen, T., Tsujimoto, N., and Li, E. (2004). The PWWP domain of Dnmt3a and Dnmt3b is required for directing DNA methylation to the major satellite repeats at pericentric heterochromatin. *Mol Cell Biol* 24, 9048–9058.

69. Watanabe, D., Suetake, I., Tada, T., and Tajima, S. (2002). Stage- and cell-specific expression of Dnmt3a and Dnmt3b during embryogenesis. *Mech Dev* 118, 187–190.

70. MacDonald, J. L., Gin, C. S., and Roskams, A. J. (2005). Stage-specific induction of DNA methyltransferases in olfactory receptor neuron development. *Dev Biol* 288, 461–473.
71. Feng, J., Chang, H., Li, E., and Fan, G. (2005). Dynamic expression of de novo DNA methyltransferases Dnmt3a and Dnmt3b in the central nervous system. *J Neurosci Res* 79, 734–746.
72. Xie, S., Wang, Z., Okano, M., Nogami, M., Li, Y., He, W. W., Okumura, K., and Li, E. (1999). Cloning, expression and chromosome locations of the human DNMT3 gene family. *Gene* 236, 87–95.
73. Hsieh, C. L. (1999). In vivo activity of murine de novo methyltransferases, Dnmt3a and Dnmt3b. *Mol Cell Biol* 19, 8211–8218.
74. Oka, M., Rodic, N., Graddy, J., Chang, L.-J., and Terada, N. (2006). CpG sites preferentially methylated by Dnmt3a in vivo. *J Biol Chem* 281, 9901–9908.
75. Takeshima, H., Suetake, I., Shimahara, H., Ura, K., Tate, S., and Tajima, S. (2006). Distinct DNA methylation activity of Dnmt3a and Dnmt3b towards naked and nucleosomal DNA. *J Biochem (Tokyo)* 139, 503–515.
76. Szyf, M., Kaplan, F., Mann, V., Giloh, H., Kedar, E., and Razin, A. (1985). Cell cycle-dependent regulation of eukaryotic DNA methylase level. *J Biol Chem* 260, 8653–8656.
77. Margot, J. B., Cardoso, M. C., and Leonhardt, H. (2001). Mammalian DNA methyltransferases show different subnuclear distributions. *J Cell Biochem* 83, 373–379.
78. Chen, T., Ueda, Y., Dodge, J. E., Wang, Z., and Li, E. (2003). Establishment and maintenance of genomic methylation patterns in mouse embryonic stem cells by Dnmt3a and Dnmt3b. *Mol Cell Biol* 23, 5594–5605.
79. Chen, T., Ueda, Y., Xie, S., and Li, E. (2002). A novel Dnmt3a isoform produced from an alternative promoter localizes to euchromatin and its expression correlates with active de novo methylation. *J Biol Chem* 277, 38746–38754.
80. Bachman, K. E., Rountree, M. R., and Baylin, S. B. (2001). Dnmt3a and Dnmt3b are transcriptional repressors that exhibit unique localization properties to heterochromatin. *J Biol Chem* 276, 32282–32287.
81. Robertson, K. D., Uzvolgyi, E., Liang, G., Talmadge, C., Sumegi, J., Gonzales, F. A., and Jones, P. A. (1999). The human DNA methyltransferases (DNMTs) 1, 3a and 3b: Coordinate mRNA expression in normal tissues and overexpression in tumors. *Nucleic Acids Res* 27, 2291–2298.
82. Weisenberger, D. J., Velicescu, M., Cheng, J. C., Gonzales, F. A., Liang, G., and Jones, P. A. (2004). Role of the DNA methyltransferase variant DNMT3b3 in DNA methylation. *Mol Cancer Res* 2, 62–72.
83. Saito, Y., Kanai, Y., Sakamoto, M., Saito, H., Ishii, H., and Hirohashi, S. (2002). Overexpression of a splice variant of DNA methyltransferase 3b, DNMT3b4, associated with DNA hypomethylation on pericentromeric satellite regions during human hepatocarcinogenesis. *Proc Natl Acad Sci USA* 99, 10060–10065.
84. Ge, Y. Z., Pu, M. T., Gowher, H., Wu, H. P., Ding, J. P., Jeltsch, A., and Xu, G. L. (2004). Chromatin targeting of de novo DNA methyltransferases by the PWWP domain. *J Biol Chem* 279, 25447–25454.
85. Brenner, C., Deplus, R., Didelot, C., Loriot, A., Vire, E., De Smet, C., Gutierrez, A., Danovi, D., Bernard, D., Boon, T., Pelicci, P. G., Amati, B., Kouzarides, T., de Launoit, Y., Di Croce, L., and Fuks, F. (2005). Myc represses transcription through recruitment of DNA methyltransferase corepressor. *EMBO J* 24, 336–346.

86. Yu, Q., Thieu, V. T., and Kaplan, M. H. (2007). Stat4 limits DNA methyltransferase recruitment and DNA methylation of the IL-18Ralpha gene during Th1 differentiation. *EMBO J* 26, 2052–2060.

87. Bourc'his, D., Xu, G.-L., Lin, C.-S., Bollman, B., and Bestor, T. H. (2001). Dnmt3L and the establishment of maternal genomic imprints. *Science* 294, 2536–2539.

88. Hata, K., Okano, M., Lei, H., and Li, E. (2002). Dnmt3L cooperates with the Dnmt3 family of de novo DNA methyltransferases to establish maternal imprints in mice. *Development* 129, 1983–1993.

89. Gowher, H., Liebert, K., Hermann, A., Xu, G., and Jeltsch, A. (2005). Mechanism of stimulation of catalytic activity of Dnmt3A and Dnmt3B DNA-(cytosine-C5)-methyltransferases by Dnmt3L. *J Biol Chem* 280, 13341–13348.

90. Suetake, I., Morimoto, Y., Fuchikami, T., Abe, K., and Tajima, S. (2006). Stimulation effect of Dnmt3L on the DNA methylation activity of Dnmt3a2. *J Biochem (Tokyo)* 140, 553–559.

91. Suetake, I., Shinozaki, F., Miyagawa, J., Takeshima, H., and Tajima, S. (2004). DNMT3L stimulates the DNA methylation activity of Dnmt3a and Dnmt3b through a direct interaction. *J Biol Chem* 279, 27816–27823.

92. Chedin, F., Lieber, M. R., and Hsieh, C. L. (2002). The DNA methyltransferase-like protein DNMT3L stimulates de novo methylation by Dnmt3a. *Proc Natl Acad Sci USA* 99, 16916–16921.

93. Chen, Z. X., Mann, J. R., Hsieh, C. L., Riggs, A. D., and Chedin, F. (2005). Physical and functional interactions between the human DNMT3L protein and members of the de novo methyltransferase family. *J Cell Biochem* 95, 902–917.

94. Nimura, K., Ishida, C., Koriyama, H., Hata, K., Yamanaka, S., Li, E., Ura, K., and Kaneda, Y. (2006). Dnmt3a2 targets endogenous Dnmt3L to ES cell chromatin and induces regional DNA methylation. *Genes Cells* 11, 1225–1237.

95. Xie, Z. H., Huang, Y. N., Chen, Z. X., Riggs, A. D., Ding, J. P., Gowher, H., Jeltsch, A., Sasaki, H., Hata, K., and Xu, G. L. (2006). Mutations in DNA methyltransferase DNMT3B in ICF syndrome affect its regulation by DNMT3L. *Hum Mol Genet* 15, 1375–1385.

96. Boyes, J., and Bird, A. (1991). DNA methylation inhibits transcription indirectly via a methyl-CpG binding protein. *Cell* 64, 1123.

97. Hendrich, B., and Bird, A. (1998). Identification and characterization of a family of mammalian methyl-CpG binding proteins. *Mol Cell Biol* 18, 6538–6547.

98. Ng, H. H., Zhang, Y., Hendrich, B., Johnson, C. A., Turner, B. M., Erdjument-Bromage, H., Tempst, P., Reinberg, D., and Bird, A. (1999). MBD2 is a transcriptional repressor belonging to the MeCP1 histone deacetylase complex. *Nat Genet* 23, 58–61.

99. Wade, P. A., Gegonne, A., Jones, P. L., Ballestar, E., Aubry, F., and Wolffe, A. P. (1999). Mi-2 complex couples DNA methylation to chromatin remodelling and histone deacetylation. *Nat Genet* 23, 62.

100. Zhang, Y., Ng, H. H., Erdjument-Bromage, H., Tempst, P., Bird, A., and Reinberg, D. (1999). Analysis of the NuRD subunits reveals a histone deacetylase core complex and a connection with DNA methylation. *Genes Dev* 13, 1924–1935.

101. Fujita, N., Watanabe, S., Ichimura, T., Tsuruzoe, S., Shinkai, Y., Tachibana, M., Chiba, T., and Nakao, M. (2003). Methyl-CpG binding domain 1 (MBD1) interacts with the Suv39h1-HP1 heterochromatic complex for DNA methylation-based transcriptional repression. *J Biol Chem* 278, 24132–24138.

102. Reese, B. E., Bachman, K. E., Baylin, S. B., and Rountree, M. R. (2003). The methyl-CpG binding protein MBD1 interacts with the p150 subunit of chromatin assembly factor 1. *Mol Cell Biol* 23, 3226–3236.

103. Kondo, E., Gu, Z., Horii, A., and Fukushige, S. (2005). The thymine DNA glycosylase MBD4 represses transcription and is associated with methylated p16(INK4a) and hMLH1 genes. *Mol Cell Biol* 25, 4388–4396.

104. Hendrich, B., Hardeland, U., Ng, H. H., Jiricny, J., and Bird, A. (1999). The thymine glycosylase MBD4 can bind to the product of deamination at methylated CpG sites. *Nature* 401, 301–304.

105. Fraga, M. F., Ballestar, E., Montoya, G., Taysavang, P., Wade, P. A., and Esteller, M. (2003). The affinity of different MBD proteins for a specific methylated locus depends on their intrinsic binding properties. *Nucleic Acids Res* 31, 1765–1774.

106. Grewal, S. I. S., and Jia, S. (2007). Heterochromatin revisited. *Nat Rev Genet* 8, 35.

107. Maison, C., and Almouzni, G. (2004). HP1 and the dynamics of heterochromatin maintenance. *Nat Rev Mol Cell Biol* 5, 296–304.

108. Maison, C., Bailly, D., Peters, A. H., Quivy, J. P., Roche, D., Taddei, A., Lachner, M., Jenuwein, T., and Almouzni, G. (2002). Higher-order structure in pericentric heterochromatin involves a distinct pattern of histone modification and an RNA component. *Nat Genet* 30, 329–334.

109. Lachner, M., O'Carroll, D., Rea, S., Mechtler, K., and Jenuwein, T. (2001). Methylation of histone H3 lysine 9 creates a binding site for HP1 proteins. *Nature* 410, 116–120.

110. Ballestar, E., and Wolffe, A. P. (2001). Methyl-CpG-binding proteins. Targeting specific gene repression. *Eur J Biochem* 268, 1–6.

111. Fujita, N., Watanabe, S., Ichimura, T., Tsuruzoe, S., Shinkai, Y., Tachibana, M., Chiba, T., and Nakao, M. (2003). Methyl-CpG binding domain 1 (MBD1) interacts with the Suv39h1-HP1 heterochromatic complex for DNA methylation-based transcriptional repression. *J Biol Chem* 278, 24132–24138.

112. Agarwal, N., Hardt, T., Brero, A., Nowak, D., Rothbauer, U., Becker, A., Leonhardt, H., and Cardoso, M. C. (2007). MeCP2 interacts with HP1 and modulates its heterochromatin association during myogenic differentiation. *Nucleic Acids Res* 35, 5402–5408.

113. Matarazzo, M. R., De Bonis, M. L., Strazzullo, M., Cerase, A., Ferraro, M., Vastarelli, P., Ballestar, E., Esteller, M., Kudo, S., and D'Esposito, M. (2007). Multiple binding of methyl-CpG and polycomb proteins in long-term gene silencing events. *J Cell Physiol* 210, 711–719.

114. Fryns, J. P., Azou, M., Jaeken, J., Eggermont, E., Pedersen, J. C., and Van den Berghe, H. (1981). Centromeric instability of chromosomes 1, 9, and 16 associated with combined immunodeficiency. *Hum Genet* 57, 108–110.

115. Tiepolo, L., Maraschio, P., Gimelli, G., Cuoco, C., Gargani, G. F., and Romano, C. (1979). Multibranched chromosomes 1, 9, and 16 in a patient with combined IgA and IgE deficiency. *Hum Genet* 51, 127–137.

116. Ehrlich, M. (2003). The ICF syndrome, a DNA methyltransferase 3B deficiency and immunodeficiency disease. *Clin Immunol* 109, 17–28.

117. Kubota, T., Furuumi, H., Kamoda, T., Iwasaki, N., Tobita, N., Fujiwara, N., Goto, Y., Matsui, A., Sasaki, H., and Kajii, T. (2004). ICF syndrome in a girl with DNA hypomethylation but without detectable DNMT3B mutation. *Am J Med Genet* 129A, 290–293.

118. Hansen, R. S., Wijmenga, C., Luo, P., Stanek, A. M., Canfield, T. K., Weemaes, C. M., and Gartler, S. M. (1999). The DNMT3B DNA methyltransferase gene is mutated in the ICF immunodeficiency syndrome. *Proc Natl Acad Sci USA* 96, 14412–14417.

119. Xu, G. L., Bestor, T. H., Bourc'his, D., Hsieh, C. L., Tommerup, N., Bugge, M., Hulten, M., Qu, X., Russo, J. J., and Viegas-Pequignot, E. (1999). Chromosome instability and immunodeficiency syndrome caused by mutations in a DNA methyltransferase gene. *Nature* 402, 187–191.

120. Tuck-Muller, C. M., Narayan, A., Tsien, F., Smeets, D. F., Sawyer, J., Fiala, E. S., Sohn, O. S., and Ehrlich, M. (2000). DNA hypomethylation and unusual chromosome instability in cell lines from ICF syndrome patients. *Cytogenet Cell Genet* 89, 121–128.

121. Gonzalo, S., Jaco, I., Fraga, M. F., Chen, T., Li, E., Esteller, M., and Blasco, M. A. (2006). DNA methyltransferases control telomere length and telomere recombination in mammalian cells. *Nat Cell Biol* 8, 416–424.

122. Vignali, M., Hassan, A. H., Neely, K. E., and Workman, J. L. (2000). ATP-dependent chromatin-remodeling complexes. *Mol Cell Biol* 20, 1899–1910.

123. Gibbons, R. J., McDowell, T. L., Raman, S., O'Rourke, D. M., Garrick, D., Ayyub, H., and Higgs, D. R. (2000). Mutations in ATRX, encoding a SWI/SNF-like protein, cause diverse changes in the pattern of DNA methylation. *Nat Genet* 24, 368–371.

124. Nan, X., Hou, J., Maclean, A., Nasir, J., Lafuente, M. J., Shu, X., Kriaucionis, S., and Bird, A. (2007). Interaction between chromatin proteins MECP2 and ATRX is disrupted by mutations that cause inherited mental retardation. *Proc Natl Acad Sci USA* 104, 2709–2714.

125. Geiman, T. M., Sankpal, U. T., Robertson, A. K., Zhao, Y., and Robertson, K. D. (2004). DNMT3B interacts with hSNF2H chromatin remodeling enzyme, HDACs 1 and 2, and components of the histone methylation system. *Biochem Biophys Res Commun* 318, 544–555.

126. Dennis, K., Fan, T., Geiman, T., Yan, Q., and Muegge, K. (2001). Lsh, a member of the SNF2 family, is required for genome-wide methylation. *Genes Dev* 15, 2940–2944.

127. Zhu, H., Geiman, T. M., Xi, S., Jiang, Q., Schmidtmann, A., Chen, T., Li, E., and Muegge, K. (2006). Lsh is involved in de novo methylation of DNA. *EMBO J* 25, 335–345.

128. Geiman, T. M., Tessarollo, L., Anver, M. R., Kopp, J. B., Ward, J. M., and Muegge, K. (2001). Lsh, a SNF2 family member, is required for normal murine development. *Biochim Biophys Acta* 1526, 211–220.

129. Xi, S., Zhu, H., Xu, H., Schmidtmann, A., Geiman, T. M., and Muegge, K. (2007). Lsh controls Hox gene silencing during development. *Proc Natl Acad Sci USA* 104, 14366–14371.

130. Loidl, P. (1994). Histone acetylation: Facts and questions. *Chromosoma* 103, 441–449.

131. Sealy, L., and Chalkley, R. (1978). The effect of sodium butyrate on histone modification. *Cell* 14, 115–121.

132. Christman, J. K., Weich, N., Schoenbrun, B., Schneiderman, N., and Acs, G. (1980). Hypomethylation of DNA during differentiation of Friend erythroleukemia cells. *J Cell Biol* 86, 366–370.

133. Fuks, F., Burgers, W. A., Brehm, A., Hughes-Davies, L., and Kouzarides, T. (2000). DNA methyltransferase Dnmt1 associates with histone deacetylase activity. *Nat Genet* 24, 88.

134. Robertson, K. D., Ait-Si-Ali, S., Yokochi, T., Wade, P. A., Jones, P. L., and Wolffe, A. P. (2000). DNMT1 forms a complex with Rb, E2F1 and HDAC1 and represses transcription from E2F-responsive promoters. *Nat Genet* 25, 338.

135. Fuks, F., Burgers, W. A., Godin, N., Kasai, M., and Kouzarides, T. (2001). Dnmt3a binds deacetylases and is recruited by a sequence-specific repressor to silence transcription. *EMBO J* 20, 2536–2544.

136. Aapola, U., Liiv, I., and Peterson, P. (2002). Imprinting regulator DNMT3L is a transcriptional repressor associated with histone deacetylase activity. *Nucleic Acids Res* 30, 3602–3608.

137. Yang, X., Phillips, D. L., Ferguson, A. T., Nelson, W. G., Herman, J. G., and Davidson, N. E. (2001). Synergistic activation of functional estrogen receptor (ER)-{alpha} by DNA methyltransferase and histone deacetylase inhibition in human ER-{alpha}-negative breast cancer cells. *Cancer Res* 61, 7025–7029.

138. Gore, S. D., Baylin, S., Sugar, E., Carraway, H., Miller, C. B., Carducci, M., Grever, M., Galm, O., Dauses, T., Karp, J. E., Rudek, M. A., Zhao, M., Smith, B. D., Manning, J., Jiemjit, A., Dover, G., Mays, A., Zwiebel, J., Murgo, A., Weng, L.-J., and Herman, J. G. (2006). Combined DNA methyltransferase and histone deacetylase inhibition in the treatment of myeloid neoplasms. *Cancer Res* 66, 6361–6369.

139. Suzuki, H., Gabrielson, E., Chen, W., Anbazhagan, R., van Engeland, M., Weijenberg, M. P., Herman, J. G., and Baylin, S. B. (2002). A genomic screen for genes upregulated by demethylation and histone deacetylase inhibition in human colorectal cancer. *Nat Genet* 31, 141–149.

140. Kuzmichev, A., Jenuwein, T., Tempst, P., and Reinberg, D. (2004). Different EZH2-containing complexes target methylation of histone H1 or nucleosomal histone H3. *Mol Cell* 14, 183–193.

141. Schlesinger, Y., Straussman, R., Keshet, I., Farkash, S., Hecht, M., Zimmerman, J., Eden, E., Yakhini, Z., Ben-Shushan, E., Reubinoff, B. E., Bergman, Y., Simon, I., and Cedar, H. (2007). Polycomb-mediated methylation on Lys27 of histone H3 pre-marks genes for de novo methylation in cancer. *Nat Genet* 39, 232–236.

142. Hernandez-Munoz, I., Taghavi, P., Kuijl, C., Neefjes, J., and van Lohuizen, M. (2005). Association of BMI1 with Polycomb bodies is dynamic and requires PRC2/EZH2 and the maintenance DNA methyltransferase DNMT1. *Mol Cell Biol* 25, 11047–11058.

143. Vire, E., Brenner, C., Deplus, R., Blanchon, L., Fraga, M., Didelot, C., Morey, L., Van Eynde, A., Bernard, D., Vanderwinden, J. M., Bollen, M., Esteller, M., Di Croce, L., de Launoit, Y., and Fuks, F. (2006). The Polycomb group protein EZH2 directly controls DNA methylation. *Nature* 439, 871–874.

144. McGarvey, K. M., Greene, E., Fahrner, J. A., Jenuwein, T., and Baylin, S. B. (2007). DNA methylation and complete transcriptional silencing of cancer genes persist after depletion of EZH2. *Cancer Res* 67, 5097–5102.

145. Jia, D., Jurkowska, R. Z., Zhang, X., Jeltsch, A., and Cheng, X. (2007). Structure of Dnmt3a bound to Dnmt3L suggests a model for de novo DNA methylation. *Nature* 449, 248–251.

146. Gowher, H., and Jeltsch, A. (2002). Molecular enzymology of the catalytic domains of the Dnmt3a and Dnmt3b DNA methyltransferases. *J Biol Chem* 277, 20409–20414.

147. Ooi, S. K. T., Qiu, C., Bernstein, E., Li, K., Jia, D., Yang, Z., Erdjument-Bromage, H., Tempst, P., Lin, S.-P., Allis, C. D., Cheng, X., and Bestor, T. H. (2007). DNMT3L connects unmethylated lysine 4 of histone H3 to de novo methylation of DNA. *Nature* 448, 714–717.

148. Appanah, R., Dickerson, D. R., Goyal, P., Groudine, M., and Lorincz, M. C. (2007). An unmethylated 3′ promoter-proximal region is required for efficient transcription initiation. *PLoS Genet* 3, e27.

149. Lehnertz, B., Ueda, Y., Derijck, A. A., Braunschweig, U., Perez-Burgos, L., Kubicek, S., Chen, T., Li, E., Jenuwein, T., and Peters, A. H. (2003). Suv39h-mediated histone H3 lysine 9 methylation directs DNA methylation to major satellite repeats at pericentric heterochromatin. *Curr Biol* 13, 1192–1200.

150. Smallwood, A., Esteve, P.-O., Pradhan, S., and Carey, M. (2007). Functional cooperation between HP1 and DNMT1 mediates gene silencing. *Genes Dev* 21, 1169–1178.

151. Wassenegger, M., Heimes, S., Riedel, L., and Sanger, H. L. (1994). RNA-directed de novo methylation of genomic sequences in plants. *Cell* 76, 567–576.

152. Mette, M. F., Aufsatz, W., van der Winden, J., Matzke, M. A., and Matzke, A. J. (2000). Transcriptional silencing and promoter methylation triggered by double-stranded RNA. *EMBO J* 19, 5194–5201.

153. Cao, X., Aufsatz, W., Zilberman, D., Mette, M. F., Huang, M. S., Matzke, M., and Jacobsen, S. E. (2003). Role of the DRM and CMT3 methyltransferases in RNA-directed DNA methylation. *Curr Biol* 13, 2212–2217.

154. Aufsatz, W., Mette, M. F., Matzke, A. J., and Matzke, M. (2004). The role of MET1 in RNA-directed de novo and maintenance methylation of CG dinucleotides. *Plant Mol Biol* 54, 793–804.

155. Zaratiegui, M., Irvine, D. V., and Martienssen, R. A. (2007). Noncoding RNAs and gene silencing. *Cell* 128, 763–767.

156. Grewal, S. I. S., and Elgin, S. C. R. (2007). Transcription and RNA interference in the formation of heterochromatin. *Nature* 447, 399–406.

157. Paul, J., and Duerksen, J. D. (1975). Chromatin-associated RNA content of heterochromatin and euchromatin. *Mol Cell Biochem* 9, 9–16.

158. Bolden, A., Ward, C., Siedlecki, J. A., and Weissbach, A. (1984). DNA methylation. Inhibition of de novo and maintenance methylation in vitro by RNA and synthetic polynucleotides. *J Biol Chem* 259, 12437–12443.

159. Jeffery, L., and Nakielny, S. (2004). Components of the DNA methylation system of chromatin control are RNA-binding proteins. *J Biol Chem* 279, 49479–49487.

160. Kanellopoulou, C., Muljo, S. A., Kung, A. L., Ganesan, S., Drapkin, R., Jenuwein, T., Livingston, D. M., and Rajewsky, K. (2005). Dicer-deficient mouse embryonic stem cells are defective in differentiation and centromeric silencing. *Genes Dev* 19, 489–501.

161. Murchison, E. P., Partridge, J. F., Tam, O. H., Cheloufi, S., and Hannon, G. J. (2005). Characterization of Dicer-deficient murine embryonic stem cells. *Proc Natl Acad Sci USA* 102, 12135–12140.

162. Aufsatz, W., Mette, M. F., van der Winden, J., Matzke, A. J., and Matzke, M. (2002). RNA-directed DNA methylation in Arabidopsis. *Proc Natl Acad Sci USA* 99 Suppl 4, 16499–16506.

163. Wassenegger, M., Heimes, S., Riedel, L., and Sanger, H. L. (1994). RNA-directed de novo methylation of genomic sequences in plants. *Cell* 76, 567–576.

164. Wutz, A., Smrzka, O. W., Schweifer, N., Schellander, K., Wagner, E. F., and Barlow, D. P. (1997). Imprinted expression of the Igf2r gene depends on an intronic CpG island. *Nature* 389, 745–749.

165. Smilinich, N. J., Day, C. D., Fitzpatrick, G. V., Caldwell, G. M., Lossie, A. C., Cooper, P. R., Smallwood, A. C., Joyce, J. A., Schofield, P. N., Reik, W., Nicholls, R. D., Weksberg, R., Driscoll, D. J., Maher, E. R., Shows, T. B., and Higgins, M. J. (1999). A maternally methylated CpG island in KvLQT1 is associated with an antisense paternal transcript and loss of imprinting in Beckwith-Wiedemann syndrome. *Proc Natl Acad Sci USA* 96, 8064–8069.

166. Tufarelli, C., Stanley, J. A., Garrick, D., Sharpe, J. A., Ayyub, H., Wood, W. G., and Higgs, D. R. (2003). Transcription of antisense RNA leading to gene silencing and methylation as a novel cause of human genetic disease. *Nat Genet* 34, 157–165.

167. Morris, K. V., Chan, S. W., Jacobsen, S. E., and Looney, D. J. (2004). Small interfering RNA-induced transcriptional gene silencing in human cells. *Science* 305, 1289–1292.

168. Kawasaki, H., and Taira, K. (2004). Induction of DNA methylation and gene silencing by short interfering RNAs in human cells. *Nature* 431, 211–217.

169. Kawasaki, H., and Taira, K. (2006). Retraction: Induction of DNA methylation and gene silencing by short interfering RNAs in human cells. *Nature* 441, 1176.

170. Weinberg, M. S., Villeneuve, L. M., Ehsani, A. L. I., Amarzguioui, M., Aagaard, L., Chen, Z.-X., Riggs, A. D., Rossi, J. J., and Morris, K. V. (2006). The antisense strand of small interfering RNAs directs histone methylation and transcriptional gene silencing in human cells. *RNA* 12, 256–262.

171. Kim, D. H., Villeneuve, L. M., Morris, K. V., and Rossi, J. J. (2006). Argonaute-1 directs siRNA-mediated transcriptional gene silencing in human cells. *Nat Struct Mol Biol* 13, 793–797.

172. Rinn, J. L., Kertesz, M., Wang, J. K., Squazzo, S. L., Xu, X., Brugmann, S. A., Goodnough, L. H., Helms, J. A., Farnham, P. J., Segal, E., and Chang, H. Y. (2007). Functional demarcation of active and silent chromatin domains in human HOX loci by noncoding RNAs. *Cell* 129, 1311–1323.

173. Lindahl, T. (1993). Instability and decay of the primary structure of DNA. *Nature* 362, 709–715.

174. Shen, J., Rideout, W. III, and Jones, P. (1994). The rate of hydrolytic deamination of 5-methylcytosine in double-stranded DNA. *Nucleic Acids Res* 22, 972–976.

175. Neddermann, P., Gallinari, P., Lettieri, T., Schmid, D., Truong, O., Hsuan, J. J., Wiebauer, K., and Jiricny, J. (1996). Cloning and expression of human G/T mismatch-specific thymine-DNA glycosylase. *J Biol Chem* 271, 12767–12774.

176. Neddermann, P., and Jiricny, J. (1993). The purification of a mismatch-specific thymine-DNA glycosylase from HeLa cells. *J Biol Chem* 268, 21218–21224.

177. Wiebauer, K., and Jiricny, J. (1989). In vitro correction of G.T mispairs to G.C pairs in nuclear extracts from human cells. *Nature* 339, 234–236.

178. Millar, C. B., Guy, J., Sansom, O. J., Selfridge, J., MacDougall, E., Hendrich, B., Keightley, P. D., Bishop, S. M., Clarke, A. R., and Bird, A. (2002). Enhanced CpG mutability and tumorigenesis in MBD4-deficient mice. *Science* 297, 403–405.

179. Griffin, S., and Karran, P. (1993). Incision at DNA G.T mispairs by extracts of mammalian cells occurs preferentially at cytosine methylation sites and is not targeted by a separate G.T binding reaction. *Biochemistry (Moscow)* 32, 13032–13039.

180. Sibghat, U., Gallinari, P., Xu, Y. Z., Goodman, M. F., Bloom, L. B., Jiricny, J., and Day, R. S. III (1996). Base analog and neighboring base effects on substrate specificity of recombinant human G:T mismatch-specific thymine DNA-glycosylase. *Biochemistry (Mosc)* 35, 12926–12932.

181. Waters, T. R., and Swann, P. F. (1998). Kinetics of the action of thymine DNA glycosylase. *J Biol Chem* 273, 20007–20014.

182. Boland, M. J., and Christman, J. K. (2008). Characterization of the dnmt3b:thymineDNA glycosylase interaction and stimulation of thymine glycosylase-mediated repair by DNA methyltransferas(es) and RNA. *J Mol Biol* 379, 492–504.

183. Li, Y. Q., Zhou, P. Z., Zheng, X. D., Walsh, C. P., and Xu, G. L. (2007). Association of Dnmt3a and thymine DNA glycosylase links DNA methylation with base-excision repair. *Nucleic Acids Res* 35, 390–400.

184. Kasten, M. B., Gowans, B. J., and Lieberman, M. W. (1984). Methylation deoxycytine incorporated by excision repair synthesis of DNA. *Cell Adhes Commun* 30, 509–516.

185. Kangapeska, S., Stride, B., Metivier, R., Polycarpou-Schwarz, M., Ibberson, D., Carmouche, R.P., Benes, V., Gannon, F., and Reid, G. (2008). Transient cyclical methylation of promoter DNA. *Nature* 452, 112–115.

186. Metivier, R., Gallais, R., Tiffoche, C., Le Peron, C., Jurkowska, R.Z., Carmouche, R.P., Ibberson, D., Barath, P., Demay, F., Reid, G., Benes, V., Jeltsch, A., Gannon, F., and Salbert, G. (2008). Cyclical DNA methylation of a transcriptionally active promoter. *Nature* 452, 45–50.

187. Ooi, S. K. T., and Bestor, T. H. (2008). The colorful history of DNA demethylation. *Cell* 133, 1145–1148.

chapter four

Chromatin remodeling and histone modifications

Gavin R. Schnitzler

Contents

The chromatin packaging of eukaryotic DNA is neither uniform nor random. In the last few decades it has become increasingly clear that the precise regulation of chromatin structures is essential for the proper control of DNA accessibility, controlling transcription, replication, recombination and repair. This chapter will provide an introduction to basic elements of chromatin structure, and then introduce the range of covalent modifications and noncovalent structural alterations that play into regulation of DNA accessibility in chromatin. As we will see, chromatin modifications have great potential as epigenetic control mechanisms, in that they can control DNA accessibility in a way that is not directly dependent on underlying DNA sequence and (at least for certain modifications) that they can persist for long periods of time. Chromatin modifications do not appear to be epigenetic marks that can be inherited from one generation of organisms to the next. Rather, they are "somatic cell epigenetic marks" that are used to control patterns of DNA accessibility through somatic cell divisions or over long periods of time in nondividing differentiated cells. That is not to say that chromatin modifications are not important for heritable epigenetic effects, such as genomic imprinting. Indeed, the functional effects of CpG methylation marks are largely caused by the differential recruitment of chromatin modifying enzymes.

4.1   Elements of chromatin structure

DNA in all eukaryotic cells is packaged into nucleosomes, in which ~147 bp of DNA is wrapped in a left-handed helix 1.65 times around an octamer of histone proteins (generally two copies each of histones H2A, H2B, H3 and H4, Figure 4.1). The histones are highly positively charged, and associate very tightly with DNA (with an approximate overall ΔG_0 of -13 kcal/mol). This strong association means that any other DNA binding factor

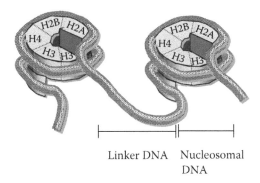

Linker DNA   Nucleosomal
                    DNA

Figure 4.1 (***A color version of this figure follows page 20***.) Basic chromatin structure. Two nucleosomes are shown, with histone octamer proteins in blue and genomic double-stranded DNA in green. Each nucleosome wraps ~146 bp of DNA, and nucleosomes are separated by linker DNA.

must effectively compete with the histones to bind its cognate sequence. As a result, the presence of a nucleosome greatly inhibits the binding of almost all tested transcription factors (for review see Reference 1), and recombination factors (e.g., see Reference 2).

4.1.1   Determinants of nucleosome positioning

Importantly, not all the DNA is bound to histones. Between every pair of nucleosomes, along the length of chromosomal DNA, are gaps of spacer, or linker, DNA. The average length of this linker DNA can vary between organisms and between cell types, but is generally on the order of ~30 to ~100 bp (see Reference 3 and references therein). In mammalian somatic cells linker DNA is ~60 bp long. Given that the nucleosome covers ~147 bp, this means that ~30% of mammalian genomic DNA sequences are not bound to histones, and are thus much more accessible.

Which DNA sequences are present in accessible linker DNA depends on the precise positioning of nucleosomes on DNA. Histones bind DNA largely via ionic interactions between positively charged amino acids and the negative charges on the DNA phosphate backbone. They do not make any clear base-specific contacts to DNA and, thus, nucleosomes might be expected to be distributed randomly on genomic sequences.[4] However, certain sequences of DNA are more amenable to being bent in a regular ~10 nm spiral around the histone octamer, and ~147 bp sequences which have this property are low-energy binding sites for nucleosomes, referred to as nucleosome positioning sequences (referred to herein as NPSes). Rather than being standard consensus sequences, NPSes tend to contain regularly repeated short sequence motifs that promote a DNA conformation favorable to histone octamer binding. For instance, NPSes are characterized (in part) by AA, AT or TT dinucleotides spaced every 10 bp (one helical turn of the DNA) which face inwards and promote DNA curvature around the octamer.[5,6] Sequences that are very resistant to wrapping around the histone octamer also exist, and are referred to as nucleosome excluding sequences.

For a long time it was thought that strong NPSes and nucleosome excluding sequences were rare, and that nucleosome positions were mostly random, despite the existence of a few notable exceptions (such as the 5S rDNA repeats). Recently, however, new genomic tiling microarray technology has been used to examine nucleosome positions throughout the yeast genome[7] and over hundreds of human gene promoters.[8] Remarkably, these studies indicated that ~50% of all yeast nucleosomes, and ~25% of tested human promoter nucleosomes, are positioned over specific genomic DNA sequences. Nucleosomes might be positioned by NPSes or by the presence of other nuclear factors—for instance, a sequence-specific factor present on the DNA before histone deposition might prevent a nucleosome from forming over it, thus restricting the nucleosome's location. To what extent are these nucleosomes being positioned by DNA sequence itself? Recent studies in the Widom and Pugh labs used known characteristics of NPSes to predict the affinity of the histone octamer for any given DNA sequence in yeast. While the resulting algorithms are still far from perfect, there was a reasonably good overlap (~50%) between predicted NPSes and observed nucleosome positions.[5,6]

Of course, nucleosome positioning by genetically encoded NPSes is not an epigenetic phenomenon. However, it is worth emphasizing here for two reasons. First, it is a poorly understood genetic factor that can give rise to effects that look "epigenetic." For instance, chromatin immuno-precipitation (ChIP) studies have shown that not all perfect transcription factor consensus binding sequences are occupied in vivo, and any number of epigenetic phenomena have been suggested as causing this effect. However, recent studies indicate that a major determinant of whether a factor will bind to a consensus site is whether or not that site is covered by a positioned nucleosome.[7,8] In addition, factors that do not interact and do not bind cooperatively to bare DNA can cooperate in binding to nucleosomes. This is because the ends of nucleosomal DNA can transiently unpeel from the octamer, allowing access of a first factor to this end-proximal site. Binding of this first factor then helps destabilize DNA further into the nucleosome, which can increase the affinity of subsequent factors for sites further from the nucleosome's edge.[9,10] Thus, positioned nucleosomes can both block factor access and also alter the functional interactions between transcription factors. Second, as discussed further in Section 4.3, the presence of genetically encoded NPSes sets the stage for specific epigenetic effects when ATP dependent remodeling complexes alter this nucleosome positioning.

4.1.2   Nucleosomes and elongation

As described above, positioned nucleosomes can inhibit transcription by blocking activator and basal factor binding sites. In addition, nucleosomes downstream of transcription start sites, largely independent of their precise positions, can strongly inhibit elongation (for review see Reference 11). In the sections below, we will see that the extent of this inhibition appears to be influenced by the specific chromatin protein composition, histone tail modifications and other factors that may aid in shuttling nucleosomal histones from in front of to behind an advancing polymerase.

4.1.3   Chromatin folding

The organization of nucleosomes spaced by linker DNA segments is only the lowest level of chromatin organization. This "beads on a string" simple chromatin fiber (which has a width of ~10 nm), has a strong propensity to fold onto itself into thicker and thicker fibers (with widths of 30 nm or more), conceptually similar to what would happen if a bead necklace is twisted. There has been much debate about the nature of folded chromatin structures, although new techniques are beginning to provide a much clearer picture (for review see Reference 12). One clear function of this chromatin folding process is compaction: allowing several meters of mammalian interphase DNA to fit inside a nucleus measuring only 10 microns in diameter, and, at an even higher level of folding, into mitotic chromosomes. Chromatin folding is also expected to play some role in regulating the accessibility of DNA sequences. In general, it appears that transcriptionally active DNA is less compacted than transcriptionally repressed DNA (e.g., see References 13 and 14, and for review see Reference 15). However, what determines chromatin compaction, and the extent to which compaction regulates factor access to DNA, are still largely open questions.

4.1.4   Histone flavors and chromatin accessories

In addition to the major core histones, H2A, H2B, H3 and H4, there are several less abundant histone variants which may have specialized functions in different regions of the genome (for review see Reference 16). The two most important variants of H3 are H3.3 (~10% to 20% of all H3 in mammalian somatic cells, and enriched on the transcribed regions of transcriptionally active genes), and Cid (which is enriched on centromeric DNA and essential for centromere formation and function). There are also several variants of H2A: H2AX, which bears a serine residue absent from normal H2A whose phosphorylation is important for functionally marking DNA damage sites; H2AZ, which marks transcriptionally active chromatin and helps it resist silencing; MacroH2A, which is associated with the inactive X chromosome in female mammalian cells and H2Abbd, which is excluded from the inactive X. Once deposited at a certain location on the DNA, histones tend to remain in place (especially H3 and H4, which form the central core of the histone octamer). Hence, the different flavors of core histones present in nucleosomes are expected to be long-lived epigenetic signals.

In addition to core histones, most nucleosomes in mammalian cells are also associated with some version of a linker histone. The most abundant of these is H1, which is estimated to be associated with ~70% of mammalian nucleosomes. H1 binds to the DNA helices as they enter and exit the core histone octamer. By doing so, H1 can change the angle of entering and exiting DNA, which can promote certain types of higher-order chromatin folding. H1 also covers an additional ~10 bp of DNA, such that the H1-bound nucleosome (referred to as the "chromatosome") covers ~155 to 160 bp of DNA instead of ~147. H1 is generally associated with transcriptional repression (although numerous counterexamples also exist). By contrast, two other chromatin proteins, HMGB1 and HMGB2, can compete with H1 for binding to the same site on the nucleosome, and are generally associated with transcriptional activation. Finally, other HMG (for "high mobility group") proteins are also present on chromatin, with functions ranging from altering the length of linker DNA between nucleosomes (HMGNs) to DNA bending (HMGAs).

4.1.5   Chromatin replication and histone chaperones

The nucleosome is assembled onto DNA by histone carrier proteins called chaperones. One class of chaperone binds to a tetramer of H3 and H4 proteins, and can transfer this tetramer to DNA. This forms the central core of the nucleosome, a left-handed spiral of H4:H3:H3:H4 proteins. A second class of histone chaperone carrying dimers of H2A and H2B then adds one dimer to each end of the H3:H4 tetramers to complete the full spiral of the histone octamer (which linearly arranged would read H2A:H2B:H4:H3:H3:H4:H2B:H2A) onto which ~147 bp of DNA is wound (Figure 4.1).

Chromatin assembly is tightly coupled to DNA replication in that the major replicative H3:H4 chaperone, CAF-1, binds directly to the PCNA sliding clamp during translocation of the DNA polymerase. This ensures that H3:H4 tetramers are deposited as soon as newly replicated DNA is made. Replicative H2A:H2B chaperones such as NAP-1 then complete the formation of the nucleosome within ~2 minutes (for review see Reference 17). In vitro, chaperones tend to position nucleosomes on DNA sequences that have a high affinity for the histone octamer (NPSes). Hence, DNA replication is expected to result in nucleosomes located in low-energy NPS-established positions.

About half the nucleosomes formed on by newly replicated DNA are made from newly synthesized histone proteins. The other half contain the same histones that were present in nucleosomes on the unreplicated DNA (although it is presently unclear if they remain associated with the DNA as the replication fork passes, or are transiently passed to chaperones, in trans, until replication is completed). One way or another, the end product is two chromatin fibers, each of which contains one strand of new DNA and one strand of old DNA (which, as you have seen is essential for propagating CpG methylation through cell divisions), as well as a mixture of new and old histone proteins. Similar to the case for CpG methylation, the distribution of some old and some new histones on each replicated DNA strand has the potential for propagating epigenetic marks encoded in chromatin, either in the form of nonstandard histone proteins or, as considered in detail below, in the form of covalent histone modifications.

Note that histone deposition is not limited only to S-phase. Recent data indicates that histone proteins can be replaced during interphase, but that this often involves both specialized chaperones and specialized histones. For instance, the normal H3 histone in highly transcribed genes can be progressively replaced by H3.3, in a process that requires the specialized HirA chaperone. Furthermore, recent studies have shown that entire nucleosomes can be removed from genes without any requirement for replication. This was first, and most convincingly, shown to occur during the activation of the yeast PHO5 promoter,[18,19] but appears to also occur during activation (or sometimes repression) of human genes (e.g., see References 20 and 21). Furthermore, recent genomewide studies of nucleosome positions show very low nucleosome occupancy over the immediate proximal promoters and transcription termination sites of highly transcribed yeast and human genes (although they do not prove that nucleosomes are lost as part of transcriptional activation).[8,22,23] Finally, fluorescence reactivation after photobleaching (FRAP) studies have indicated that, while H3 and H4 histones do not exchange rapidly on and off the DNA, H2A, H2B and H1 linker histones are all in surprisingly rapid exchange (for review see Reference 24). H2A/B exchange is also increased in actively transcribed regions, consistent with observations that elongation factors, such as FACT, can function as H2A/B chaperones.[25] These studies challenge the notion that nucleosomes are permanent barriers that are only briefly disrupted during DNA replication, and suggest new models for regulation via controlled exchange of histones in a dynamic chromatin environment.

4.1.6 Heterochromatin versus euchromatin

Early studies showed that areas of metaphase chromosomes which appeared dark after Giemsa staining often corresponded to transcriptionally silent, late replicating, gene poor regions of the genome, while light staining regions were transcriptionally active, early replicating and gene rich. The dark staining chromatin was referred to as "heterochromatin" and the light staining chromatin as "euchromatin" (or good chromatin). Over the last several years, we have learned a great deal about the nature of these distinct chromatin types and the proteins that are required for their formation and maintenance.

Mammalian cells appear to contain three principal types of transcriptionally silenced chromatin: HP1-mediated heterochromatin, Polycomb-silenced chromatin and the inactive X chromosome in female mammalian cells. Each of these provides a mechanism of epigenetic control of transcription that can be maintained for long periods of time and through several cell divisions. Here, I will present a brief introduction to these types of repressive chromatin, with an emphasis on the noncatalytic protein components that define them. The importance of histone tail modifications and ATP-dependent chromatin remodeling complexes in establishing and maintaining these chromatin structures will then be explored in the latter half of this chapter.

4.1.7   HP1-mediated heterochromatin

The HP1 protein ("heterochromatin protein 1") has long been associated with heterochromatin. However, it is only relatively recently that the molecular mechanisms by which HP1 contributes to transcriptional silencing have begun to be revealed. The emerging picture (from humans down to the yeast *Saccharomyces pombe*, but not *Saccharomyces cerevisiae*— which lacks this type of heterochromatin structure) is that tandem repeat sequences characteristic of pericentromeric heterochromatin are transcribed by RNA polymerase II to give overlapping sense and antisense transcripts. These transcripts form RNA duplexes that are processed by dicer to give short double-stranded RNAs. Note that similar short interfering RNAs, when bound to a complex called RISC, can recognize mRNA sequences and either target those mRNAs for degradation or block their translation. By contrast, the short double-stranded RNAs resulting from pericentromeric heterochromatin repeats bind to a different protein complex, called RITS, containing proteins from the Argonaut family (which bind to the siRNA) and Chromodomain families (which are homologous to HP1).[26] The siRNAs then allow the RITS complex to be targeted to the same pericentromeric heterochromatin repeats via interactions with nascent transcripts.[27] Once there, the complex promotes certain histone tail modifications (as described further in Section 4.2), as well as HP1 binding, which altogether results in the formation of a domain of chromatin that is repressive for most transcription (with the exception of low levels of transcripts from the repeat sequences themselves). Characteristics of HP1-mediated heterochromatin are illustrated in Figure 4.2a.

HP1-mediated silencing, while nucleated at transcribed repeat regions (or at other sequences targeted by siRNAs), can spread to adjacent chromatin, resulting in silencing of nearby genes. This gives rise to one of the best studied examples of an epigenetic effect, position effect variegation (or PEV) in *Drosophila*. In one classic experimental system, the white gene (which, when expressed gives red pigment to *Drosophila* eye cells, but when silenced gives white eye cells) was inserted near centromeric heterochromatin. This resulted in a variegated color phenotype in which some eye cells were red and others white, indicating that this location near heterochromatin caused the white gene to be randomly silenced and activated during the development of the eye. Furthermore, red cells and white cells were seen to be clustered together, indicating that once the on or off state of the gene was established this state could be maintained clonally through many cell divisions. The current explanation for this is that HP1-mediated heterochromatin varies in the distance it spreads from pericentric heterochromatin repeats, sometimes extending far enough to silence the white gene, and sometimes not (Figure 4.2b). The clonal heritability of HP1-mediated heterochromatic silencing is likely to be maintained by two mechanisms. First, as soon as the heterochromatic silencing weakens, more dsRNA is made from the repeat sequences, enforcing silencing in a feedback loop. Second, the HP1 proteins and other heterochromatin components may be distributed between the two DNA strands after replication, which would help maintain a particular zone of silenced chromatin through cell divisions.

4.1.8   Polycomb and trithorax group genes maintain silenced and active chromatin domains

In early *Drosophila* development sequence-specific activators and repressors establish the transcription state of a group of developmental control genes which are arrayed one after the other at two chromosomal loci (the Hox gene clusters). In the anterior of the embryo, only the leftmost gene in each cluster is active, while more and more genes (proceeding rightwards across the cluster) are active the closer cells are to the anterior of the embryo. Strikingly, as development proceeds, most of the transcription factors that set up this expression pattern are lost, yet the anterior to posterior gradient of gene activation is maintained. This is one of the classic examples of somatic cell epigenetic effect—where the expression pattern in adult somatic cells is not determined by direct DNA sequence elements, but by the embryonic history of gene expression.

The proteins required to maintain repressed Hox cluster genes in their "off" state are encoded by the Polycomb group genes. Mutations in these genes results in an abnormal expansion of active genes in the cluster, causing anterior body segments to become more posterior-like

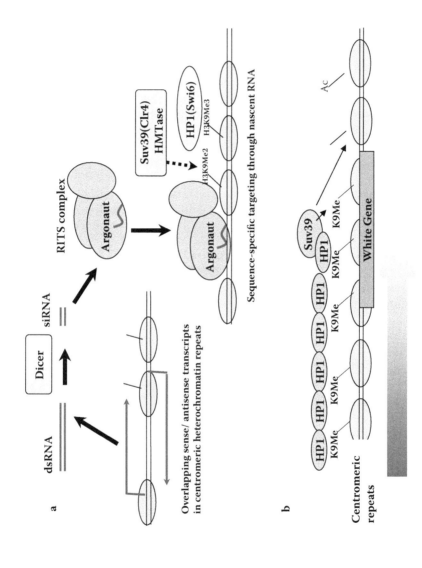

Figure 4.2.

(anterior to posterior transformation). Conversely, the proteins required to maintain Hox genes in their on state are encoded by the Trithorax group genes, and mutations in these result in abnormal retraction of the zone of active gene expression in the clusters, causing posterior to anterior transformations. Similar sets of Hox gene clusters are also important for mammalian development, and are regulated by a very similar set of Polycomb and Trithorax genes. Furthermore, it has become apparent that far more than just the Hox gene clusters are regulated by Polycomb and Trithorax proteins. For instance, Polycomb proteins are involved in silencing of the female mammalian inactive X chromosome[28–30] and in silencing (but also allowing the activation of) differentiation-specific regulatory genes in mammalian embryonic stem cells[31,32] (for review see Reference 32).

Polycomb group proteins (and also some Trithorax group proteins) are recruited to specific regions of the Hox clusters called Polycomb Response Elements, or PREs.[33] The nature of PREs and mechanisms by which Polycomb proteins are recruited to them and stabilized are not fully understood. Certain DNA binding proteins, such as the Trithorax group protein GAGA play a role, as do proteins that bind specific types of modified chromatin. Recent studies also indicate a role for noncoding RNAs and the RNAi pathway (similar to HP1-mediated heterochromatin; for review see Reference 34). One model of how the enzymatic and nonenzymatic components of Polycomb and Trithorax complexes may antagonize each other to maintain inactive and active chromatin domains is shown in Figure 4.3. Some additional details of how the enzymatic activities of some Polycomb and Trithorax proteins function to modulate chromatin and regulate transcription will be given in the following sections.

4.1.9   X inactivation

One of the most dramatic examples of an epigenetic effect is the almost complete silencing of one of the two copies of female mammalian X chromosomes (for recent review see Reference 35). This silencing accomplishes dosage compensation such that the effective gene dose of X-linked genes is the same in XX female and XY male cells. X inactivation is initiated in early development. In trophoblasts, zygote-derived cells that go on to form extra-embryonic tissues, this silencing is imprinted, such that the sperm-derived paternal X chromosome is always inactivated. By contrast,

Figure 4.2 **(Opposite)** (*A color version of this figure follows page 20.*) Model for HP1-mediated heterochromatin. (a) Model for the mechanism by which double-stranded DNA from pericentromeric repeats results in formation of HP1-containing silent heterochromatin over these same repeats. (b) Model for the spread of heterochromatin to variably cover or uncover nearby loci, resulting in position effect variegation.

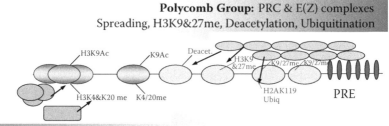

Figure 4.3 (A color version of this figure follows page 20.) Model for functional antagonism of Polycomb and Thrithorax complexes. Polycomb group complexes nucleated at PREs may spread by deacetylating H3K9 and H3K27 and then methylating these residues. Methyl H3K9 and H3K27 is a signal that is then bound by other Polycomb group proteins. Polycomb-mediated heterochromatin also requires enzymes that ubiquitinate H2A at K119. Trithorax group proteins may counter this repressive effect by rearranging nucleosome positions with SWI/SNF (nucleosome on the right), and by laying down activating histone methylation marks (H3K4me and H3K20me).

in embryonic cells, the paternal and maternal X are inactivated at equal frequencies. Since this occurs randomly at the 16 to 64 cell stage, female mammals become functional mosaics for X-linked genes, with about half their cells expressing paternal X-linked genes and half expressing maternal X-linked genes. Once this silencing is established, it is maintained throughout the lifetime of the organism.

X inactivation is initiated when a long noncoding RNA polymerase II transcript called Xist is expressed from the X inactivation center (Xic). Xist expression is countered by expression of an antisense RNA called Tsix, and the X chromosome that most effectively blocks Xist expression with Tsix becomes the active X chromosome. On the inactive X, Xist is expressed in large amounts. While the RNA is spliced and processed it does not exit the nucleus (or even the vicinity of the X chromosome where it is expressed), but instead coats the full length of the inactive X chromosome. This then leads to many other markers of inactive chromatin, including CpG hypermethylation, association of Polycomb group proteins, as well as a variety of repression-associated covalent histone modifications.

4.2   Covalent histone tail modifications

Only about 70% of the mass of the core histones is involved in forming the spiral of histone octamer proteins onto which DNA is wrapped. The remainder of these proteins are largely unstructured N- and C-terminal tails that extend outward from the nucleosome. Even though they are unstructured, the histone tails are extremely well conserved throughout eukaryotic evolution. The reason for this conservation is that many of the amino acids in the histone tails are sites for a variety of posttranslational modifications with essential roles in modulating the effects of chromatin. These posttranslational modifications include phosphorylation, acetylation, methylation and ubiquitination. In Figure 4.4, the sequence of the human histone tails is shown, with each site of modification noted. For a good general review of covalent histone modifications, see Reference 36.

There are three general mechanisms that have been proposed for how these histone modifications might regulate transcription (which are largely analogous to mechanisms by which covalent modifications of other proteins, such as phosphorylation, can alter their function). First, the covalent modification might cause a structural change in the nucleosome or the resulting higher-order chromatin structures which might alter the accessibility properties of chromatin. As described further below, this is certainly the case for one specific location of histone acetylation. However, the strong regulatory effects of all other covalent histone modifications have not been directly linked to changes in nucleosome or chromatin structure. Instead, most functions of histone tail modifications appear to arise from two other mechanisms, which together make up the "histone code hypothesis" first proposed by Strahl and Allis in 2000.[37] The first of these two mechanisms is that modified (or unmodified) histone tails function

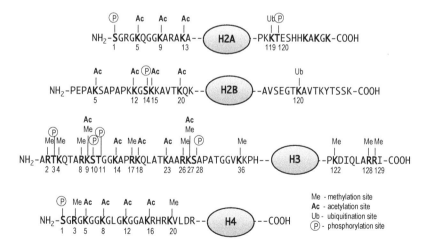

Figure 4.4 Sites of histone tail modification. Major sites for histone methylation, acetylation, ubiquitination and phosphorylation are shown. One that is not shown is the nontail H3K79 site which is methylated by Dot1. The variant histone, H2AX, has a serine at position 129, which is phosphorylated during DNA damage.

as ligands that bind and recruit a variety of factors which can regulate chromatin accessibility and transcription. Thus, histone tail modifications can be seen as markers that regulate protein-protein interactions. The second of these mechanisms is that some histone tail modifications can regulate subsequent histone tail modifications. This might occur because the first modification acts as a signal that recruits a subsequent modifying enzyme, or because the first modification increases or decreases the ability of the histone tail substrate to be productively modified by subsequent enzymes. In this way one type of epigenetic marker can regulate the type and amino acid preference of subsequent epigenetic markers.

In the sections below, I will review the known effects of each major histone tail modification, the enzymes that make these modifications and remove them, and the potential of each of these modifications for epigenetic regulation.

4.2.1   *Histone acetylation*

Histone tail acetylation occurs on conserved lysines (single letter abbreviation K) on the N-terminal tails of all four core histones. Acetylation of chromosomal histones has long been associated with transcriptionally active chromatin domains.[38] Indeed, one of the first applications of elementary chromatin immunoprecipitation techniques showed that the active chicken beta-globin locus in red blood cells contained highly acetylated histones, while the histones in surrounding inactive chromatin and other inactive loci were hypoacetylated.[39,40]

4.2.1.1   *HATs*

The histone acetyltransferase (HAT) enzymes function to transfer an acetyl ($-CH_3-COO^-$) group from acetyl-CoA to lysine residues. HATs fall in two broad classes. The cytoplasmic, type B HATs modify tails of newly synthesized histone proteins, which may help prepare these proteins for association with chaperones and deposition during DNA replication. By contrast nuclear, type A HATs acetylate nucleosomal histones present on nuclear genomic chromatin. The first nuclear HAT was identified in 1996 by Brownell et al.,[41] and this discovery was rapidly followed by the identification of many more nuclear HATs. Strikingly, some factors that had long been associated with transcriptional coactivation, such as CBP/p300 and the SRC1/ACTR nuclear hormone coactivators, were found to have HAT activity. Some basal transcription factors were also found to be HATs, including the TBP-associated factor TAF250 and the PolIII factor TFIIIC. We now know of more than 50 type A HATs, many of which are conserved across evolution (Table 4.1; for review see Reference 42). The two largest HAT families, conserved from yeast to man, are the GNAT family (typified by GCN5) and the MYST family (typified by

Table 4.1 Histone acetylation and deacetylation enzymes

Family/Type	Examples	Functions and other details
HATs (Histone acetyl transferases)		
GNAT (many)	Yeast and human GCN5 yeast Elp3	Mostly coactivators, in large complexes, H3 > H4
MYST (many)	Yeast Sas3 and Esa1	Silencing, dosage comp., transcriptional activation, in complexes, H4 > H3
p300/CBP	p300 and CBP	Coactivators, acetylate all four histones
SRCs	SRC1, ACTR	Nuclear receptor coactivators, H3 > H4
TAF250	TAFII250	Basal factor, part of TFIID, H3 > H4
TFIIIC	TFIIIC	RNA polymerase III activator, H3 > H4
HDACs (Histone deacetylases)		
Type I	Human HDACs 1–3, yeast Rpd3	Transcriptional repression, constitutively nuclear, in large complexes, cofactor independent
Type II	Human HDACs 4–6, yeast Hda1	Transcriptional repression, shuttles between nucleus and cytoplasm, cofactor independent
Type III, sirtuins	Human SIRTs, yeast SIR2	Repression of telomeres and silent mating loci in yeast, requires NAD cofactor

Esa1). Most HATs display some level of specificity for the lysines they acetylate, although they usually affect multiple lysines. HATs also frequently show a preference for the histone tail they work on (e.g., GNAT HATs prefer the H3 tail, while MYST HATs prefer the H4 tail). Many HAT enzymes exist as part of multisubunit complexes, such as yeast or human GCN5 in the SAGA/PCAF complex. The other subunits in these complexes can influence the choice of lysines to be acetylated, the efficiency of histone acetylation in chromatin and the targeting of the HAT to specific regions of chromatin through interaction with sequence-specific transcription factors.

HATs have also been shown to acetylate other transcription factors, and this acetylation can alter the binding and activation properties of these factors.[43] While these effects are certainly important, it is also clear that chromatin is a functional target for acetylation. This was first demonstrated clearly in 1999, in in vitro transcription experiments showing that a pre-acetylated chromatin template would support transcription in the absence of continued HAT activity.[44]

4.2.1.2   HDACs

Acetyl lysine is not a naturally labile species, and the acetyl group must be actively removed. The enzymes that perform this function are histone deacetylases (or HDACs) (for a more extensive review see Reference 45). HDACs come in three major varieties (Table 4.1). The type I and II HDACs remove the acetyl group by hydrolyzing the amide bond, and do not require a cofactor for this reaction. Both are inhibited by classical HDAC inhibitory drugs such as trichostatin A (TSA) and butyrate. Type I HDACs (typified by human HDACs 1, 2 and 3 and the yeast Rpd3) are constitutively nuclear. By contrast, type II HDACs (typified by human HDACs 4, 5 and 6, and the yeast Hda1) can shuttle in and out of the nucleus in response to signal transduction cascades. Type III HDACs, called sirtuins after the prototypical family member yeast SIR2, are NAD-dependent deacetylases that perform deacetylation by breaking down a nicotinamide adenine dinucleotide (NAD) cofactor and releasing nicotinamide and *O*-acetyl ADP-ribose. Because of their dependence on NAD, there is considerable interest in the potential for sirtuin function to be regulated by dietary and other controls on NAD^+ levels.[46] In yeast and the nematode *Caenorhabditis elegans* surtuins also function to promote longevity.[47] As would be expected by their ability to antagonize HATs, many HDACs function as transcriptional corepressors, recruited to DNA by sequence-specific repressor proteins (such as the yeast Ume6 protein) or by other corepressors (such as the NCoR nuclear receptor corepressor, which recruits both type I and type II HDACs).

4.2.1.3   Acetylation is a short-duration epigenetic mark

HDACs are abundant in the nucleus, even in the absence of specific signals, and are continuously removing acetyl groups from histone tail lysines. Thus, even in the absence of HDAC recruitment by sequence-specific transcription factors, acetyl lysine marks are rapidly removed (for review see Reference 48). For instance, one study in yeast showed that an H3 acetylation mark was removed with a half time of 1.5 minutes after loss of the SAGA HAT complex from the locus.[49] Conversely, HATs are also abundant throughout the nucleus, and even without recruitment by sequence-specific activators, histone tails cannot remain fully deacetylated for long (a region that was deacetylated by HDAC recruitment returned to a partially acetylated state with a half time of 6 minutes).[49] Thus, the level of histone tail acetylation at any chromosomal location depends on the local balance of both recruited and background HAT and HDAC activities. Once this balance changes, the rapid turnover of acetyl lysines ensures that the acetylation state adjusts rapidly to the new balance.

Because of its rapid turnover, histone acetylation/deacetylation is a short-term epigenetic mark that must be continually maintained by localized recruitment of HATs or HDACs. This is in contrast to epigenetic marks such as CpG methylation, which can be stable for long periods of time after the enzyme that introduced them leaves the area. Acetylation can still be thought of as an epigenetic mark, however, since its function is not *directly* linked to DNA sequences. Instead, it is an epiphenomenon that arises from factors that bind to those sequences, which then can alter the functions of surrounding chromatin. Indeed, HATS or HDACs recruited to a specific site on DNA have been shown to modify the histone tails of nucleosomes covering 3kb or more of DNA sequence (e.g., see Reference 50 and for review see Reference 51).

4.2.1.4   Specific acetylation of H4K16 prevents chromatin folding

The addition of the acetyl group (from acetyl CoA) forms an amide bond that neutralizes the charge of the lysine. It is generally expected that (despite the lack of structure in the histone tails) the positive charges of the histone tail lysines will bind to the negative charges of the DNA phosphate backbone. This could potentially help hold DNA more tightly to the nucleosome, reduce the accessibility of linker DNA or create bridges between separate nucleosomes that might promote chromatin folding. Thus, early on it was proposed that histone acetylation would promote transcription by altering DNA histone affinities or chromatin folding. Most biochemical studies that tried to test this hypothesis, however, showed only minor effects of acetylation. Recently, however, a process which allowed quantitative site-specific modification of individual histone tail lysines showed that one specific acetylation at H4K16 greatly inhibits chromatin folding (while other tested lysines had little effect).[52] As folded chromatin is hypothesized to present a much greater barrier to DNA accessibility, this structural effect could potentially greatly facilitate transcription.

4.2.1.5   Acetylated lysines are protein-protein interaction surfaces

Perhaps the major mechanism by which acetylation promotes transcriptional activation is binding to and recruiting transcriptional coactivators. Acetyl lysine is specifically bound by bromodomains, which are present in a variety of coactivators, including the SWI/SNF ATP-dependent chromatin remodeling complex. Furthermore, bromodomains are present in several HAT proteins and complexes, including on GCN5/PCAF, TAFII250 and CPB/p300. Thus, acetylation recruits HATs, providing a positive feedback loop that can serve to maintain a domain of active-acetylated chromatin. This also provides a mechanism by which patterns of acetylated chromatin might be maintained after DNA replication: the acetylated histones that were present on the chromatin before replication are equally distributed on both strands after replication, and can then recruit HATs to acetylate the newly synthesized histones that were also deposited after replication. In addition to promoting the binding of coactivators, acetylation can also inhibit the binding of some repressors, such as the yeast Tup1 repressor. Finally, as described further below, acetylated lysines cannot be methylated (and vice versa). Thus, in keeping with the histone code hypothesis, acetylation can function both as a protein-protein interaction signal and as a regulator of other histone modifications.

4.2.2   Histone methylation

Histone methylation has emerged as a modification that is used widely for both transcriptional activation and repression (for review see Reference 53). In contrast to histone acetylation, methylation is a relatively long-lived mark which is likely to remain for hours after the enzymes that introduce it have moved on. Methylation can occur on the primary NH_3^+ amine group of lysine, which can accept up to three methyl groups (monomethyl -$NH_2(CH_3)_1^+$, dimethyl -$NH (CH_3)_2^+$, and trimethyl -$N(CH_3)_3^+$). Note that, unlike acetylation, methylation does not change the charge of the lysine, and is thus less likely to alter histone tail-DNA backbone interactions. Methylation can also occur on the terminal $H_2N-C=NH_2^+$ group of arginine (where the C is linked to the rest of the arginine side chain), to give monomethyl $H(CH_3)N-C=NH_2^+$, asymmetrical dimethyl $(CH_3)_2N-C=NH_2^+$ or symmetrical dimethyl $H(CH_3)N-C=N(CH_3)H^+$ arginine. The methylation states of lysine (K) and arginine (R) are often abbreviated as Kme1, Kme2, Kme3, Rme1 and Rme2.

4.2.2.1   Lysine and arginine methyltransferases

Histone methylation is performed by methyltransferases that use the methyl donor cofactor S-adenosyl methionine (AdoMet, SAM), see Table 4.2. The histone methyltransferases (HMTs) specialize in methylation of lysine, and include a large family of proteins containing a conserved SET domain, as well as a few other HMTs that lack SET domains (such as the evolutionarily conserved DOT1 protein). Arginine methylation is performed by a family of protein arginine methyl transferases (PRMTs). Unlike the somewhat loose specificity displayed by HATs, both HMTs and PRMTs tend to be very specific about the residue that is methylated (generally only modifying one or two histone tail residues). For instance the Suv39 HMT methylates only H3 K9, while the MLL HMT methylates only H3K4. Furthermore, methylases can distinguish between different levels of methylation on the same residue and are often limited to performing a subset of methylation reactions. For instance, the yeast Set2 HMT can make H3K4me1 and me2, but not me3, while the Set1 HMT is specialized in converting H3K4me2 to H3K4me3.

Table 4.2 Histone methylation and demethylation enzymes

Family/Type	Examples	Functions and other details
HMTs (Histone lysine methytransferases)		
SET domain	Suv39, ALL/Trithorax, etc.	Activation, repression, depending on specific lysine targeted and me level, AdoMet cofactor
Non-SET domain	yeast Dot1	Telomeric silencing, AdoMet cofactor, methylates nontail H3K79
PRMTs (Protein argenine methyl transferases)		
Type I	CARM1, most PRMTs	Transcriptional activation, AdoMet cofactor, does asymmetric R me2
Type II	PRMT5/JBP1	AdoMet cofactor, only one that does symmetric R me2
Lysine demethylases		
JARID/ Jumonji	Human JARID1A, yeast Yjr119c	Transcriptional repression and activation, different lysines, some can remove Kme3 mark, Fe(II) α-ketoglutarate dependent
LSD1	LSD1	Transcriptional repression, riboflavin dependent, removes H3K4 me1 or me2
Argenine demethylases		
PADs	PAD4	Transcriptional repression, peptidyl arginine deiminases, leave citrulline product

4.2.2.2 Lysine and arginine demethylases

Early studies indicated that lysine methylation was a much longer lived mark than lysine acetylation (with half lives in the range of hours). For several years it was hypothesized that the mark might be effectively permanent, and that the only way to remove it from chromatin would be to degrade the histone and replace it, or dilute it through successive rounds of DNA replication. That all changed in 2004, with the discovery of the first enzymes capable of demethylating lysine and arginine.[54,55] Similar to the methyltransferases, demethylases also tend to work only on specific residues and are limited to specific demethylation events (Table 4.2; for a more detailed review see Reference 56). Intriguingly, the same demethylase can have different effects when recruited by disparate factors. For instance, the LSD1 lysine demethylase (an FAD-dependent amine oxidase that creates formaldehyde as part of the demethylation reaction) demethylates H3K4 when recruited to chromatin via interaction with the CoREST corepressor[57] but demethylates H3K9me3 when recruited by androgen receptor.[58]

4.2.2.3   Histone methylation controls protein recruitment to chromatin

Specific kinds of histone methylation have been shown to function as signals that bind to different transcriptional regulators, recruiting them to chromatin. At least four types of protein domains can recognize and bind to specific methylated lysines: chromodomains, tudor domains, PhD fingers and WD40-repeat domains.[59,60] In any given protein, these domains can be remarkably specific for the methylated lysine that is recognized (e.g., the PHD finger in NURF binds primarily to H3K4me3).[61] The effect of the histone methylation signal (to either repress or activate transcription) is then determined by the nature and function of these proteins and others they recruit.

In HP1-mediated heterochromatin formation, the Suv39 methyltransferase (*S. pombe* Clr4) promotes mono-, di- and trimethylation of H3K9. The H3K9me3 mark is then bound by a combination of chromo- and chromoshadow domains in HP1 (*S. pombe* Swi6). This is required for HP1 recruitment to chromatin and for transcriptional silencing of pericentromeric heterochromatin (for review see Reference 62). Suv39 can also be recruited to specific sites on promoters (e.g., by Rb bound to E2F at cell cycle regulated genes), which can promote localized transcriptional silencing by formation of H3K9me3 and HP1 recruitment. A similar but distinct pattern of histone methylation is used for transcriptional repression mediated by Polycomb. The enhancer of zeste E(Z) HMT methylates H3K9 and H3K27, and this combined signal then binds to the Polycomb protein, which facilitates the recruitment of other Polycomb repressor proteins.[34] H3K9 and K27 methylation and Polycomb proteins are also associated with the inactive X chromosome. Thus, histone lysine methylation is associated with all three major classes of somatic-cell epigenetic silencing in mammals. Importantly, there appears to be an efficient means for maintaining the H3K9 methylation mark after DNA replication, in that certain H3K9-specific methyltransferases (SETDB1 and G9a) are localized to DNA replication forks (together with the maintenance DNA methyltransferase).[63,64]

Whereas H3K9 and K27 methylation are involved in transcriptional silencing, other histone methylation marks are important for the formation and maintenance of transcriptionally active chromatin. Indeed, arginine methylation through PRMTs generally functions in transcriptional activation (e.g., PRMT1, which methylates H4R3 and CARM1/PRMT4 which methylates H3 R2, R17 and R26 are both recruited by the p160 steroid receptor coactivator to activate transcription). This effect can be countered by recruitment of an enzyme that performs a demethylimination reaction, converting Rme1 to citrulline.[65] Note that while lysine methylation marks tend to be very long lasting, arginine methylation appears to be more like histone acetylation, with strong methylation or demethylation marks rapidly returning to an intermediate default state unless continually refreshed.[66]

Some forms of lysine methylation, most prominently H3K4me, are also involved in transcriptional activation. Indeed, H3K4 methylation tends to co-localize with histone acetylation and be broadly associated with transcriptionally active chromatin (for review, see Reference 67). In yeast, H3K4 HMTs specific for different levels of methylation are recruited by the polymerase II transcription machinery and play roles in elongation control, and an H3K4/H3K20 HMT is recruited via p300/CBP HAT coactivators. In flies and humans, the Trithorax/MLL H3K4 methylase is an essential member of the Trithorax group genes, which antagonizes Polycomb-mediated transcriptional silencing. The functions of H3K4 methylation are mediated, in part, by binding to proteins that contain PHD fingers.

4.2.2.4   Interplay between acetylation and methylation

The second half of the histone code hypothesis states that histone modifications might function, at least in part, by positively or negatively influencing other histone modifications. This is clearly the case for histone acetylation and methylation. As mentioned above, the presence of one of these modifications blocks the formation of the other. One residue where this functional competition occurs is H3K9, and given that this residue is essential for establishing both HP1 and Polycomb-mediated silencing, its acetylation would be expected to effectively prevent these forms of epigenetic silencing. Other forms of cross-talk between acetylation and methylation have also been shown. For instance, H3K14 acetylation blocks H3K9 methylation, H4R3 methylation promotes H4 K8 and K12 acetylation, and H4 tail acetylation prevents H4R3 methylation.

4.2.3   Histone phosphorylation, ubiquitination, and other modifications

While acetylation and methylation are the predominant forms of histone tail modification (at least in terms of the variety of the functional effects and the number of residues involved), histone tails are also subject to many other modifications. Chief among these are ubiquitination and phosphorylation.

Histones can be ubiquitinated on the H2A and H2B C-terminal tails at K119 and K120, respectively. The ubiquitin ligases involved tend to stop at mono-ubiquitination, and it is thought that the major function of histone ubiquitination is not to target histones for proteosomal degradation, but to serve as a signal to other factors (for review see Reference 68). For instance, in yeast, H2B ubiquitination by Rad6 is required for the subsequent methylation of H3K4 by SET1. Histone ubiquitination is important for silencing by Polycomb group proteins[69,70] and also for X inactivation.[28,71]

Histones can be phosphorylated at H3Serine10 (S10) and S28, H4 S1 and H2A S1. H3 S10 phosphorylation can function in transcriptional activation of immediate early genes in response to phorbal esters. Abundant H3 S10 phosphorylation is also associated with chromatin compaction during mitosis. H3 S10 phosphorylation can also control and be controlled by other histone modifications. For instance it blocks H3K9 methylation while enhancing H3K14 acetylation by the SAGA or p300 HATs. Conversely, H3K9 methylation inhibits H3S10 phosphorylation (for review see Reference 72). Phosphorylation of the C-terminal tail of the H2AX variant of H2A (at Ser139) is also an essential early step in DNA damage repair (for review see Reference 73).

Lastly, histones had long been hypothesized to be functional targets of poly-ADP ribosylation by poly-ADP ribose polymerase (PARP). Recent studies, however, have shown that histones are not detectably poly-ADP-ribosylated (although PARPs can mono-ribosylate H2B glu2 and several residues on H1 linker histones). Indeed, several studies indicate that auto-ribosylated PARP may promote unfolding/decompaction of chromatin without needing to covalently modify histones (for review see Reference 74). Furthermore, unmodified PARP binds strongly to chromatin and has the ability to greatly enhance chromatin folding.[75] The implication is that auto-ribosylation causes PARP release from chromatin, and this might function to convert chromatin from a condensed inaccessible conformation to an uncondensed conformation. Thus, the stimulation of PARP activity at sites of DNA damage might contribute to facilitating access of the DNA repair machinery.

4.3   ATP-dependent chromatin remodeling complexes

In addition to the covalent modifications described above, chromatin can be modulated by the action of ATP-dependent chromatin remodeling complexes. These multisubunit enzymes use the energy of ATP hydrolysis to cause noncovalent changes in nucleosomes and chromatin. Each remodeling complex has at its core an ATPase subunit that is related, to a greater or lesser degree, to the yeast SWI2/SNF2 ATPase. Several subfamilies of remodeling complex exist, as defined by sequence similarities and differences in their ATPase subunits. These include the SWI/SNF, ISWI, CHD/NuRD, Ino80, Swr1, Rad54, CSB and DDM1 subfamilies (Table 4.3). The largest of these are the SWI/SNF and ISWI families. In addition to a core ATPase/remodeling domain (which is related to the DEAD/H DNA and RNA helicases, although remodeling complexes do not possess DNA or RNA unwinding activities), each ATPase subunit has distinctive N- and C-terminal domains, which can confer differential functionalities

Table 4.3 ATP-dependent chromatin remodeling complexes[a]

Family/Type	Examples	Functions and other details
SWI/SNF	Human and yeast SWI/SNF, yeast RSC	Activation and repression, DNA repair, can form altered structures, in addition to moving nucleosomes
ISWI	Human SNF2L and H, yeast ISW1 and 2	Mostly repression, chromatin deposition and compaction, varied effects depending on other complex subunits
Mi2/CHD	Human NuRD	Repression, associated with HDACs
Rad54	*Drosophila* and yeast Rad54	DNA damage repair
Swr1 and Ino80	Yeast and human Swr1 and Ino80	Activation and DNA repair, Swr1 replaces nucleosomal H2A with H2AZ, characterized by "split" ATPase domain
DDM1	*Arabidopsis* DDM1	Required for CpG and H3K9 methylation
CSB	Human Cockayne's syndrome B	Transcription coupled DNA repair

[a] These represent the major families of complexes, based on the homology of their ATPase domains. Several other remodeling ATPases that do not fit well into any of these families also exist.

to complexes that contain it. For instance, the bromodomain of the SWI/SNF ATPases (which include yeast SWI2/SNF2) can help to stabilize the association of the complex with acetylated chromatin.[76] Each complex is also associated with one or more additional protein subunits, some of which can modulate the activity and effects of the ATPase subunit, and others of which can bind to sequence-specific transcriptional regulators or their coregulators, and recruit the complex to specific sites on chromatin. The general model for how chromatin remodeling complexes function is similar to that for the histone tail-modifying enzymes: a transcription factor bound at a specific site in chromatin (perhaps by virtue of having its site be in a linker region between two positioned nucleosomes) recruits the remodeling complex, which then alters surrounding chromatin structure to activate or repress transcription. The details of what these remodeling complexes do to cellular chromatin, or how these effects regulate transcription, are largely unknown. However, a reasonably good understanding of the basic biochemistry of remodeling is starting to give insights into the mechanisms of transcriptional control by these complexes.

4.3.1   Nucleosome movement and spacing

All tested ATP-dependent remodeling complexes have the ability to alter the positions of nucleosomes on DNA. One way of looking at nucleosome movement is by a spacing assay, where a polynucleosomal template (a long piece of DNA assembled into an array of nucleosomes) is treated with the remodeling complex, followed by light digestion with a nuclease that cuts between adjacent nucleosomes (such as micrococcal nuclease, MNAse). If nucleosomes are regularly spaced (having invariant linker DNA length between nucleosomes) this treatment results in a regular ladder of bands. If nucleosomes are not evenly spaced, this treatment results in a smear of DNA. Using this assay, it was found that some remodeling complexes, particularly several complexes of the ISWI subfamily, are adept at generating regularly spaced chromatin. Others, including all tested SWI/SNF complexes and a minority of ISWI complexes do the opposite, causing well-spaced chromatin to become disorganized.[77] Biophysical studies strongly imply that regular spacing between nucleosomes can be important for efficient chromatin folding. Thus, complexes that evenly space nucleosomes might be important for creating highly folded, transcriptionally silent chromatin. This is consistent with studies in flies showing that the loss of the sole fly ISWI ATPase or the major non-ATPase subunit in the efficient-spacing CHRAC and ACF complexes caused defects in nucleosome spacing and/or chromatin condensation.[78,79]

A second way of looking at movement is to consider the position of the nucleosomes relative to the underlying DNA. As detailed in Section 4.1, nucleosomes are frequently found positioned on DNA sequences that have a high affinity for the histone octamer (NPSes). This NPS-established arrangement of nucleosomes leaves specific DNA sequences covered by nucleosomes while other specific sequences are in accessible linker regions. This default arrangement of nucleosomes might be permissive for transcription (if activator and basal factor binding sites are present in linker regions) or might be repressive (if transcription factor binding sites are covered by nucleosomes). Thus, the regulatory function of a remodeling complex will depend greatly on how it affects this default distribution of nucleosomes. Does it reinforce the default positions, sliding nucleosomes to their lowest energy positions on DNA? Does it override DNA sequence effects and randomize positions? Or, does it move nucleosomes to some complex- and sequence-specific position? Studies that examined linear mononucleosomal templates in vitro suggested that the positions of remodeled nucleosomes might depend on sequence. However, for the SWI/SNF complexes, at least, sequence-specific effects were largely hidden by a strong propensity of the complex to move nucleosomes to DNA ends. Strikingly, recent studies on nucleosomal templates lacking ends showed that human SWI/

SNF prefers to move nucleosomes away from NPSes and to place them on other complex-preferred sequences.[80] This gives rise to a new model for SWI/SNF function, that it might regulate transcription by switching nucleosome positions from an NPS-specified default state to a distinct SWI/SNF-preferred remodeled state. Furthermore, nucleosomes that have been moved out of their default positions by SWI/SNF appear to remain out of place for many hours.[81] Thus, this sort of sequence- and complex-specific nucleosome movement has the potential to serve as a long-lasting epigenetic signal—such that nucleosome positions at any given locus are controlled by a combination of DNA sequence and the history of remodeling complex exposure. The functional consequences of this effect are still largely unknown. Furthermore, it is not yet known whether different remodeling complexes might compete with each other by creating distinct patterns of repositioned nucleosomes. Note that DNA replication promotes deposition of old and new nucleosomes in NPS-favored locations. Thus, it would be expected to erase remodeler-specific position changes, unless the remodeling complex is maintained at the locus throughout DNA replication.

4.3.2   *Formation of structurally altered nucleosomes*

Certain remodeling complexes, most notably the SWI/SNF complexes, have the additional ability to create stable structurally altered nucleosomes. Early studies showed that SWI/SNF complexes could create altered structures from mononucleosomes assembled onto short linear DNA fragments: attaching two mononucleosomes together in an altered dimer, sliding the histone octamer up to ~70 bp off the edge of the DNA and (apparently) looping exiting DNA from one end of the octamer around to enter again on the other end of the octamer. They also showed that SWI/SNF complexes could reduce the number of nucleosome-constrained negative supercoils (normally one negative supercoil per nucleosome) on circular templates (see Reference 77 for a review). Recently, it was shown that SWI/SNF complexes could convert about 40% of the nucleosomes on polynucleosomal templates into altered dinucleosomes, termed altosomes, and that this altered structure could explain the SWI/SNF-dependent loss of supercoiling.[81] While SWI/SNF-dependent reduction of supercoiling has been linked to transcriptional activation in vivo (for review see Reference 77), the detailed regulatory functions of altosomes are still largely unclear. Interestingly, altosomes revert to being a pair of normal nucleosomes with a half time of ~1 hr under conditions that approximate mammalian nuclear salt concentrations.[81] Thus, if (for instance) altosome formation activated transcription, this reversion would provide an automatic shut off switch (a time-dependent epigenetic mechanism for transcriptional attenuation).

4.3.3   General roles in nucleosome deposition

Several remodeling complexes, especially those of the ISWI subfamily, have been shown to assist histone chaperones in the formation of nucleosomes in vitro.[82–84] Proper assembly of nucleosomes is likely to be an important aspect of their function in vivo, as suggested by the observation that ISWI mutant *Drosophila* embryos have pronounced defects in chromosome condensation.[78,85] As noted above, some remodeling complexes have the ability to enforce an even spacing between nucleosomes, and this activity could potentially override some nucleosome position preferences encoded in the DNA itself as NPSes.

4.3.4   Targeted histone removal and redeposition

While traditional models of interphase chromatin have argued against histone and nucleosome removal as regulatory mechanisms, recent studies have shown that histone octamers can be entirely removed from the yeast *PHO5* promoter, in trans, during transcriptional activation.[19,86,87] In mammalian cells, recent reports also indicate that promoter histones are lost from the *IL-2* gene during T-cell activation,[21] and that the histones from two repressive promoter nucleosomes on *cyclin A* are lost upon transcriptional activation[20] (although it is unclear whether these effects represent histone removal in trans or simply sliding of octamers in cis). Note that these effects are also reversible, with nucleosomes over PHO5 and *cyclin A* rapidly reestablished during transcriptional repression of these genes.

The emerging picture is that locus-specific histone removal and redeposition events are controlled, at least in part, by a combination of ATP-dependent remodeling complexes and specific histone chaperones. For instance, nucleosome depletion from the active *PHO5* and *SUC2* promoters, as well as nucleosome restoration during *PHO5* repression was slower in yeast cells lacking functional SWI/SNF[86,88–91], and the two repressive *cyclin A* promoter nucleosomes were found to be absent in mammalian cells lacking the hBRM hSWI/SNF ATPase.[20] At *PHO5*, nucleosome removal was also partially dependent on the specific histone chaperone Asf1.[92,93] Furthermore, biochemical evidence has shown that certain ATP-dependent chromatin remodeling complexes can mediate the loss of H2A/H2B dimers from nucleosomes (leaving an H3/H4 tetramer associated with DNA) as well as the complete removal of nucleosomal histones from DNA. Early studies showed that H2A/H2B dimers or complete histone octamers could be transferred in trans to acceptor DNA or chromatin, although these effects were weak relative to other remodeling activities.[94–96] However, a combination of the specific histone chaperone protein NAP1 (whose normal function is the deposition of H3/H4 tetramers) and the yeast SWI/SNF-family complex, RSC, could efficiently remove all histones from a mononucleosome template.[97] Other studies indicate that histone removal by remodeling complexes might be promoted by specific DNA sequences[98] or by transcriptional activation domains.[99]

4.3.5   Histone replacement

Lastly, certain chromatin remodeling complexes can promote the targeted replacement of one core histone for a variant core histone. Htz1, the yeast H2AZ variant, copurifies with the SWR1 complex, and chromatin binding of Htz1 in vivo requires functional Swr1. This suggested that Swr1 may act as a histone exchanger in vivo, replacing canonical H2A with Htz1. In vitro studies using nucleosomal arrays confirmed the ability of SWR1 to replace H2A with Htz1.[100–102] By contrast, the SWI/SNF, RSC and INO80 complexes showed extremely weak histone exchange activity, if at all.[100]

Each of these three chromatin remodeling functions, histone deposition, histone removal and histone replacement, would be expected to have long-lasting epigenetic effects. Of course, as for changes in nucleosome positions, DNA replication followed by new histone deposition would be expected to decrease the fractional occupancy of variant histones and to restore the default nucleosome density. Thus, these remodeling complex-driven changes would be expected to function as epigenetic marks only during interphase and/or in nondividing G0 cells. Alternatively, the remodeling complex (as well as required chaperones and other factors) would have to remain present throughout the S phase, so as to reestablish the remodeled structure after replication.

4.3.6   Cooperation between chromatin remodeling complexes and other chromatin effects

The existing evidence indicates that, in most cases, ATP-dependent chromatin remodeling factors work together with histone tail modifying complexes to create active versus inactive chromatin configurations. Some well-studied examples of genes in which phased recruitment of remodeling and modifying complexes control transcriptional activation are the yeast HO promoter[103] and the human interferon β and PS2 promoters.[104–106] The emerging picture from these systems, as well as from dozens of other chromatin immunoprecipitation and genetic studies, is that a large fraction of genes is regulated by both types of chromatin modifications. There are several possible ways that these complexes might work together. First, ATP-dependent remodeling complexes might help make the histone tails more accessible to factors that make covalent modifications. For instance, the NuRD complex contains both a remodeling ATPase subunit and HDAC subunits, and ATP can stimulate HDAC activity.[107] Second, histone modifications can help remodeling complexes function. For instance, acetylated histone tails bind to bromo-domains in the yeast SWI/SNF complex, which can stabilize the complex's association with chromatin, allowing it to resist competition to other chromatin.[76] Third, histone modifications or ATP-dependent remodeling might both act to alter chromatin folding, which could increase or decrease the accessibility of the locus to all other factors. Remodeling and modifying complexes must also cooperate with other structural or noncatalytic chromatin components, such as HP1 or the Polycomb complexes, in order to establish active and inactive chromatin states. Finally, remodelers and histone modifying enzymes can alter and be regulated by the presence of different core histone variants. For instance, Swr1 can replace H2A with H2AZ,[100] and chromatin containing the H2A variant, macroH2A (which is abundant on the inactive X chromosome), is completely refractory to remodeling by SWI/SNF.[108]

4.3.7   Remodeling complexes in epigenetic regulation?

As mentioned above, changes in histone composition, nucleosome abundance and/or nucleosome positions are all expected to be erased or diluted during DNA replication. Thus, the epigenetic effects of ATP-dependent remodeling complexes are expected to be most relevant for the control of transcription in interphase or in differentiated nondividing cells. However, there is one example of a chromatin remodeling complex that is known to function in long-term epigenetic regulation that can survive many somatic cell divisions: the fly SWI/SNF complex is an important member of the Trithorax group genes that is required to prevent silencing of active Homeobox cluster genes by Polycomb. How this works is largely unknown. SWI/SNF could, for instance, aid the Trithorax/MLL HMTase in methylation of H3K4, or it could act to dislodge or disrupt Polycomb complexes from chromatin. Intriguingly, in vitro studies have shown that the PRC1 Polycomb complex can prevent human SWI/SNF from remodeling chromatin, but only if it is preincubated with chromatin before SWI/SNF is added.[109]

4.4   Conclusions

In summary, chromatin is much more than a neutral system for packaging and condensing genomic DNA. It is a critical player in controlling the accessibility of DNA for transcription and other reactions. Modifications to chromatin can give rise to a variety of epigenetic effects. Some effects are relatively local, such as the loss of one or two promoter nucleosomes, while others can be far-reaching, such as the spread of histone acetylation when a HAT is recruited to a promoter or the variable spreading of

HP1-mediated heterochromatin. Some effects, such as histone tail acetylation, are very short lived and must be continually reinforced, while others, such as histone lysine methylation can last for many hours and can contribute to long-term epigenetic effects (such as X-inactivation and Polycomb heterochromatin) that persist through all the cell divisions in an organism's lifetime.

4.4.1   Maintenance of chromatin modifications

It is clear that at least some kinds of chromatin structures and histone tail modifications can be maintained through DNA replication and cell division. In a few cases these mechanisms are reasonably well defined, for example, double-stranded RNA expressed from pericentric heterochromatin repeats continuously reinforces HP1-mediated heterochromatin. However, in most cases we do not know precisely how these chromatin patterns are maintained, nor how faithfully they are maintained. Many of these chromatin patterns may be maintained at a level that is only one step removed from the direct DNA sequence. For instance, maintenance of a specific pattern of nucleosome positions after DNA replication may require a sequence-specific transcription factor to recruit a remodeling complex to push nucleosomes out of the default positions favored by nucleosome assembly factors. Other chromatin patterns may be maintained without needing to be reinforced by sequence-specific factors. For instance, acetylated histone tails could recruit bromodomain containing HATs to promote acetylation of newly deposited histones, and H3K9 HMTs have been seen to be recruited to DNA replication forks.

4.4.2   Cooperation between CpG methylation
and chromatin changes

Even though mechanisms to maintain chromatin-based epigenetic marks exist, or are suspected to exist, in no case are these mechanisms as simple and precise as the ability of maintenance DNA methyltransferases to preserve the pattern of CpG methylation. Furthermore, while there is some evidence in flies that HP1- and Polycomb-mediated heterochromatin can have effects across generations,[110,111] CpG methylation is the only epigenetic mark that can be clearly linked to heritable epigenetic effects, such as genomic imprinting in mammals. Does this mean that chromatin modifications are ineffectual relative to CpG methylation? Not at all. In fact, CpG methylation is expected to be effective, in large part, only because it promotes changes in chromatin.

A small percentage of regulatory factors whose binding sites contain CGs can distinguish between the methylated and unmethylated states (notably the activator SP1[112] and the insulator protein CTCF[113]). Thus, for the fraction of genes that are regulated by these factors, CpG methylation might directly contribute to transcriptional regulation. In most cases, however, methyl CpG works by binding a class of methyl-CpG binding proteins, which function to recruit chromatin modifying enzymes (for reviews see References 114 and 115). For instance, the prototypical Me-CpG binding protein, MeCP2, binds to Sin3 which binds to HDAC1 and HDAC2, resulting in deacetylation of local chromatin. MeCP2 can also recruit the SWI/SNF chromatin remodeling complex. Another Me-CpG binding protein, MBD1 recruits the SETDB1 HMTase which lays down the repressive H3K9 methylation mark. Lastly, the MBD3 protein recruits the NuRD complex which has both ATP-dependent remodeling and histone deacetylation functions. Thus, while CpG methylation may be an initial, stably maintained epigenetic mark, it usually relies on additional chromatin-mediated epigenetic marks for its function. Conversely, chromatin-based epigenetic marks can also regulate CpG methylation. For instance, H3K9 methylation in *Arabidopsis* and *Tetrahymena* is essential for CpG methylation. Proper CpG methylation in *Arabidopsis* also requires an ATP-dependent chromatin remodeling factor called DDM1. Thus, CpG methylation, histone modifying enzymes, ATP-dependent chromatin remodeling complexes and other chromatin proteins all appear to contribute to an integrated web of epigenetic control mechanisms.

References

1. Beato, M., and Eisfeld, K. (1997). Transcription factor access to chromatin. *Nucleic Acids Res* 25, 3559–3563.
2. Kwon, J., Imbalzano, A. N., Matthews, A., and Oettinger, M. A. (1998). Accessibility of nucleosomal DNA to V(D)J cleavage is modulated by RSS positioning and HMG1. *Mol Cell* 2, 829–839.
3. Blank, T. A., and Becker, P. B. (1995). Electrostatic mechanism of nucleosome spacing. *J Mol Biol* 252, 305–313.
4. Luger, K., Mader, A. W., Richmond, R. K., Sargent, D. F., and Richmond, T. J. (1997). Crystal structure of the nucleosome core particle at 2.8 A resolution. *Nature* 389, 251–260.
5. Segal, E., Fondufe-Mittendorf, Y., Chen, L., Thastrom, A., Field, Y., Moore, I. K., Wang, J. P., and Widom, J. (2006). A genomic code for nucleosome positioning. *Nature* 442, 772–778.
6. Ioshikhes, I. P., Albert, I., Zanton, S. J., and Pugh, B. F. (2006). Nucleosome positions predicted through comparative genomics. *Nat Genet* 38, 1210–1215.
7. Yuan, G. C., Liu, Y. J., Dion, M. F., Slack, M. D., Wu, L. F., Altschuler, S. J., and Rando, O. J. (2005). Genome-scale identification of nucleosome positions in S. cerevisiae. *Science* 309, 626–630.
8. Ozsolak, F., Song, J. S., Liu, X. S., and Fisher, D. E. (2007). High-throughput mapping of the chromatin structure of human promoters. *Nat Biotechnol* 25, 244–248.

9. Adams, C. C., and Workman, J. L. (1995). Binding of disparate transcriptional activators to nucleosomal DNA is inherently cooperative. *Mol Cell Biol* 15, 1405–1421.
10. Polach, K. J., and Widom, J. (1996). A model for the cooperative binding of eukaryotic regulatory proteins to nucleosomal target sites. *J Mol Biol* 258, 800–812.
11. Wolffe, A. P. (2001). Transcriptional regulation in the context of chromatin structure. *Essays Biochem* 37, 45–57.
12. Tremethick, D. J. (2007). Higher-order structures of chromatin: The elusive 30 nm fiber. *Cell* 128, 651–654.
13. Tumbar, T., Sudlow, G., and Belmont, A. S. (1999). Large-scale chromatin unfolding and remodeling induced by VP16 acidic activation domain. *J Cell Biol* 145, 1341–1354.
14. Nye, A. C., Rajendran, R. R., Stenoien, D. L., Mancini, M. A., Katzenellenbogen, B. S., and Belmont, A. S. (2002). Alteration of large-scale chromatin structure by estrogen receptor. *Mol Cell Biol* 22, 3437–3449.
15. Henikoff, S. (2004). Visualizing gene expression: An unfolding story. *Cell* 116, 633–634.
16. Pusarla, R. H., and Bhargava, P. (2005). Histones in functional diversification. Core histone variants. *FEBS J* 272, 5149–5168.
17. Tabancay, A. P., Jr., and Forsburg, S. L. (2006). Eukaryotic DNA replication in a chromatin context. *Curr Top Dev Biol* 76, 129–184.
18. Korber, P., Luckenbach, T., Blaschke, D., and Horz, W. (2004). Evidence for histone eviction in trans upon induction of the yeast PHO5 promoter. *Mol Cell Biol* 24, 10965–10974.
19. Boeger, H., Griesenbeck, J., Strattan, J. S., and Kornberg, R. D. (2004). Removal of promoter nucleosomes by disassembly rather than sliding in vivo. *Mol Cell* 14, 667–673.
20. Coisy, M., Roure, V., Ribot, M., Philips, A., Muchardt, C., Blanchard, J. M., and Dantonel, J. C. (2004). Cyclin A repression in quiescent cells is associated with chromatin remodeling of its promoter and requires Brahma/SNF2alpha. *Mol Cell* 15, 43–56.
21. Chen, X., Wang, J., Woltring, D., Gerondakis, S., and Shannon, M. F. (2005). Histone dynamics on the interleukin-2 gene in response to T-cell activation. *Mol Cell Biol* 25, 3209–3219.
22. Lee, C. K., Shibata, Y., Rao, B., Strahl, B. D., and Lieb, J. D. (2004). Evidence for nucleosome depletion at active regulatory regions genome-wide. *Nat Genet* 36, 900–905.
23. Ercan, S., Carrozza, M. J., and Workman, J. L. (2004). Global nucleosome distribution and the regulation of transcription in yeast. *Genome Biol* 5, 243.
24. Kimura, H. (2005). Histone dynamics in living cells revealed by photobleaching. *DNA Repair (Amst)* 4, 939–950.
25. Reinberg, D., and Sims, R. J. III. (2006). De facto nucleosome dynamics. *J Biol Chem* 9, 9.
26. Ekwall, K. (2004). The RITS complex: A direct link between small RNA and heterochromatin. *Mol Cell* 13, 304–305.
27. Buhler, M., Verdel, A., and Moazed, D. (2006). Tethering RITS to a nascent transcript initiates RNAi- and heterochromatin-dependent gene silencing. *Cell* 125, 873–886.

28. Hernandez-Munoz, I., Lund, A. H., van der Stoop, P., Boutsma, E., Muijrers, I., Verhoeven, E., Nusinow, D. A., Panning, B., Marahrens, Y., and van Lohuizen, M. (2005). Stable X chromosome inactivation involves the PRC1 Polycomb complex and requires histone MACROH2A1 and the CULLIN3/SPOP ubiquitin E3 ligase. *Proc Natl Acad Sci USA* 102, 7635–7640.

29. Kalantry, S., Mills, K. C., Yee, D., Otte, A. P., Panning, B., and Magnuson, T. (2006). The Polycomb group protein EED protects the inactive X-chromosome from differentiation-induced reactivation. *Nat Cell Biol* 8, 195–202.

30. Kalantry, S., and Magnuson, T. (2006). The Polycomb group protein EED is dispensable for the initiation of random X-chromosome inactivation. *PLoS Genet* 2, e66.

31. Jorgensen, H. F., Giadrossi, S., Casanova, M., Endoh, M., Koseki, H., Brockdorff, N., and Fisher, A. G. (2006). Stem cells primed for action: Polycomb repressive complexes restrain the expression of lineage-specific regulators in embryonic stem cells. *Cell Cycle* 5, 1411–1414.

32. Pasini, D., Bracken, A. P., Hansen, J. B., Capillo, M., and Helin, K. (2007). The Polycomb group protein Suz12 is required for embryonic stem cell differentiation. *Mol Cell Biol* 27, 3769–3779.

33. Muller, J., and Kassis, J. A. (2006). Polycomb response elements and targeting of Polycomb group proteins in Drosophila. *Curr Opin Genet Dev* 16, 476–484.

34. Schuettengruber, B., Chourrout, D., Vervoort, M., Leblanc, B., and Cavalli, G. (2007). Genome regulation by polycomb and trithorax proteins. *Cell* 128, 735–745.

35. Chang, S. C., Tucker, T., Thorogood, N. P., and Brown, C. J. (2006). Mechanisms of X-chromosome inactivation. *Front Biosci* 11, 852–866.

36. Nightingale, K. P., O'Neill, L. P., and Turner, B. M. (2006). Histone modifications: Signalling receptors and potential elements of a heritable epigenetic code. *Curr Opin Genet Dev* 16, 125–136.

37. Strahl, B. D., and Allis, C. D. (2000). The language of covalent histone modifications. *Nature* 403, 41–45.

38. Kimura, A., Matsubara, K., and Horikoshi, M. (2005). A decade of histone acetylation: marking eukaryotic chromosomes with specific codes. *J Biochem (Tokyo)* 138, 647–662 .

39. Hebbes, T. R., Thorne, A. W., and Crane-Robinson, C. (1988). A direct link between core histone acetylation and transcriptionally active chromatin. *EMBO J* 7, 1395–1402.

40. Hebbes, T. R., Clayton, A. L., Thorne, A. W., and Crane-Robinson, C. (1994). Core histone hyperacetylation co-maps with generalized DNase I sensitivity in the chicken beta-globin chromosomal domain. *EMBO J* 13, 1823–1830.

41. Brownell, J. E., Zhou, J., Ranalli, T., Kobayashi, R., Edmondson, D. G., Roth, S. Y., and Allis, C. D. (1996). Tetrahymena histone acetyltransferase A: A homolog to yeast Gcn5p linking histone acetylation to gene activation. *Cell* 84, 843–851.

42. Lee, K. K., and Workman, J. L. (2007). Histone acetyltransferase complexes: One size doesn't fit all. *Nat Rev Mol Cell Biol* 8, 284–295.

43. Glozak, M. A., Sengupta, N., Zhang, X., and Seto, E. (2005). Acetylation and deacetylation of non-histone proteins. *Gene* 363, 15–23.

44. Ikeda, K., Steger, D. J., Eberharter, A., and Workman, J. L. (1999). Activation domain-specific and general transcription stimulation by native histone acetyltransferase complexes. *Mol Cell Biol* 19, 855–863.

45. Hildmann, C., Riester, D., and Schwienhorst, A. (2007). Histone deacetylases: An important class of cellular regulators with a variety of functions. *Appl Microbiol Biotechnol* 75, 487–497.

46. Grubisha, O., Smith, B. C., and Denu, J. M. (2005). Small molecule regulation of Sir2 protein deacetylases. *FEBS J* 272, 4607–4616.

47. Trapp, J., and Jung, M. (2006). The role of NAD+ dependent histone deacetylases (sirtuins) in ageing. *Curr Drug Targets* 7, 1553–1560.

48. Waterborg, J. H. (2002). Dynamics of histone acetylation in vivo. A function for acetylation turnover? *Biochem Cell Biol* 80, 363–378.

49. Katan-Khaykovich, Y., and Struhl, K. (2002). Dynamics of global histone acetylation and deacetylation in vivo: Rapid restoration of normal histone acetylation status upon removal of activators and repressors. *Genes Dev* 16, 743–752.

50. Vignali, M., Steger, D. J., Neely, K. E., and Workman, J. L. (2000). Distribution of acetylated histones resulting from Gal4-VP16 recruitment of SAGA and NuA4 complexes. *EMBO J* 19, 2629–2640.

51. Calestagne-Morelli, A., and Ausio, J. (2006). Long-range histone acetylation: Biological significance, structural implications, and mechanisms. *Biochem Cell Biol* 84, 518–527.

52. Shogren-Knaak, M., Ishii, H., Sun, J. M., Pazin, M. J., Davie, J. R., and Peterson, C. L. (2006). Histone H4-K16 acetylation controls chromatin structure and protein interactions. *Science* 311, 844–847.

53. Trievel, R. C. (2004). Structure and function of histone methyltransferases. *Crit Rev Eukaryot Gene Expr* 14, 147–169.

54. Shi, Y., Lan, F., Matson, C., Mulligan, P., Whetstine, J. R., Cole, P. A., and Casero, R. A. (2004). Histone demethylation mediated by the nuclear amine oxidase homolog LSD1. *Cell* 119, 941–953.

55. Wang, Y., Wysocka, J., Sayegh, J., Lee, Y. H., Perlin, J. R., Leonelli, L., Sonbuchner, L. S., McDonald, C. H., Cook, R. G., Dou, Y., Roeder, R. G., Clarke, S., Stallcup, M. R., Allis, C. D., and Coonrod, S. A. (2004). Human PAD4 regulates histone arginine methylation levels via demethylimination. *Science* 306, 279–283.

56. Shi, Y., and Whetstine, J. R. (2007). Dynamic regulation of histone lysine methylation by demethylases. *Mol Cell* 25, 1–14.

57. Lee, M. G., Wynder, C., Cooch, N., and Shiekhattar, R. (2005). An essential role for CoREST in nucleosomal histone 3 lysine 4 demethylation. *Nature* 437, 432–435.

58. Metzger, E., Wissmann, M., Yin, N., Muller, J. M., Schneider, R., Peters, A. H., Gunther, T., Buettner, R., and Schule, R. (2005). LSD1 demethylates repressive histone marks to promote androgen-receptor-dependent transcription. *Nature* 437, 436–439.

59. Mellor, J. (2006). It takes a PHD to read the histone code. *Cell* 126, 22–24.

60. Torok, M. S., and Grant, P. A. (2006). The generation and recognition of histone methylation. *Results Probl Cell Differ* 41, 25–46.

61. Wysocka, J., Swigut, T., Xiao, H., Milne, T. A., Kwon, S. Y., Landry, J., Kauer, M., Tackett, A. J., Chait, B. T., Badenhorst, P., Wu, C., and Allis, C. D. (2006). A PHD finger of NURF couples histone H3 lysine 4 trimethylation with chromatin remodelling. *Nature* 21, 21.

62. Grewal, S. I., and Jia, S. (2007). Heterochromatin revisited. *Nat Rev Genet* 8, 35–46.

63. Esteve, P. O., Chin, H. G., Smallwood, A., Feehery, G. R., Gangisetty, O., Karpf, A. R., Carey, M. F., and Pradhan, S. (2006). Direct interaction between DNMT1 and G9a coordinates DNA and histone methylation during replication. *Genes Dev* 20, 3089–3103.

64. Sarraf, S. A., and Stancheva, I. (2004). Methyl-CpG binding protein MBD1 couples histone H3 methylation at lysine 9 by SETDB1 to DNA replication and chromatin assembly. *Mol Cell* 15, 595–605.

65. Klose, R. J., and Zhang, Y. (2007). Regulation of histone methylation by demethylimination and demethylation. *Nat Rev Mol Cell Biol* 8, 307–318.

66. Wysocka, J., Allis, C. D., and Coonrod, S. (2006). Histone arginine methylation and its dynamic regulation. *Front Biosci.* 11, 344–355.

67. Ruthenburg, A. J., Allis, C. D., and Wysocka, J. (2007). Methylation of lysine 4 on histone H3: Intricacy of writing and reading a single epigenetic mark. *Mol Cell* 25, 15–30.

68. Osley, M. A., Fleming, A. B., and Kao, C. F. (2006). Histone ubiquitylation and the regulation of transcription. *Results Probl Cell Differ* 41, 47–75.

69. Cao, R., Tsukada, Y. I., and Zhang, Y. (2005). Role of Bmi-1 and Ring1A in H2A ubiquitylation and Hox gene silencing. *Mol Cell* 20, 845–854.

70. Wang, H., Wang, L., Erdjument-Bromage, H., Vidal, M., Tempst, P., Jones, R. S., and Zhang, Y. (2004). Role of histone H2A ubiquitination in Polycomb silencing. *Nature* 431, 873–878.

71. Fang, J., Chen, T., Chadwick, B., Li, E., and Zhang, Y. (2004). Ring1b-mediated H2A ubiquitination associates with inactive X chromosomes and is involved in initiation of X-inactivation. *J Biol Chem* 26, 26.

72. Johansen, K. M., and Johansen, J. (2006). Regulation of chromatin structure by histone H3S10 phosphorylation. *Chromosome Res* 14, 393–404.

73. Foster, E. R., and Downs, J. A. (2005). Histone H2A phosphorylation in DNA double-strand break repair. *FEBS J* 272, 3231–3240.

74. Petermann, E., Keil, C., and Oei, S. L. (2005). Importance of poly(ADP-ribose) polymerases in the regulation of DNA-dependent processes. *Cell Mol Life Sci* 62, 731–738.

75. Nusinow, D. A., Hernandez-Munoz, I., Fazzio, T. G., Shah, G. M., Kraus, W. L., and Panning, B. (2007). Poly (ADP-ribose) polymerase 1 is inhibited by a histone H2A variant, MACROH2A, and contributes to silencing of the inactive X chromosome. *J Biol Chem* 282, 12851–12859.

76. Hassan, A. H., Prochasson, P., Neely, K. E., Galasinski, S. C., Chandy, M., Carrozza, M. J., and Workman, J. L. (2002). Function and selectivity of bromodomains in anchoring chromatin-modifying complexes to promoter nucleosomes. *Cell* 111, 369–379.

77. Ramachandran, A., and Schnitzler, G. (2004). Regulating transcription one nucleosome at a time: Nature and function of chromatin remodeling complex products. *Recent Res Devel Mol Cell Biol* 5, 149–170.

78. Deuring, R., Fanti, L., Armstrong, J. A., Sarte, M., Papoulas, O., Prestel, M., Daubresse, G., Verardo, M., Moseley, S. L., Berloco, M., Tsukiyama, T., Wu, C., Pimpinelli, S., and Tamkun, J. W. (2000). The ISWI chromatin-remodeling protein is required for gene expression and the maintenance of higher order chromatin structure in vivo. *Mol Cell* 5, 355–365.

79. Fyodorov, D. V., Blower, M. D., Karpen, G. H., and Kadonaga, J. T. (2004). Acf1 confers unique activities to ACF/CHRAC and promotes the formation rather than disruption of chromatin in vivo. *Genes Dev* 18, 170–183.

80. Sims, H. I., Lane, J. M., Ulyanova, N. P., and Schnitzler, G. R. (2007). Human SWI/SNF drives sequence-directed repositioning of nucleosomes on C-myc promoter DNA minicircles. *Biochemistry* 46, 11377–11388.

81. Ulyanova, N. P., and Schnitzler, G. R. (2005). Human SWI/SNF generates abundant, structurally altered dinucleosomes on polynucleosomal templates. *Mol Cell Biol* 25, 11156–11170.

82. Corona, D. F., Langst, G., Clapier, C. R., Bonte, E. J., Ferrari, S., Tamkun, J. W., and Becker, P. B. (1999). ISWI is an ATP-dependent nucleosome remodeling factor. *Mol Cell* 3, 239–245.

83. Fyodorov, D. V., and Kadonaga, J. T. (2002). Dynamics of ATP-dependent chromatin assembly by ACF. *Nature* 418, 897–900.

84. Ito, T., Levenstein, M. E., Fyodorov, D. V., Kutach, A. K., Kobayashi, R., and Kadonaga, J. T. (1999). ACF consists of two subunits, Acf1 and ISWI, that function cooperatively in the ATP-dependent catalysis of chromatin assembly. *Genes Dev* 13, 1529–1539.

85. Corona, D. F., and Tamkun, J. W. (2004). Multiple roles for ISWI in transcription, chromosome organization and DNA replication. *Biochim Biophys Acta* 1677, 113–119.

86. Reinke, H., and Horz, W. (2003). Histones are first hyperacetylated and then lose contact with the activated PHO5 promoter. *Mol Cell* 11, 1599–1607.

87. Boeger, H., Griesenbeck, J., Strattan, J. S., and Kornberg, R. D. (2003). Nucleosomes unfold completely at a transcriptionally active promoter. *Mol Cell* 11, 1587–1598.

88. Schermer, U. J., Korber, P., and Horz, W. (2005). Histones are incorporated in trans during reassembly of the yeast PHO5 promoter. *Mol Cell* 19, 279–285.

89. Adkins, M. W., Williams, S. K., Linger, J., and Tyler, J. K. (2007). Chromatin disassembly from the PHO5 promoter is essential for the recruitment of the general transcription machinery and coactivators. *Mol Cell Biol* 27, 6372–6382.

90. Barbaric, S., Luckenbach, T., Schmid, A., Blaschke, D., Horz, W., and Korber, P. (2007). Redundancy of chromatin remodeling pathways for the induction of the yeast PHO5 promoter in vivo. *J Biol Chem* 282, 27610–27621.

91. Schwabish, M. A., and Struhl, K. (2007). The Swi/Snf complex is important for histone eviction during transcriptional activation and RNA polymerase II elongation in vivo. *Mol Cell Biol* 27, 6987–6995.

92. Korber, P., Barbaric, S., Luckenbach, T., Schmid, A., Schermer, U. J., Blaschke, D., and Horz, W. (2006). The histone chaperone Asf1 increases the rate of histone eviction at the yeast PHO5 and PHO8 promoters. *J Biol Chem* 281, 5539–5545.

93. Adkins, M. W., Howar, S. R., and Tyler, J. K. (2004). Chromatin disassembly mediated by the histone chaperone Asf1 is essential for transcriptional activation of the yeast PHO5 and PHO8 genes. *Mol Cell* 14, 657–666.

94. Phelan, M. L., Schnitzler, G. R., and Kingston, R. E. (2000). Octamer transfer and creation of stably remodeled nucleosomes by human SWI-SNF and its isolated ATPases. *Mol Cell Biol* 20, 6380–6389.

95. Bruno, M., Flaus, A., Stockdale, C., Rencurel, C., Ferreira, H., and Owen-Hughes, T. (2003). Histone H2A/H2B dimer exchange by ATP-dependent chromatin remodeling activities. *Mol Cell* 12, 1599–1606.

96. Lorch, Y., Zhang, M., and Kornberg, R. D. (1999). Histone octamer transfer by a chromatin-remodeling complex. *Cell* 96, 389–392.

 97. Lorch, Y., Maier-Davis, B., and Kornberg, R. D. (2006). Chromatin remodeling by nucleosome disassembly in vitro. *Proc Natl Acad Sci USA* 103, 3090–3093.
 98. Vicent, G. P., Nacht, A. S., Smith, C. L., Peterson, C. L., Dimitrov, S., and Beato, M. (2004). DNA instructed displacement of histones H2A and H2B at an inducible promoter. *Mol Cell* 16, 439–452.
 99. Gutierrez, J. L., Chandy, M., Carrozza, M. J., and Workman, J. L. (2007). Activation domains drive nucleosome eviction by SWI/SNF. *EMBO J* 26, 730–740.
100. Mizuguchi, G., Shen, X., Landry, J., Wu, W. H., Sen, S., and Wu, C. (2004). ATP-driven exchange of histone H2AZ variant catalyzed by SWR1 chromatin remodeling complex. *Science* 303, 343–348.
101. Krogan, N. J., Keogh, M. C., Datta, N., Sawa, C., Ryan, O. W., Ding, H., Haw, R. A., Pootoolal, J., Tong, A., Canadien, V., Richards, D. P., Wu, X., Emili, A., Hughes, T. R., Buratowski, S., and Greenblatt, J. F. (2003). A Snf2 family ATPase complex required for recruitment of the histone H2A variant Htz1. *Mol Cell* 12, 1565–1576.
102. Kobor, M. S., Venkatasubrahmanyam, S., Meneghini, M. D., Gin, J. W., Jennings, J. L., Link, A. J., Madhani, H. D., and Rine, J. (2004). A protein complex containing the conserved Swi2/Snf2-related ATPase Swr1p deposits histone variant H2A.Z into euchromatin. *PLoS Biol* 2, E131.
103. Cosma, M. P., Tanaka, T., and Nasmyth, K. (1999). Ordered recruitment of transcription and chromatin remodeling factors to a cell cycle- and developmentally regulated promoter. *Cell* 97, 299–311.
104. Agalioti, T., Lomvardas, S., Parekh, B., Yie, J., Maniatis, T., and Thanos, D. (2000). Ordered recruitment of chromatin modifying and general transcription factors to the IFN-beta promoter. *Cell* 103, 667–678.
105. Metivier, R., Penot, G., Hubner, M. R., Reid, G., Brand, H., Kos, M., and Gannon, F. (2003). Estrogen receptor-alpha directs ordered, cyclical, and combinatorial recruitment of cofactors on a natural target promoter. *Cell* 115, 751–763.
106. Reid, G., Hubner, M. R., Metivier, R., Brand, H., Denger, S., Manu, D., Beaudouin, J., Ellenberg, J., and Gannon, F. (2003). Cyclic, proteasome-mediated turnover of unliganded and liganded ERalpha on responsive promoters is an integral feature of estrogen signaling. *Mol Cell* 11, 695–707.
107. Tong, J. K., Hassig, C. A., Schnitzler, G. R., Kingston, R. E., and Schreiber, S. L. (1998). Chromatin deacetylation by an ATP-dependent nucleosome remodeling complex. *Nature* 395, 917–921.
108. Angelov, D., Molla, A., Perche, P. Y., Hans, F., Cote, J., Khochbin, S., Bouvet, P., and Dimitrov, S. (2003). The histone variant macroH2A interferes with transcription factor binding and SWI/SNF nucleosome remodeling. *Mol Cell* 11, 1033–1041.
109. Shao, Z., Raible, F., Mollaaghababa, R., Guyon, J. R., Wu, C. T., Bender, W., and Kingston, R. E. (1999). Stabilization of chromatin structure by PRC1, a Polycomb complex. *Cell* 98, 37–46.
110. Bantignies, F., Grimaud, C., Lavrov, S., Gabut, M., and Cavalli, G. (2003). Inheritance of Polycomb-dependent chromosomal interactions in Drosophila. *Genes Dev* 17, 2406–2420.
111. Joanis, V., and Lloyd, V. K. (2002). Genomic imprinting in Drosophila is maintained by the products of suppressor of variegation and trithorax group, but not Polycomb group, genes. *Mol Genet Genomics* 268, 103–112.

112. Zhu, W. G., Srinivasan, K., Dai, Z., Duan, W., Druhan, L. J., Ding, H., Yee, L., Villalona-Calero, M. A., Plass, C., and Otterson, G. A. (2003). Methylation of adjacent CpG sites affects Sp1/Sp3 binding and activity in the p21(Cip1) promoter. *Mol Cell Biol* 23, 4056–4065.
113. Hark, A. T., Schoenherr, C. J., Katz, D. J., Ingram, R. S., Levorse, J. M., and Tilghman, S. M. (2000). CTCF mediates methylation-sensitive enhancer-blocking activity at the H19/Igf2 locus. *Nature* 405, 486–489.
114. Klose, R. J., and Bird, A. P. (2006). Genomic DNA methylation: The mark and its mediators. *Trends Biochem Sci* 31, 89–97.
115. Fuks, F. (2005). DNA methylation and histone modifications: Teaming up to silence genes. *Curr Opin Genet Dev* 15, 490–495.

chapter five

Nutrients and DNA methylation

Sang-Woon Choi, Roberto Corrocher, and Simonetta Friso

Contents

5.1 Introduction

In order to maintain normal function and homeostasis, appropriate gene expression is critical in individual cells. Aberrant gene expression can induce disordered conditions. Regulation of gene expression is not fully known yet but current evidence indicates that epigenetics, a phenomenon that affects gene expression without changes in DNA base pairs,[1] is an important mechanism in gene expression control. A body of evidence has accumulated in recent years pointing out that DNA methylation, a major epigenetic phenomenon, is critical for embryonic development, aging and the process of certain diseases such as cancer.

Epidemiologic and animal studies have demonstrated increased carcinogenesis associated with diets containing low methyl donor nutrients such as methionine, choline and folate,[2,3] evoking the idea that altered methylation of DNA due to diminished methyl availability in one-carbon metabolism is a plausible candidate mechanism through which diet facilitates carcinogenesis. Moreover, in an animal model, diets containing different levels of methyl donors[4] or bioactive food compounds[5] altered the expression of a specific gene for embryonic development by modifying DNA methylation. More studies regarding the relationship between nutrients and DNA methylation will shed light on the nature of gene regulation as well as nutritional chemoprevention.

In contrast to mutation, which implies irreversibly altered base sequence, DNA methylation is reversible and can be modified by nutrients. This characteristic initiated the research for nutritional prevention of diseases by modulating DNA methylation. In this chapter we briefly describe the role of DNA methylation in embryonic development, aging and carcinogenesis, and thereafter address specific roles of nutrients on DNA methylation as well as associated physiologic and pathologic processes.

5.1.1   DNA methylation

Methylation of cytosine is a unique endogenous modification of DNA in mammalian cells. DNA methyltransferases catalyze the transfer of methyl group from *S*-adenosylmethionine (AdoMet) to the carbon-5′ position of cytosine in CpG dinucleotides.[6] Except for a few rare cases (e.g., non-CpG methylation), 5′-methylcytosine in mammalian DNA is present in 5′-CpG-3′ dinucleotides. DNA methylation has a number of functions. Methylation within gene regulatory elements such as promoters, enhancers, insulators and repressors generally suppresses the function of the gene. Methylation within gene-deficient regions, such as in pericentromeric heterochromatin, is critical for maintaining the structure and integrity of the chromosome.[7,8] Methylation has also been proposed as a genome defense mechanism against parasitic sequences in DNA.[9]

Among the many functions of DNA methylation, evidence for an active role of promoter methylation in gene silencing is the most convincing. In vitro methylation of promoter-reporter constructs inhibits their subsequent expression in transfected cells.[10] Demethylation by

5-azadeoxycytidine, a methyltransferase inhibitor, leads to reexpression of previously methylated genes.[11] Homozygous embryos with a germline deletion of the DNA methyltransferase 1 (*Dnmt1*) gene that encodes a maintenance DNA methyltransferase, express normally silenced genes, including several imprinted genes, and repressed endogenous retroviral sequences, which are methylated and silent in heterozygous littermates.[12] DNA binding proteins that selectively bind to methylated CpG residues seems to be involved in CpG island-associated gene silencing by the recruitment of silencing complexes including histone deacetylases.[13,14]

5.1.2   DNA methylation for embryonic development and aging

DNA methylation is a vital mechanism for normal embryonic development. Methylation of the mammalian genome undergoes notable changes during early development and appears to be an integral mechanism for the differentiation and formation of various tissues and organs. At fertilization, the paternal genome undergoes DNA demethylation, while the maternal genome appears epigenetically more static.[15] During preimplantation development, genome-wide demethylation occurs followed by de novo global remethylation after implantation prior to organ development.[16] This epigenetic reprogramming is likely to be needed for totipotency, correct initiation of embryonic gene expression and early lineage development in the embryo. Therefore, each cell type establishes its own epigenetic pattern, which reflects its genotype and is ultimately reflected in the phenotype of the cell and the organism as a whole. These DNA methylation patterns in a particular cell type are stably maintained within a narrow margin during later development as well as later life.

However, these patterns are not immutable: aging in mammals is associated with alterations in the amount and patterns of DNA methylation in somatic cells.[17] Emerging observations suggest that these changes may have pathologic consequences, contributing to cell proliferation with aging and the development of malignancies. Aging changes DNA methylation status in a complex fashion. In general, genomic DNA methylation tends to decrease with aging.[18] Mammalian brain, liver, small intestine mucosa, heart and spleen all undergo genomic DNA hypomethylation with aging, while kidney reveals increased genomic DNA methylation and lung shows no changes with aging.[19,20] Aging also affects site-specific DNA methylation.[21] Restriction sites in the *c-myc* gene showed decreased methylation with aging in rodent spleen, while other CpG dinucleotides in this gene develop age-associated hypermethylation in the liver along with decreased mRNA expression.[22] Age-dependent methylation changes in CpG islands, where methylation correlates strongly with suppression of gene expression, have been the subject of multiple recent reports.[23] CpG islands in the promoter region of the estrogen receptor gene are not methylated in young individuals, but are partially methylated in older individuals and invariably hypermethylated in colonic adenomas and cancers. Exogenous introduction of an unmethylated promoter of this gene into colon carcinoma cells suppresses growth, suggesting that this methylation is responsible for regulating gene expression.[24] To date, mechanisms by which aging induces alterations in genomic and promoter DNA methylation are not clear, although altered expression of DNA methyltransferase genes and dietary factors in the elderly have been implicated.

5.1.3   DNA methylation in cancer

A decreased level of genomic DNA methylation is a common finding in tumorigenesis, which appears early in carcinogenesis and usually precedes the mutation and deletion events that occur later in the evolution of cancer.[25,26] Evidence indicates that hypomethylation might contribute to genomic instability, structural changes in chromosomes and enhancement of gene expression. However, the exact implication of genomic hypomethylation in human carcinogenesis is not known yet. In rodent studies genomic hypomethylation directly causes tumorigenesis. Genetically engineered mice carrying a hypomorphic *Dnmt1* allele, which reduces *Dnmt1* expression and results in substantial genome-wide hypomethylation in all tissues, developed aggressive T cell lymphomas.[27] In rat models, diets that are deficient in methionine, choline, folate and vitamin B12 (lipotropes) promote chemical carcinogenesis. In certain strains of mice, prolonged intake of such diets leads to the spontaneous development of liver cancer along with rapid appearance of hypomethylated DNA in the liver.[28] In an old rat study, treatment with 5-azacytidine, a potent DNA methyltransferase inhibitor, induced many different types of tumors in rats.[29]

Current evidence indicates that DNA methylation is associated with cancer initiation, progression and even mutation and metastasis through epigenetic silencing of critical genes such as tumor suppressor or DNA repair genes, so called gate keeper or caretaker genes. Among several candidate mechanisms by which altered DNA methylation increases carcinogenesis, aberrations in DNA methylation at critical loci are most relevant.[30] Interestingly, experimental deficiency of one-carbon nutrients in animals may also cause a paradoxical hypermethylation at selected loci,[31] which is of interest because the promoter regions of several tumor suppressor genes such as *p16*, *p53* and *APC* and DNA repair genes such as *MGMT* and *hMLH1* are frequently found to be hypermethylated in cancer.[32–34] In carcinogenesis, hypermethylation of CpG islands in the promoter region is clearly associated with transcriptional silencing of gene expression, providing an important alternative pathway by which tumor suppressor genes are inactivated without mutation or allele deletion. On the other hand, hypomethylation of CpG islands is associated with gene activation, which appears to be a significant mechanism by which proto-oncogenes may be activated.[35]

5.2 Nutrients modifying DNA methylation

Many dietary components are known to modulate DNA methylation, and imbalance of nutrients in the diet can alter DNA methylation status. Moreover, it is expected that dietary modification may reverse disordered DNA methylation induced by the disease process. Four different types of nutrients are considered to affect DNA methylation: (1) B vitamins as coenzymes of one-carbon metabolism, (2) dietary methyl donor nutrients, (3) micronutrients that can modify one-carbon metabolism and (4) bioactive food compounds that can modify the activity of DNA methyltransferases (Table 5.1).

Table 5.1 Nutrients that affect DNA methylation

	Nutrients	Action
B vitamins	Folate	Methyl acceptors and donors in one-carbon metabolism
	Vitamin B12	Coenzyme for MS
	Vitamin B6	Coenzyme for SHMT, CBS, and cystathionase
	Vitamin B2	Coenzyme for MTHFR
Dietary methyl donor nutrients	Methionine	Precursor of AdoMet
	Choline	Homocysteine remethylation after converting to betaine
	Betaine	Homocysteine remethylation by BHMT
	Serine	Methyl donor to tetrahydrofolate by SHMT
Micronutrients	Retinoic acid	Increases the activity of GNMT
	Zinc	Coenzyme for MAT
	Selenium	Increases the transsulfuration pathway
Bioactive food components	Genistein	Inhibition of DNA methyltransferases
	Tea polyphenols	Inhibition of DNA methyltransferases

5.2.1   B vitamins, coenzymes of one-carbon metabolism

One-carbon metabolism is a network of interrelated biochemical reactions in which a one-carbon unit is received from methyl donor nutrients (serine, methionine, choline and betaine) and transferred into biochemical and molecular pathways essential for DNA synthesis; thymidylate and purine synthesis and biological methylation of DNA, RNA, protein, phospholipids and small molecules (see Figure 5.1). Since one-carbon metabolism synthesizes AdoMet, a unique methyl donor for DNA methylation, and S-adenosylhomocysteine (AdoHcy), an inhibitor of DNA methylation, any dietary components that affect one-carbon metabolism can potentially affect DNA methylation status. It is already well known that dietary folate alters DNA methylation status in both human and animal studies.[36–38] Other B vitamins, vitamin B12, B6 and B2, can also affect DNA methylation as coenzymes in one-carbon metabolism.[39]

Folate coenzymes act as acceptors or donors of one-carbon units (methyl groups) in one-carbon metabolism.[40,41] Serine hydroxymethyltransferase, a pyridoxal-5′-phosphate (vitamin B6) containing enzyme, catalyzes the reversible transfer of a one-carbon unit from serine to tetrahydrofolate (THF) to generate glycine and 5,10 methylene THF. Then methylenetetrahydrofolate reductase (MTHFR), a flavin adenine dinucleotide (vitamin B2) containing enzyme, irreversibly catalyzes 5,10 methylene THF to 5-methyl THF, the primary methyl donor for the remethylation of homocysteine to methionine by methionine synthase (remethylation pathway). The methionine synthase reaction allows for the reutilization of the homocysteine backbone to be used as a carrier of methyl groups derived primarily from serine. The enzyme contains a cobalamin (vitamin B12) cofactor and the

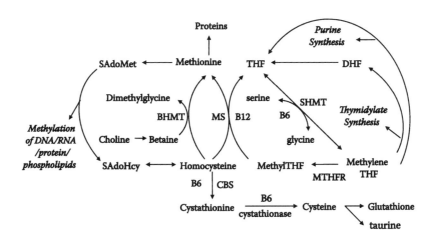

Figure 5.1 One-carbon metabolism.

reaction proceeds via a methyl-cobalamin intermediate.[42] Homocysteine can also be methylated to regenerate methionine by the betaine-homocysteine methyltransferase reaction using choline and betaine in liver and kidney.[43]

Methionine, which is regenerated from homocysteine or obtained directly from the diet, is converted to AdoMet. AdoMet then donates the labile methyl groups from 5-methyl THF to over 80 biological methylation reactions, including the methylation of DNA, RNA, proteins, phospholipids and small molecules and is converted to AdoHcy, which inhibits methyltransferases by binding to the enzymes with a higher affinity than AdoMet. Thus, the efficiency of methyltransferase reactions is dependent on the efficient product removal of AdoHcy. Under normal conditions, AdoHcy is hydrolyzed by AdoHcy hydrolase to adenosine and homocysteine. However, this reaction is readily reversible and causes a chronic elevation in plasma homocysteine levels. Usually this has an indirect and negative effect on cellular methylation reactions through a concomitant increase in intracellular AdoHcy levels.[44,45]

Through a transsulfuration pathway, homocysteine condenses with serine to form cystathionine in an irreversible reaction catalyzed by the pyridoxal-5'-phosphate (vitamin B6)-containing enzyme, cystathionine-β-synthase.[46] Cystathionine is subsequently hydrolyzed to form cysteine by cystathionase, another pyridoxal-5'-phosphate (vitamin B6)-containing enzyme. Cysteine may in turn be utilized to produce taurine and glutathione (Figure 5.1).

5.2.1.1 Folate and DNA methylation

Since the folate-derived methyl group is a main methyl donor for homocysteine remethylation and thereby determines the status of AdoMet, a unique methyl donor for DNA methyltransferases, and AdoHcy, an inhibitor of DNA methyltransferases, it is not surprising that folate is a major determinant of DNA methylation.

Jacob et al.[36] demonstrated the induction of genomic hypomethylation in human lymphocytic DNA when healthy human volunteers were placed on a long-term folate-deficient diet (56 µg folate/day) in a metabolic unit and showed that the effect was reversible when the deficiency was corrected. Rampersaud et al.[37] also reproduced the induction of genomic hypomethylation in lymphocytic DNA of postmenopausal women after 7 weeks with an even less restrictive diet (120 µg folate/day). Supporting evidence from an observational study exists as well: Fowler et al.[47] reported that serum folate levels, as well as folate concentrations in the uterine cervix, were significantly correlated with genomic DNA methylation in a study of cervical intraepithelial neoplasia. Friso et al.[48] also reported decreased genomic DNA methylation in low folate status among subjects with the homozygote variant of *MTHFR 677 C* to *T* polymorphism.

In 1993 Balaghi and Wagner demonstrated that hepatic DNA from folate-deficient rats was hypomethylated on a genomic level compared to DNA from pair-fed control animals.[49] Thereafter, studies performed in rodents fed diets deficient in folate generally have not shown significant changes in genomic DNA methylation, indicating that the rodent is less dependent on folate as a methyl source compared to humans. Also, juvenile animals, which most studies use, are more resistant to folate depletion than old animals. A recent rat study demonstrated that folate supplementation (four times higher than baseline) significantly increased the levels of hepatic DNA methylation in elder rats compared with folate-deplete and folate-replete groups. In addition, liver folate concentrations and genomic DNA methylation were significantly correlated in elder rats ($p = 0.004$).[38] Most recent mice studies also demonstrated that both genomic and *p16* promoter methylation of colonic DNA are in parallel with dietary folate levels in old mice, which was not found from the young ones.[50]

Collectively, it appears that high folate status increases and low folate status decreases DNA methylation status but the effect is specific for species, age, genotype and tissue.

5.2.1.2   *Vitamin B12 and DNA methylation*

Since vitamin B12 serves as a cofactor in the synthesis of methyl precursors for biological methylation, B12 deficiency has been known to induce hyperhomocysteinemia along with a "methylfolate trap" phenomenon which limits methyl availability for homocysteine remethylation and DNA methylation. However, direct evidence for the association between vitamin B12 and DNA methylation is weak.

A recent animal study demonstrated that a vitamin B12 deplete diet disturbed the normal homeostasis of one-carbon metabolism in the colonic mucosa and resulted in diminished genomic DNA methylation.[39] Thirty weanling male Sprague-Dawley rats were divided into two groups and fed either a vitamin B12-deplete diet (0 µg vitamin B12/kg diet) or a similar diet containing adequate amounts of the vitamin (50 µg vitamin B12/kg diet) along with 50 g pectin/kg diet to facilitate vitamin B12 excretion for 10 weeks. By the end of the experiment the colonic DNA of the deplete rats displayed a 35% decrease in genomic DNA methylation ($p < .05$). Brunaud et al.[51] also reported that vitamin B12 is a determinant of DNA methylation in gastrectomized rats devoid of intrinsic factor for vitamin B12 absorption.

Piyathilake et al.[52] compared tissue vitamin B12 concentrations and genomic DNA methylation status in twelve paired tissue samples of squamous cell lung cancer and adjacent grossly normal appearing uninvolved bronchial mucosa. In the cancer tissue both vitamin B12 concentrations and genomic DNA methylation were significantly lower than those in uninvolved tissues ($p = 0.03$ and $p = 0.02$) and the correlation between

vitamin B12 and genomic DNA methylation also was statistically significant ($p = 0.009$), indicating that vitamin B12 deficiency is associated with
genomic DNA hypomethylation.

5.2.1.3   Combined B vitamin deficiency and DNA methylation

In contrast to folate and vitamin B12, to date there is no report which
indicates that either vitamin B6 or vitamin B2 individually affects
DNA methylation status. Since vitamin B6 is a coenzyme for the serine
hydroxymethyltransferase reaction, unique methyl source for folate coenzymes, and cystathionine β-synthase reaction (transsulfuration pathway),
hyperhomocysteinemia and altered DNA methylation are expected with
vitamin B6 depletion. However, vitamin B6 deficiency leads to postpran-
dial rises in homocysteine[53] but has less of an effect on fasting hyperhomocysteinemia, lending to the theory that the adverse effect of vitamin
B6 deficiency on DNA methylation is well compensated. Vitamin B2 is a
coenzyme for MTHFR as flavin adenine dinucleotide. Even though vitamin B2 affects MTHFR activity and decreased MTHFR activity is known
to reduce genomic DNA methylation, until now there is no report indicating that the vitamin B2 affects DNA methylation status.

Nevertheless, most recently in the mice colon, Liu et al.[54] reported
that mild combined deficiency of these B vitamins induces genomic DNA
hypomethylation, even though individual deficiencies of folate, vitamin
B12, vitamin B6, and vitamin B2 did not alter genomic DNA methylation
status. Additionally, mild combined deficiency of these B vitamins alters
multiple components of the Wnt pathway, a signal transduction pathway
that is well known for its role in embryogenesis and cancer. This observation indicates that reduced status of each B vitamin can interact and
synergistically derange one-carbon metabolism significantly enough to
induce genomic DNA hypomethylation.

5.2.2   Methyl donor nutrients for one-carbon metabolism

Theoretically, dietary methyl donors for one-carbon metabolism such
as methionine, choline, betaine and serine can affect DNA methylation
status through methyl group availability,[55] even though evidence regarding the association between individual deficiency of these methyl donor
nutrients and DNA methylation is few.[56]

5.2.2.1   Dietary methyl donor deficiency induces cancer

Based on the observations that diets deficient in methionine, choline,
folic acid and vitamin B12 (lipotropes) promote chemical carcinogenesis in rodents[2,3] and prolonged intake of such diets can lead to the
development of liver cancers,[57] Wainfan et al.[28] investigated whether
methyl-deficient diets can alter DNA methylation. In this rat model

hypomethylation of DNA was detected within one week after initiation of the methyl-deficient diet and it persisted throughout the whole four week study, indicating that low methyl-donor diets may induce cancer by diminishing genomic DNA methylation as found in the other rodent models: both *Dnmt1* gene-deficient mice[27] and demethylating agent aza-cytidine-treated rats[29] developed cancer along with profound genome-wide DNA hypomethylation.

Interestingly, Pogribny et al. investigated the effect of a methyl-deficient diet on hepatic *p53* gene-specific DNA methylation during hepatic carcinogenesis. Increased *p53* gene hypomethylation was found after one week on the methyl-deficient diet[58] and progressive demethylation was observed at cytosine residues despite a paradoxical increase in DNA methyltransferase activity,[59] while specific 5-methyl cytosines within the hepatic *p53* gene from methyl-deficient rats were resistant to demethylation despite the diet-induced decrease in AdoMet, indicating that the demethylating effect of the methyl-deficient diet is CpG site specific. In a prolonged observation study of this animal model, a progressive loss of methyl groups was observed at most CpG sites on both coding and noncoding strands within exons 6 to 7 of the *p53* gene during the first 36 weeks of the methyl-deficient diet, while DNA from tumors developed after 54 weeks of methyl-deficient diet demonstrated remethylation of cytosines. CpG sites that had previously lost methyl groups on both strands during preneoplasia, as well as CpG sites that had been constitutively nonmethylated, had undergone de novo methylation in DNA of tumors in which de novo methyltransferase activity was increased more than fourfold relative to the control or preneoplastic lesion.[31]

5.2.2.2 Dietary methyl donor deficiency alters embryonic development

Epigenetically determined characteristics produce interesting developmental patterns in many animals. Among them is the epigenetic variation in expression of the *agouti* gene in mice.[60] The mouse *agouti* alleles, A^w and A, regulate the alternative production of black (eumelanin) and yellow (pheomelanin) pigments in individual hair follicles. Due to mutations in the regulatory region of the *agouti* locus, mice bearing the dominant "viable yellow" (A^{vy}), "IAPyellow" (A^{iapy}), or "hyperviable yellow" (A^{hvy}) alleles synthesize much more pheomelanin than eumelanin.[4] These mutations arise through spontaneous insertion of single intracisternal A particle (IAP) sequence in different regions of the *agouti* gene, all preceding the first coding exon. Unlike most other *agouti* mutations, expressivity of A^{vy} is variable and subject to parental imprinting effects.[61] The *nonagouti* (*a*) allele is caused by a loss-of-function mutation in A; a/a homozygotes are therefore black. Dietary methyl donor supplementation of a/a dams with extra folic acid, vitamin B12, choline and betaine alters the phenotype of their A^{vy}/a offspring via increased CpG methylation at the A^{vy}, as indicated by increased agouti/black mottling in the direction of pseudoagouti phenotype (black).

Nutrition is the major intrauterine environmental factor that alters expression of the fetal genome and may have lifelong consequences. Uteroplacental insufficiency induced by ligating both uterine arteries of the pregnant rats alters DNA methylation in postnatal rat liver by increased AdoHcy, homocysteine and methionine in association with decreased mRNA levels of methionine adenosyltransferase and cystathionine-β-synthase.[62] Since AdoHcy is an inhibitor of DNA methyltransferase and AdoMet is a methyl donor for the histone methylation reaction,[63,64] one might speculate that any nutritional conditions that alter AdoHcy and AdoMet levels are able to affect DNA methylation, which is associated with DNA methyltransferase activity.[65] By the same token, folate insufficiency in pregnancy is well recognized as a risk factor for neural tube defects in humans and altered DNA methylation by folate insufficiency during early embryonic stage has been regarded as a responsible mechanism.[66,67] Most recently Niculescu et al.[68] reported that during fetal development of the mouse brain, dams fed a no choline diet, had induced alterations in genomic and gene-specific DNA methylation, especially specific CpG sites within genes that regulate cell cycling. Kovacheva et al.[69] also reported that choline deficiency induces hypomethylation of CpGs islands within the *Dnmt1* gene, resulting in increased expression as well as global and gene-specific DNA methylation.

5.2.3   *Other micronutrients modifying one-carbon metabolism*

Fell and Steele[70] reported that vitamin A deficiency decreases 10-formyl THF dehydrogenase activity and increases MTHFR activity in the rat liver. At the follow-up studies,[71,72] they also reported that rats fed a diet containing excess retinol (1000 IU of retinol/g diet) showed decreased synthesis of 5-methyl THF and AdoMet and increases in THF concentrations with reduced MTHFR activity. These observations indicate that retinoic acid can alter one-carbon metabolism as well as methylation reactions. Thereafter, Rowling et al.[73] demonstrated that in the rat liver, retinoic acid as well as retinoic acid derivatives, 13-*cis*- and all-*trans*-retinoic acid, increase the activity of glycine *N*-methyltransferase, which is essential in optimizing the methyl group supply in one-carbon metabolism, thereby inducing hepatic DNA hypomethylation. Inappropriate induction of glycine *N*-methyltransferase can lead to a biologically important loss of methyl groups and the subsequent impairment of essential transmethylation processes. Since retinoic acid can affect DNA methylation by altering the methyl availability, this characteristic might be useful against aberrant DNA methylation induced by carcinogenesis.

Deficiency of zinc, a coenzyme for methionine adenosyltransferases which catalyze the conversion from methionine to AdoMet, can reduce the utilization of methyl groups from AdoMet in the rodent liver and results in genomic DNA hypomethylation as well as histone hypomethylation.[74,75]

Selenium does not directly affect the function of enzymes that are associated with one-carbon metabolism but enhances the transsulfuration pathway. Selenium is needed for glutathione recycling and under selenium deficiency one-carbon metabolism needs to produce more glutathione by accelerating the transsulfuration pathway, which results in reduced methyl availability. Dietary deficiency of selenium decreased genomic DNA methylation in Caco-2 cells, and in rat liver and colon.[76,77]

5.2.4 Bioactive food components modifying DNA methyltransferases

Bioactive food components are defined nonessential biomolecules that are present in foods and exhibit the capacity to modulate metabolic processes, which secure better health. Since these bioactive food components can influence a number of molecular events for maintaining health and disease resistance,[78] it is not surprising that bioactive components such as genistein, tea polyphenols and lycopene can affect DNA methylation.

Genistein, one of the phytoestrogens contained in soy, has been known to inhibit the proliferation of breast and prostate cancer cell lines[79] and to compete with estrogen, playing a role in cell growth through a pathway mediated by estrogen receptor.[80] Day et al.[81] reported that dietary genistein is positively associated with changes in prostate DNA methylation at CpG islands of mouse genes. Fang et al.[82] reported that genistein can reduce hypermethylation status of *RARβ*, *p16*, and *MGMT* genes in cultured cells and dose-dependently inhibit the activity of DNA methyltransferases, lending that genistein can reactivate methylation-silenced genes, through an inhibition of DNA methyltransferase. Dolinoy et al.[5] reported the supplementation effect of maternal dietary genistein during the gestation period on site-specific DNA methylation of offspring and phenotypic expression using the *agouti* mouse model. Maternal dietary supplementation of genistein at levels comparable with humans consuming high-soy diets changed the coat color of heterozygous yellow *agouti* (A^{vy}/a) pups toward black pseudoagouti by reducing the DNA methylation status of the *agouti* locus.

In the 4-(methylnitrosamino)-1-(3-pyridyl)-1-butanone (NNK)-induced lung cancer model of A/J female mice, Shi et al.[83] described that decaffeinated green tea and black tea extracts can inhibit NNK-induced DNA methylation and among many tea components (-)-epigallocatechin-3-gallate (EGCG) is the most potent inhibitor of DNA methylation. Fang et al.[84] also reported that EGCG, a major polyphenol from green tea, can inhibit the enzyme activity of DNA methyltransferase and reactivate methylation-silenced genes in cancer cells, suggesting the potential use of EGCG to reverse the epigenetically silenced genes during carcinogenesis. Lee et al.[85] demonstrated that each of the tea polyphenols (catechin, epicatechin and EGCG) and bioflavonoids (quercetin, fisetin and myricetin) can inhibit Dnmt 1-mediated DNA methylation in a concentration-dependent manner but among them EGCG is the most potent inhibitor.

King-Batoon et al.[86] reported that lycopene, a potent antioxidant carotenoid that can modulate expression of many genes associated with the cell cycle, DNA repair and apoptosis, can alter DNA methylation of the *GSTP1* gene and upregulate this gene in the breast cancer cell line. They also reported that methylated *RARβ2* and *HIN-1* genes can be partially demethylated by lycopene. It appears that lycopene affects gene expression by modifying gene-specific methylation.

5.3   Nutrient-gene interactions on DNA methylation

On the premise that nutrients alter DNA methylation by modifying one-carbon metabolism, we can easily speculate that a certain polymorphism that alters methyl availability in one-carbon metabolism may affect DNA methylation according to the status of one-carbon nutrients. Among several combinations of nutrients and genes, folate and the *MTHFR 677 C to T* polymorphism is a paradigm for nutrient and gene interactions on DNA methylation.[8,48,87] The biological significance of the interaction between folate and this gene is predominantly associated with the reduced availability of 5-methyl THF due to reduced MTHFR activity by the polymorphic site. The methyl moiety of 5-methyl THF is utilized for homocysteine remethylation and ultimately AdoMet synthesis (Figure 5.1).

Jacques et al.[88] first showed that individuals with the thermolabile *MTHFR* variant (*MTHFR 677TT* genotype) may have a higher folate requirement for the regulation of plasma homocysteine concentrations, highlighting the presence of an interaction between this common polymorphism and folate in homocysteine metabolism and theorizing that this interaction can subsequently affect DNA methylation due to decreased methyl availability. Thereafter, in a small group of subjects Stern et al.[87] reported that DNA from subjects with *MTHFR 677TT* genotype had a significantly higher methyl group acceptance capacity compared to wild-type (*MTHFR 677CC*) individuals ($p < .05$). This result was seen only among subjects with low plasma folate concentrations. In 2002 Friso et al.[48] determined the effect of folate status on genomic DNA methylation with an emphasis on the interaction with the common *677 C to T* polymorphism in the *MTHFR* gene. A newly developed liquid chromatography/mass spectrometry method for the analysis of nucleotide bases was used to assess genomic DNA methylation in peripheral blood mononuclear cell DNA from 105 subjects homozygous for this polymorphism (*MTHFR 677TT*) and 187 homozygous for the wild type (*MTHFR 677CC*). The results of the study showed that subjects with *MTHFR 677TT* genotype had a decreased genomic DNA methylation compared to those with the wild-type genotype ($p < .0001$). When analyzed according to folate status, however, only the subjects with *MTHFR 677TT* genotype and low folate accounted for the decreased DNA methylation ($p < .0001$). Intriguingly, in subjects with *MTHFR 677TT* genotype, DNA methylation status correlated with the methylated proportion of red blood cell folate ($p < .03$). These results indicate that the *MTHFR 677 C* to *T* polymorphism influences genomic DNA methylation status through an interaction with folate status.[48]

In the same cohort, the researchers also evaluated whether the interaction between the other common *1298 A* to *C* polymorphism in the *MTHFR* gene and folate also affect genomic DNA methylation.[89] Interestingly, subjects with *MTHFR 1298AA* wild-type genotype showed decreased genomic DNA methylation compared to subjects with *1298 AC* or *1298 CC* genotypes ($p < .0001$ and $p = .007$, respectively). When DNA methylation was evaluated according to plasma folate status, only subjects with *MTHFR 1298 AA* wild type and low folate levels revealed decreased DNA methylation ($p < .0001$). Moreover, when the two *MTHFR* polymorphisms were concomitantly evaluated at the low folate status, DNA methylation was reduced only in *1298AA/677TT* compared to *1298AA/677CC* ($p = .001$) and to *1298CC/677CC* genotypes ($p = .004$). However, the high prevalence of *677TT* variants within the *1298AA* group (79%) and the similar biochemical features of *1298AA/677CC* and *1298CC/677CC* combined genotypes, suggest that the nutrient-gene interaction affecting DNA methylation in subjects with *MTHFR 1298AA* genotype is mainly due to the coexistence of the *MTHFR 677TT* genotype. [89]

In brief, a nutrient-gene interaction phenomenon can affect DNA methylation status and further studies will verify underlying mechanisms for nutrition-associated diseases, such as neural tube defects, cardiovascular disease and cancer, as well as enable individually tailored chemoprevention using nutrients.

5.4   Conclusions

In recent years, epigenetics has been among the most rapidly growing fields in molecular science. In fact, epigenetics has revealed new mechanisms responsible for development, aging, and disease process such as cancer development. One major epigenetic phenomenon in the eukaryote cell is DNA methylation, which attributes to gene expression and integrity. Deepening the knowledge on one-carbon metabolism is very important to understanding DNA methylation because DNA methylation is directly associated with the status of AdoMet, a unique methyl donor, and SAdoHcy, an inhibitor of methyltransferases, both of which are metabolites of one-carbon metabolism and can be influenced by dietary nutrients, such as methionine, choline, betaine, folate and vitamin B12.

Due to its reversibility, DNA methylation is more attractive to the field of nutritional intervention in cancer rather than irreversible phenomena such as mutations or loss of heterozygosity. Furthermore, inhibitors of DNA methyltransferases, which have been used to investigate epigenetic mechanisms, are now tested in several on-going clinical trials of cancer chemotherapy. Thus, studies on DNA methylation, especially the modulation of DNA methyltransferase activity using bioactive food compounds such as genistein or catechin, will lead us to potentially safe and effective nutritional intervention strategy against cancer disease.

Based on the currently available data, this chapter discussed the effect of nutrients on DNA methylation. However, evidence is still limited, especially in regard to the combined effects of nutrients with other factors, such as gene polymorphisms and/or therapeutic drugs, on DNA methylation. Although important questions wait to be answered, studies regarding the modulation of epigenetic systems with nutrients, especially through one-carbon metabolism or by modifying associated enzymes, will provide new insights for physiologic and pathologic processes, and consequently new preventive or therapeutic intervention modalities.

Abbreviations

AdoHcy: *S*-adenosylhomocysteine
AdoMet: *S*-adenosylmethionine
BHMT: betaine homocysteine methyltransferase
CBS: cystathionine β-synthase
Dnmt1: DNA methyltransferase 1
EGCG: (-)-epigallocatechin-3-gallate
GNMT: glycine *N*-methyltransferase
MAT: methionine adenosyltransferase
MS: methionine synthase
MTHFR: methylenetetrahydrofolate reductase
NNK: 4-(methylnitrosamino)-1-(3-pyridyl)-1-butanone
SHMT: serine hydroxymethyltransferase
THF: tetrahydrofolate

References

1. Sansam, C. G., and Roberts, C. W. (2006). Epigenetics and cancer: Altered chromatin remodeling via Snf5 loss leads to aberrant cell cycle regulation. *Cell Cycle* 5, 621–624.
2. Newberne, P. M., and Rogers, A. E. (1986). Labile methyl groups and the promotion of cancer. *Annu Rev Nutr* 6, 407–432.

3. Mikol, Y. B., Hoover, K. L., Creasia, D., and Poirier, L. A. (1983). Hepatocarcinogenesis in rats fed methyl-deficient, amino acid-defined diets. *Carcinogenesis* 4, 1619–1629.

4. Wolff, G. L., Kodell, R. L., Moore, S. R., and Cooney, C. A. (1998). Maternal epigenetics and methyl supplements affect agouti gene expression in Avy/a mice. *FASEB J* 12, 949–957.

5. Dolinoy, D. C., Weidman, J. R., Waterland, R. A., and Jirtle, R. L. (2006). Maternal genistein alters coat color and protects Avy mouse offspring from obesity by modifying the fetal epigenome. *Environ Health Perspect* 114, 567–572.

6. Costello, J. F., and Plass, C. (2001). Methylation matters. *J Med Genet* 38, 285–303.

7. Robertson, K. D., and Jones, P. A. (2000). DNA methylation: Past, present and future directions. *Carcinogenesis* 21, 461–467.

8. Friso, S., and Choi, S. W. (2002). Gene-nutrient interactions and DNA methylation. *J Nutr* 132, 2382S–2387S.

9. O'Neill, R. J., O'Neill, M. J., and Graves, J. A. (1998). Undermethylation associated with retroelement activation and chromosome remodelling in an interspecific mammalian hybrid. *Nature* 393, 68–72.

10. Stein, R., Razin, A., and Cedar, H. (1982). In vitro methylation of the hamster adenine phosphoribosyltransferase gene inhibits its expression in mouse L cells. *Proc Natl Acad Sci USA* 79, 3418–3422.

11. Chen, Z. J., and Pikaard, C. S. (1997). Epigenetic silencing of RNA polymerase I transcription: A role for DNA methylation and histone modification in nucleolar dominance. *Genes Dev* 11, 2124–2136.

12. Li, E., Bestor, T. H., and Jaenisch, R. (1992). Targeted mutation of the DNA methyltransferase gene results in embryonic lethality. *Cell* 69, 915–926.

13. Jones, P. L., Veenstra, G. J., Wade, P. A., Vermaak, D., Kass, S. U., Landsberger, N., Strouboulis, J., and Wolffe, A. P. (1998). Methylated DNA and MeCP2 recruit histone deacetylase to repress transcription. *Nat Genet* 19, 187–191.

14. Nan, X., Ng, H. H., Johnson, C. A., Laherty, C. D., Turner, B. M., Eisenman, R. N., and Bird, A. (1998). Transcriptional repression by the methyl-CpG-binding protein MeCP2 involves a histone deacetylase complex. *Nature* 393, 386–389.

15. Morgan, H. D., Santos, F., Green, K., Dean, W., and Reik, W. (2005). Epigenetic reprogramming in mammals. *Hum Mol Genet* 14 (Special issue no. 1), R47–R58.

16. McKay, J. A., Williams, E. A., and Mathers, J. C. (2004). Folate and DNA methylation during in utero development and aging. *Biochem Soc Trans* 32, 1006–1007.

17. Liu, L., Wylie, R. C., Andrews, L. G., and Tollefsbol, T. O. (2003). Aging, cancer and nutrition: The DNA methylation connection. *Mech Ageing Dev* 124, 989–998.

18. Holliday, R. (1987). The inheritance of epigenetic defects. *Science* 238, 163–170.

19. Vanyushin, B. F., Mazin, A. L., Vasilyev, V. K., and Belozersky, A. N. (1973). The content of 5-methylcytosine in animal DNA: The species and tissue specificity. *Biochim Biophys Acta* 299, 397–403.

20. Richardson, B. (2003). Impact of aging on DNA methylation. *Ageing Res Rev* 2, 245–261.

21. Slagboom, P. E., de Leeuw, W. J., and Vijg, J. (1990). Messenger RNA levels and methylation patterns of GAPDH and beta-actin genes in rat liver, spleen and brain in relation to aging. *Mech Ageing Dev* 53, 243–257.
22. Ono, T., Uehara, Y., Kurishita, A., Tawa, R., and Sakurai, H. (1993). Biological significance of DNA methylation in the ageing process. *Age Ageing* 22, S34–S43.
23. Issa, J. P. (2000). CpG-island methylation in aging and cancer. *Curr Top Microbiol Immunol* 249, 101–118.
24. Issa, J. P., Ottaviano, Y. L., Celano, P., Hamilton, S. R., Davidson, N. E., and Baylin, S. B. (1994). Methylation of the oestrogen receptor CpG island links ageing and neoplasia in human colon. *Nat Genet* 7, 536–540.
25. Goelz, S. E., Vogelstein, B., Hamilton, S. R., and Feinberg, A. P. (1985). Hypomethylation of DNA from benign and malignant human colon neoplasms. *Science* 228, 187–190.
26. Counts, J. L., and Goodman, J. I. (1994). Hypomethylation of DNA: An epigenetic mechanism involved in tumor promotion. *Mol Carcinog* 11, 185–188.
27. Gaudet, F., Hodgson, J. G., Eden, A., Jackson-Grusby, L., Dausman, J., Gray, J. W., Leonhardt, H., and Jaenisch, R. (2003). Induction of tumors in mice by genomic hypomethylation. *Science* 300, 489–492.
28. Wainfan, E., Dizik, M., Stender, M., and Christman, J. K. (1989). Rapid appearance of hypomethylated DNA in livers of rats fed cancer-promoting, methyl-deficient diets. *Cancer Res* 49, 4094–4097.
29. Carr, B. I., Reilly, J. G., Smith, S. S., Winberg, C., and Riggs, A. (1984). The tumorigenicity of 5-azacytidine in the male Fischer rat. *Carcinogenesis* 5, 1583–1590.
30. Wainfan, E., and Poirier, L. A. (1992). Methyl groups in carcinogenesis: Effects on DNA methylation and gene expression. *Cancer Res* 52, 2071s–2077s.
31. Pogribny, I. P., Miller, B. J., and James, S. J. (1997). Alterations in hepatic p53 gene methylation patterns during tumor progression with folate/methyl deficiency in the rat. *Cancer Lett* 115, 31–38.
32. Herman, J. G., Merlo, A., Mao, L., Lapidus, R. G., Issa, J. P., Davidson, N. E., Sidransky, D., and Baylin, S. B. (1995). Inactivation of the CDKN2/p16/MTS1 gene is frequently associated with aberrant DNA methylation in all common human cancers. *Cancer Res* 55, 4525–4530.
33. Schroeder, M., and Mass, M. J. (1997). CpG methylation inactivates the transcriptional activity of the promoter of the human p53 tumor suppressor gene. *Biochem Biophys Res Commun* 235, 403–406.
34. Hiltunen, M. O., Alhonen, L., Koistinaho, J., Myohanen, S., Paakkonen, M., Marin, S., Kosma, V. M., and Janne, J. (1997). Hypermethylation of the APC (adenomatous polyposis coli) gene promoter region in human colorectal carcinoma. *Int J Cancer* 70, 644–648.
35. Choi, S. W., and Mason, J. B. (2000). Folate and carcinogenesis: An integrated scheme. *J Nutr* 130, 129–132.
36. Jacob, R. A., Gretz, D. M., Taylor, P. C., James, S. J., Pogribny, I. P., Miller, B. J., Henning, S. M., and Swendseid, M. E. (1998). Moderate folate depletion increases plasma homocysteine and decreases lymphocyte DNA methylation in postmenopausal women. *J Nutr* 128, 1204–1212.
37. Rampersaud, G. C., Kauwell, G. P., Hutson, A. D., Cerda, J. J., and Bailey, L. B. (2000). Genomic DNA methylation decreases in response to moderate folate depletion in elderly women. *Am J Clin Nutr* 72, 998–1003.

38. Choi, S. W., Friso, S., Keyes, M. K., and Mason, J. B. (2005). Folate supplementation increases genomic DNA methylation in the liver of elder rats. *Br J Nutr* 93, 31–35.

39. Choi, S. W., Friso, S., Ghandour, H., Bagley, P. J., Selhub, J., and Mason, J. B. (2004). Vitamin B-12 deficiency induces anomalies of base substitution and methylation in the DNA of rat colonic epithelium. *J Nutr* 134, 750–755.

40. MacKenzie, R. (1984). *Biogenesis and Interconversion of Substituted Tetrahydrofolates,* Vol. 1. New York: Wiley.

41. Shane, B. (1989). Folylpolyglutamate synthesis and role in the regulation of one-carbon metabolism. *Vitam Horm* 45, 263–335.

42. Weiss, A., Keshet, I., Razin, A., and Cedar, H. (1996). DNA demethylation in vitro: Involvement of RNA *Cell* 86, 709–718 [published erratum appears in *Cell* 95, no. 4 (1998): following 573].

43. Craig, S. A. (2004). Betaine in human nutrition. *Am J Clin Nutr* 80, 539–549.

44. Yi, P., Melnyk, S., Pogribna, M., Pogribny, I. P., Hine, R. J., and James, S. J. (2000). Increase in plasma homocysteine associated with parallel increases in plasma S-adenosylhomocysteine and lymphocyte DNA hypomethylation. *J Biol Chem* 275, 29318–29323.

45. Coppola, A., Davi, G., De Stefano, V., Mancini, F. P., Cerbone, A. M., and Di Minno, G. (2000). Homocysteine, coagulation, platelet function, and thrombosis. *Semin Thromb Hemost* 26, 243–254.

46. Martinez, M., Cuskelly, G. J., Williamson, J., Toth, J. P., and Gregory, J. F. III. (2000). Vitamin B-6 deficiency in rats reduces hepatic serine hydroxymethyltransferase and cystathionine beta-synthase activities and rates of in vivo protein turnover, homocysteine remethylation and transsulfuration. *J Nutr* 130, 1115–1123.

47. Fowler, B. M., Giuliano, A. R., Piyathilake, C., Nour, M., and Hatch, K. (1998). Hypomethylation in cervical tissue: Is there a correlation with folate status? *Cancer Epidemiol Biomarkers Prev* 7, 901–906.

48. Friso, S., Choi, S. W., Girelli, D., Mason, J. B., Dolnikowski, G. G., Bagley, P. J., Olivieri, O., Jacques, P. F., Rosenberg, I. H., Corrocher, R., and Selhub, J. (2002). A common mutation in the 5,10-methylenetetrahydrofolate reductase gene affects genomic DNA methylation through an interaction with folate status. *Proc Natl Acad Sci USA* 99, 5606–5611.

49. Balaghi, M., and Wagner, C. (1993). DNA methylation in folate deficiency: Use of CpG methylase. *Biochem Biophys Res Commun* 193, 1184–1190.

50. Keyes, M. K., Jang, H., Mason, J. B., Liu, Z., Crott, J. W., Smith, D. E., Friso, S., and Choi, S. W. (2007). Older age and dietary folate are determinants of genomic and p16-specific DNA methylation in mouse colon. *J Nutr* 137, 1713–1717.

51. Brunaud, L., Alberto, J. M., Ayav, A., Gerard, P., Namour, F., Antunes, L., Braun, M., Bronowicki, J. P., Bresler, L., and Gueant, J. L. (2003). Vitamin B12 is a strong determinant of low methionine synthase activity and DNA hypomethylation in gastrectomized rats. *Digestion* 68, 133–140.

52. Piyathilake, C. J., Johanning, G. L., Macaluso, M., Whiteside, M., Oelschlager, D. K., Heimburger, D. C., and Grizzle, W. E. (2000). Localized folate and vitamin B-12 deficiency in squamous cell lung cancer is associated with global DNA hypomethylation. *Nutr Cancer* 37, 99–107.

53. Poirier, L. A., Wise, C. K., Delongchamp, R. R., and Sinha, R. (2001). Blood determinations of S-adenosylmethionine, S-adenosylhomocysteine, and homocysteine: correlations with diet. *Cancer Epidemiol Biomarkers Prev* 10, 649–655.

54. Liu, Z., Choi, S. W., Crott, J. W., Keyes, M. K., Jang, H., Smith, D. E., Kim, M., Laird, P. W., Bronson, R., and Mason, J. B. (2007). Mild depletion of dietary folate combined with other B vitamins alters multiple components of the Wnt pathway in mouse colon. *J Nutr* 137, 2701–2708.
55. Davis, C. D., and Uthus, E. O. (2004). DNA methylation, cancer susceptibility, and nutrient interactions. *Exp Biol Med (Maywood)* 229, 988–995.
56. Waterland, R. A. (2006). Assessing the effects of high methionine intake on DNA methylation. *J Nutr* 136, 1706S–1710S.
57. Ghoshal, A. K., and Farber, E. (1984). The induction of liver cancer by dietary deficiency of choline and methionine without added carcinogens. *Carcinogenesis* 5, 1367–1370.
58. Pogribny, I. P., Basnakian, A. G., Miller, B. J., Lopatina, N. G., Poirier, L. A., and James, S. J. (1995). Breaks in genomic DNA and within the p53 gene are associated with hypomethylation in livers of folate/methyl-deficient rats. *Cancer Res* 55, 1894–1901.
59. Pogribny, I. P., Poirier, L. A., and James, S. J. (1995). Differential sensitivity to loss of cytosine methyl groups within the hepatic p53 gene of folate/methyl deficient rats. *Carcinogenesis* 16, 2863–2867.
60. Cooney, C. A., Dave, A. A., and Wolff, G. L. (2002). Maternal methyl supplements in mice affect epigenetic variation and DNA methylation of offspring. *J Nutr* 132, 2393S–2400S.
61. Duhl, D. M., Vrieling, H., Miller, K. A., Wolff, G. L., and Barsh, G. S. (1994). Neomorphic agouti mutations in obese yellow mice. *Nat Genet* 8, 59–65.
62. MacLennan, N. K., James, S. J., Melnyk, S., Piroozi, A., Jernigan, S., Hsu, J. L., Janke, S. M., Pham, T. D., and Lane, R. H. (2004). Uteroplacental insufficiency alters DNA methylation, one-carbon metabolism, and histone acetylation in IUGR rats. *Physiol Genomics* 18, 43–50.
63. Zhang, X., Yang, Z., Khan, S. I., Horton, J. R., Tamaru, H., Selker, E. U., and Cheng, X. (2003). Structural basis for the product specificity of histone lysine methyltransferases. *Mol Cell* 12, 177–185.
64. Kim, K. C., Geng, L., and Huang, S. (2003). Inactivation of a histone methyltransferase by mutations in human cancers. *Cancer Res* 63, 7619–7623.
65. Kishikawa, S., Ugai, H., Murata, T., and Yokoyama, K. K. (2002). Roles of histone acetylation in the Dnmt1 gene expression. *Nucleic Acids Res Suppl*, 209–210.
66. Rogner, U. C., Danoy, P., Matsuda, F., Moore, G. E., Stanier, P., and Avner, P. (2002). SNPs in the CpG island of NAP1L2: A possible link between DNA methylation and neural tube defects? *Am J Med Genet* 110, 208–214.
67. Al-Gazali, L. I., Padmanabhan, R., Melnyk, S., Yi, P., Pogribny, I. P., Pogribna, M., Bakir, M., Hamid, Z. A., Abdulrazzaq, Y., Dawodu, A., and James, S. J. (2001). Abnormal folate metabolism and genetic polymorphism of the folate pathway in a child with Down syndrome and neural tube defect. *Am J Med Genet* 103, 128–132.
68. Niculescu, M. D., Craciunescu, C. N., and Zeisel, S. H. (2006). Dietary choline deficiency alters global and gene-specific DNA methylation in the developing hippocampus of mouse fetal brains. *FASEB J* 20, 43–49.
69. Kovacheva, V. P., Mellott, T. J., Davison, J. M., Wagner, N., Lopez-Coviella, I., Schnitzler, A. C., and Blusztajn, J. K. (2007). Gestational choline deficiency causes global and Igf2 gene DNA hypermethylation by up-regulation of Dnmt1 expression. *J Biol Chem* 282, 31777–31788.

70. Fell, D., and Steele, R. D. (1985). The effects of vitamin A deficiency on hepatic folate metabolism in rats. *Arch Biochem Biophys* 240, 843–850.
71. Fell, D., and Steele, R. D. (1986). Modification of hepatic folate metabolism in rats fed excess retinol. *Life Sci* 38, 1959–1965.
72. Fell, D., and Steele, R. D. (1987). Effect of retinol toxicity on hepatic S-adenosylmethionine-dependent transmethylation in rats. *Drug Nutr Interact* 5, 1–7.
73. Rowling, M. J., McMullen, M. H., and Schalinske, K. L. (2002). Vitamin A and its derivatives induce hepatic glycine N-methyltransferase and hypomethylation of DNA in rats. *J Nutr* 132, 365–369.
74. Wallwork, J. C., and Duerre, J. A. (1985). Effect of zinc deficiency on methionine metabolism, methylation reactions and protein synthesis in isolated perfused rat liver. *J Nutr* 115, 252–262.
75. Dreosti, I. E. (2001). Zinc and the gene. *Mutat Res* 475, 161–167.
76. Davis, C. D., Uthus, E. O., and Finley, J. W. (2000). Dietary selenium and arsenic affect DNA methylation in vitro in Caco-2 cells and in vivo in rat liver and colon. *J Nutr* 130, 2903–2909.
77. El-Bayoumy, K. (2001). The protective role of selenium on genetic damage and on cancer. *Mutat Res* 475, 123–139.
78. Milner, J. A. (2004). Molecular targets for bioactive food components. *J Nutr* 134, 2492S–2498S.
79. Moyad, M. A. (1999). Soy, disease prevention, and prostate cancer. *Semin Urol Oncol* 17, 97–102.
80. Wang, T. T., Sathyamoorthy, N., and Phang, J. M. (1996). Molecular effects of genistein on estrogen receptor mediated pathways. *Carcinogenesis* 17, 271–275.
81. Day, J. K., Bauer, A. M., DesBordes, C., Zhuang, Y., Kim, B. E., Newton, L. G., Nehra, V., Forsee, K. M., MacDonald, R. S., Besch-Williford, C., Huang, T. H., and Lubahn, D. B. (2002). Genistein alters methylation patterns in mice. *J Nutr* 132, 2419S–2423S.
82. Fang, M. Z., Chen, D., Sun, Y., Jin, Z., Christman, J. K., and Yang, C. S. (2005). Reversal of hypermethylation and reactivation of p16INK4a, RARbeta, and MGMT genes by genistein and other isoflavones from soy. *Clin Cancer Res* 11, 7033–7041.
83. Shi, S. T., Wang, Z. Y., Smith, T. J., Hong, J. Y., Chen, W. F., Ho, C. T., and Yang, C. S. (1994). Effects of green tea and black tea on 4-(methylnitrosamino)-1-(3-pyridyl)-1-butanone bioactivation, DNA methylation, and lung tumorigenesis in A/J mice. *Cancer Res* 54, 4641–4647.
84. Fang, M. Z., Wang, Y., Ai, N., Hou, Z., Sun, Y., Lu, H., Welsh, W., and Yang, C. S. (2003). Tea polyphenol (-)-epigallocatechin-3-gallate inhibits DNA methyltransferase and reactivates methylation-silenced genes in cancer cell lines. *Cancer Res* 63, 7563–7570.
85. Lee, W. J., Shim, J. Y., and Zhu, B. T. (2005). Mechanisms for the inhibition of DNA methyltransferases by tea catechins and bioflavonoids. *Mol Pharmacol* 68, 1018–1030.
86. King-Batoon, A., Leszczynska, J. M., and Klein, C. B. (2008). Modulation of gene methylation by genistein or lycopene in breast cancer cells. *Environ Mol Mutagen* 49, 36–45.

87. Stern, L. L., Mason, J. B., Selhub, J., and Choi, S. W. (2000). Genomic DNA hypomethylation, a characteristic of most cancers, is present in peripheral leukocytes of individuals who are homozygous for the C677T polymorphism in the methylenetetrahydrofolate reductase gene. *Cancer Epidemiol Biomarkers Prev* 9, 849–853.
88. Jacques, P. F., Bostom, A. G., Williams, R. R., Ellison, R. C., Eckfeldt, J. H., Rosenberg, I. H., Selhub, J., and Rozen, R. (1996). Relation between folate status, a common mutation in methylenetetrahydrofolate reductase, and plasma homocysteine concentrations. *Circulation* 93, 7–9.
89. Friso, S., Girelli, D., Trabetti, E., Olivieri, O., Guarini, P., Pignatti, P. F., Corrocher, R., and Choi, S. W. (2005). The MTHFR 1298A>C polymorphism and genomic DNA methylation in human lymphocytes. *Cancer Epidemiol Biomarkers Prev* 14, 938–943.

chapter six

Nutrients, histone modifications, and chromatin remodeling in chronic inflammation

Barbara Delage and Roderick H. Dashwood

Contents

6.1   The epigenetic language

In the nucleus of eukaryotic cells, chromosomal DNA is wrapped around octamers of histone proteins; these octamers consist of paired histones H2A, H2B, H3, and H4. Another histone, called H1 linker, serves to anchor the DNA to each histone octamer, thereby stabilizing the nucleosome. Such packaged DNA around proteins is referred to as the chromatin. The genome is further organized into cytologically distinct and high-order structures called euchromatin and heterochromatin. Euchromatin, usually referred to as being an "open" chromatin conformation, is characterized by its high gene density and transcriptional activity. Heterochromatin contains few genes and is associated with centromeric and telomeric structures. Additionally, heterochromatin consists of the repetitive DNA and transposable elements that are silenced by chromatin condensation. Chromatin conformation correlates with the distinct functions attributed to euchromatin and heterochromatin. Moreover, the structural and functional complexities of chromatin are governed by epigenetic mechanisms that involve, in particular, the addition of chemical groups (e.g., methyl groups) to cytosine residues in DNA and to amino acid residues on histone tails.

Although the importance of posttranslational modifications of histone tails is well recognized in chromatin structure and function, the underlying mechanisms are currently unclear. It was first thought that addition and removal of chemical groups, such as acetyl groups, may modify the charge of lysines and thus regulate histone-protein and histone-DNA interactions.[1] However, histone modifications may also serve to recruit and bind histone-associated proteins that contain highly conserved protein domains, including bromodomain,[2] chromodomain,[3,4] Tudor domain,[5] SET domain,[6] and WD40-repeat domain.[7] These conserved domains are often integrated into complexes that function to effectively "read" modified histones, further altering the epigenome and ultimately affecting a wide range of biological processes. Thus, through dynamic adjustments of the structure and accessibility of chromatin, DNA and histone modifications can change the folding of chromatin and allow the regulation of various cellular processes, such as replication, transcription, and repair. Indeed, the dynamic regulation of chromatin results from the intrinsic lability of histone modifications; this allows cells to adapt rapidly, via changes in gene expression and regulation.[8] Unwrapped DNA requires the specific binding of transcription factors, and condensed chromatin represses transcription. Open chromatin regions, also designated as "active" or "permissive," are sensitive to DNAse I digestion due to the absence of nucleosomes upstream of transcription start sites.[9,10] Indeed, the remodeling of nucleosomes is thought to increase the accessibility to DNA of transcriptional coactivator complexes, which help to initiate transcription.[11] The regulation of gene transcription is, therefore, not only the result of combinatorial interactions of multiple transcription factors able to bind to their specific binding sites in the 5′-promoter regions of genes, but also highly dependent on chromatin conformation.

Histone modifications have been known for about 50 years.[12] However, a growing interest from the scientific community emerged in the 1980s when epigenetic deregulations were associated with carcinogenesis.[13] Alterations in DNA methylation were further correlated with histone modifications in tumor tissues.[14] During the last decade, a number of epigenetic regulatory mechanisms that involve histone modifications and histone-modifying enzymes have been identified and correlated with physiological and pathological processes. The ultimate aim of such research is to decode the epigenetic information. Acetylation, phosphorylation, and methylation of histones have been studied most extensively. Other modifications, such as ubiquitination, SUMOylation,

ADP-ribosylation, carbonylation, deimination, and hydroxylation have been researched, but these modifications need to be better characterized. The interplay between histone modifications has led to the hypothesis of a "histone code,"[15] capable of affecting distinct transcriptional states, although this notion has been open to some debate.[16–18]

Nevertheless, specific patterns of modified histones have been correlated with gene transcription in euchromatin, or with chromatin condensation in heterochromatin. Indeed, hyperacetylated histones, including H3, H4, H2A, and H2B, have been localized in transcriptionally active chromatin, which is also enriched in mono-, di-, and trimethylated H3 at lysine 4 (H3K4) and trimethylated H3K36 and H3K79.[19] The presence of hypermethylated H3K4 reportedly prevents the recruitment of DNA methyltransferase 3-like protein (DNMT3L),[20] a protein that promotes DNA methylation and gene silencing.[21,22] In fact, DNMT3L may only be able to interact with histone H3 when the tail is unmethylated at lysine 4. Under this condition, DNMT3L may facilitate the recruitment of other DNMTs[20] and thereby enhance DNA hypermethylation. Moreover, the active deubiquitination of H2AK119 by 2A-deubiquitinase (2A-DUB) has been related to the increased histone acetylation and histone H1 phosphorylation, which promotes nucleosome displacement and gene activation.[23]

Conversely, ubiquitinated H2A has been co-localized with another repressive modification, hypermethylated H3K27, and could inhibit transcription initiation by preventing H3K4 di- and tri-methylation.[24] The demethylation of trimethylated H3K27 by the ubiquitously transcribed tetratricopeptide repeat, X chromosome (UTX) was logically associated with deubiquitination of H2A, hypermethylation of H3K4, and transcription activation.[25] In contrast, the depletion of UTX was able to induce gene repression and correlated with the presence of polycomb repressive complex 1 (PRC1) together with trimethylated H3K27 in the promoter.[25] H3K27 di- and trimethylation is catalyzed by enhancer of zeste homologue 2 (EZH2), a core protein of polycomb repressive complex 2 (PRC2). H3K27 is further recognized by PRC1,[26] which ensures the maintenance of a silent chromatin state and also promotes H2A ubiquitination.[27] Another PRC2 subunit, suppressor of zeste 12 (SUZ12), has been found to be not only required for H3K27 hypermethylation by EZH2 but also involved in the methylation of H3K9.[28]

Hypermethylated H3K9 is also well known to serve as a recognition mark for the recruitment of heterochromatin protein 1 (HP1) at pericentromeric heterochromatin. G9a histone methyl transferase (HMT) catalyses H3K9 methylation in euchromatin;[29] the HMT Suv39h1 and Suv39h2 methylate H3K9 in heterochromatic regions.[30] Methylated H3K9 is recognized by the bromodomain of HP1, along with other cofactors.[31,32] Although originally thought to have a structural role in heterochromatin assembly,

HP1 accumulation at pericentromeric regions might not be necessary to maintain heterochromatin organization,[33] or for transcription silencing mediated by methylated H3K9 in euchromatin.[31] On the contrary, loss of Suv39h1/h2 can lead to the loss of H3K9 trimethylation and to aberrant heterochromatic organization, as well as defects in chromosome segregation during mitosis and meiosis.[34] Depletion of DNMT1 or DNMT3a/3b has also resulted in loss of hypermethylated H3K9 and alterations in global genome methylation,[35] centromeric function,[36] and telomere integrity.[37] Suv39h1/h2 and methylated H3K9 may be responsible for recruiting DNMTs at pericentromeric heterochromatin[38] and may also prevent the establishment of "permissive" modifications, such as phosphorylation of H3S10 and H3 acetylation.[6,34]

6.2   *Epigenetic deregulation and cancer*

Knudson's two-hit model[39] suggests that cancer initiation requires two somatic mutations in one tumor suppressor gene, leading to a "loss-of-function" phenotype, as epitomized by p53 and adenomatous polyposis coli (APC) in human colorectal cancer. This concept has been revisited in light of the new evidence implicating epigenetic deregulations and chromosome instability in cancer development.[40] Indeed, tumor suppressor genes are often silenced by loss of heterozygosity and promoter hypermethylation, which represent alternative mechanisms for inactivation.

6.2.1   *DNA methylation in cancers*

Changes in the pattern of DNA methylation have been found consistently in tumor tissues.[41,42] Specifically, cytosines in CpG island-enriched promoters, located in nearly half of all genes, are unmethylated in normal tissues; however, they are often highly methylated in tumors. 5-Methylcytosines may be easily deaminated to thymines, which facilitate gene mutation. Moreover, DNA hypermethylation of promoters is associated with condensed chromatin and can efficiently silence tumor suppressor genes, such as those encoding DNA repair proteins, cell cycle regulators, and pro-apoptotic proteins. Accumulating evidence suggests that abnormal DNA methylation and promoter silencing can be detected very early in precancerous tissues, as well as in histologically normal tissues from individuals predisposed to cancer.[43,44] Contrasting with promoter-associated CpG islands, methylated CpG dinucleotides are found in the bulk of the genome (i.e., more than 95% to 98% of DNA) and can be progressively demethylated during the cancer process.[45] Global hypomethylation of this large part of the genome, which mainly consists in noncoding and repetitive sequences, is thought to generate chromatin decondensation and chromosomal instability, thereby predisposing to chromosomal rearrangements associated with cancer.[46] A great deal more work is needed, however, to fully substantiate the generality of this hypothesis.

Although aberrations in DNA methylation are recognized as hallmarks of cancer, the specific mechanisms driving such events are unclear. In tumors, alterations in DNA methylation are likely caused by deregulations in DNMT recruitment, expression, or activity. In mammals, DNA methylation is established by five DNMTs: DNMT1, 2, 3a, 3b, and 3L. De novo DNA methylation is mainly carried out by DNMT3a and 3b, while DNMT1 and, to a certain extent, DNMT3b[35,47] ensure the maintenance of methylation. Aberrant expression of DNMTs has been observed in certain cancers[48,49] and may be responsible for promoter hypermethylation.[50] This also includes DNMT1, although the enzyme has a preference for hemimethylated DNA. Overexpression of DNMT1 induces regional DNA hypermethylation.[35,51] The rare deficiency in DNMT3b activity, detected in the syndrome immunodeficiency, centromeric region instability, facial anomalies (ICF), has been associated with pericentromeric hypomethylation and a predisposition to loss of heterochromatin and corresponding genome instability.[52]

However, not all tumors exhibit altered levels of DNMTs, and recent findings strongly suggest that DNMTs can be mistargeted to specific DNA sequences by other proteins. For example, hypermethylated CpG islands in silent promoters were associated with "repressive" histone modifications, such as hypoacetylated histones, hypomethylated H3K4, and hypermethylated H3K27 and H4K20. Co-localization of methylated CpG and modified histones at the same promoter suggests coordination or communication between DNMTs and histone-modifying enzymes in order to trigger and stabilize gene silencing. Several publications have documented that "repressive" histone modifications may precede DNA methylation within regulatory regions, and even be a prerequisite for DNMT recruitment. While Suv39h1 may certainly play an essential role for DNMT recruitment at heterochromatin,[38] the PRC2 subunit EZH2 targets DNMTs to promoters, leading to the methylation of CpG islands and aberrant gene repression.[53,54] Likewise, G9a HMT deficiency can induce hypomethylation of CpG islands;[55] this suggests that the enzyme may direct DNA methylation by promoting H3K9 methylation and HP1 binding.[56] These data also imply that deregulation and mistargeting of HMTs may lead to aberrant DNA methylation. Moreover, the interplay between epigenetic changes[22,57] may drive histone-modifying enzymes to recruit repressive complexes that remodel chromatin and promote aberrant gene silencing.

6.2.2   Histone acetylation and cancers

Deregulation of histone acetylation has been shown to contribute to the neoplastic process. For instance, global genome deacetylation has been correlated recently with a high risk of prostate tumor recurrence.[58] As mentioned earlier, silent chromatin is enriched in deacetylated histones, whereas active chromatin is hyperacetylated. The removal of an acetyl group from histone tails is catalyzed by histone deacetylases (HDACs); in contrast, histone acetyl transferases (HATs) add acetyl groups to lysines on histone tails. To date, 18 HDAC members have been identified and classified into four groups depending on their homology with yeast proteins: class I, class II, class III, and class IV. Class I (HDAC1–3 and HDAC8), class II (HDAC4–7 and HDAC9–10), and class IV (HDAC11) constitute the classical HDACs, because they share sequence similarity and also the need of Zn^{2+} for deacetylase activity. In contrast, class III HDACs (SIRT1–7), often called sirtuins, catalyze deacetylation in an NAD^+-dependent manner and are generally nonresponsive to inhibitors of classical HDACs (e.g., trichostatin A, TSA). Under certain conditions, histone deacetylation by HDACs may antagonize or block the transcriptional activation of tumor suppressor genes, thereby promoting cancer development. This has been well documented in various cancers[59–61] and has been attributed to the overexpression of class I HDACs in tumor tissues and cancer cell lines.[62] HDAC2 was implicated, for example, in the development of spontaneous intestinal polyps in *Apc*[min] mice.[63]

Aberrant promoter deacetylation also may be attributed to HDAC mistargeting, which leads to inappropriate inhibition of gene expression. Mistargeted HDACs have been implicated in a variety of leukemias that are characterized by the lack of myeloid differentiation. For example, acute promyelocytic leukemia (APL) is caused by the expression of proteins resulting from the fusion of promyelocytic leukemia gene (PML) or promyelocytic zinc-finger gene (PLZF) to RARα gene encoding the retinoic acid-activated receptor alpha (reviewed elsewhere[64]). Wild-type RAR_ protein, activated by retinoic acid (RA), can induce expression of target genes involved in promyeloblast differentiation, but the fusion proteins appear insensitive to RA and block myeloblast differentiation by recruiting corepressors such as NcoR/SMRT, mSin3 and HDACs,[65] as well as HMTs[66,67] and DNMTs.[68] Inappropriate recruitment of HDACs also has been implicated in other translocation-induced leukemias.[69]

Alterations in acetylation-related gene expression may also be associated with aberrant HAT activity. HAT enzymes are classified into several families. These include the GNAT (Gcn5-related *N*-acetyltransferase) family with GCN5 and p/CAF (p300/CBP-associated factor), the MYST (MOZ, YBF2/SAS3 and TIP60) family, p300/CBP (cAMP response element-binding protein), and nuclear receptor coactivators, such as SRC-1 and TIF-2. A recent report provided an elegant account of the structural basis of protein acetylation by the p300/CBP transcriptional coactivator.[70]

Rubenstein-Taybi syndrome, characterized by mental retardation and skeletal abnormalities, has been associated with predisposition to some types of cancer.[71] This dominant disorder is usually caused by heterozygous mutation of the CBP-encoding gene, with loss of CBP acetyltransferase activity,[72] and, in rare cases, by mutation of p300.[73] Opposed to HDACs, CBP and p300 HAT activity appear to be required for the transcriptional activation of tumor suppressor genes.[74–76] However, their overexpression may also contribute to tumor development.[77] In fact, as with HDACs, chromosomal rearrangements involving HATs have been associated with defects in hematopoietic cell maturation. The expression of a number of fusion proteins combining the MYST family proteins MOZ and MORF, or MLL (HMT homologous to *Drosophila* Trithorax), to CBP,[78,79] p300[80,81] or TIF2[82] has been found to prevent leukemogenesis, although the mechanisms are not yet understood.

Various reports have also implicated different HAT enzymes in the transcription mediated by viral proteins exhibiting cancer-promoting properties. Indeed, the replication of viruses, oncogenic or not, is usually achieved through the corruption of the host transcriptional machinery for the benefit of the viral gene expression and virus multiplication. Examples given by the Epstein-Barr virus nuclear protein 2 (Epstein-Barr virus),[83] the viral oncoprotein SV40 large T antigen (SV40 virus),[84] the adenoviral oncoprotein E1A (adenovirus),[85] and the proviral protein Tax (human T cell leukemia virus type-1)[86] illustrate the efficient regulation of viral and cellular gene expression via the recruitment of coactivators p300, CBP, or PCAF to target promoters. This is in direct support of HAT activity in coactivator complexes that regulate genes involved in diverse cellular functions, such as proliferation, differentiation, and apoptosis. Depending on the target genes, the gain of HAT function may induce the expression of oncoproteins, while a loss of activity can lead to improper gene silencing. The recruitment of multiple HATs, such as Gnc5, p/CAF, and p300, by Ada3 to estrogen-responsive promoters has been associated with the hormone-dependent proliferation of breast cancer cells.[87] Ada3, together with Gnc5 and p/CAF in coactivator complexes, was also required for tumor suppressor p53 transcriptional activity, because p53 acetylation increases its promoter-binding activity.[88]

Histones are not exclusive targets for HAT enzymes, which also catalyze the acetylation of a number of coactivators, corepressors, and transcription factors. P300-dependent acetylation of E2F1 has been involved in increasing E2F1 half-life in response to DNA damage[89] and might initiate E2F1-induced cell death.[90] However, elevated expression of E2F1 has also been associated with neoplastic transformation. Interestingly, the presence of highly expressed E2F1 may increase cell sensitivity to HDAC inhibitor (HDACi)-induced apoptosis.[91] However, although the HDACi suberoylanilide hydroxamic acid (SAHA) and TSA did not enhance E2F1 acetylation, it is not known if HDACi-induced apoptosis is mediated by an increased recruitment of HATs at E2F1-responsive promoters. This is, however, the proof-of-concept that targeting HAT or/and HDAC enzymes therapeutically may constitute an efficient strategy to oppose deregulations in pathways that lead to cancer.

6.3   Epigenetic deregulation, chronic inflammation, and natural therapeutics

6.3.1   Chronic inflammation: The cradle of cancer

Chronic inflammation has been implicated in a large variety of disorders, including cardiovascular diseases, diabetes mellitus, arthritis, Alzheimer's disease, pulmonary diseases, and autoimmune diseases. Inflammation also appears to be a risk factor for a great number of cancers. Some conditions, such as infection by the bacteria *Helicobacter pylori* or ulcerative colitis, illustrate the role of inflammation in the occurrence of digestive cancers.[92] Pro-inflammatory mediators have been associated with every step of cancer development, from initiation and promotion to progression and metastasis.[93,94] Leukocytes are immune cells that produce a number of pro-inflammatory, growth-stimulating, and pro-angiogenic factors; leukocytes also generate oxygen intermediates and metalloproteinases, which promote tumorigenesis.

Pro-inflammatory stimuli, such as endotoxins (lipopolysaccharide, LPS) and tumor necrosis factor alpha (TNF-α) regulate several key genes through two transcription factors that mediate the pro-inflammatory response: NFκB and AP-1. Because these transcription factors are critical in orchestrating the immune response, they are also potential therapeutic targets for diseases involving chronic inflammation, including neurodegenerative diseases, autoimmune diseases, and cancers. Recently, chromatin remodeling has been implicated in the regulation of gene expression mediated by NFκB and AP-1.[95,96] In a number of inflammation-associated pathologies, alterations in the expression and recruitment of histone-modifying enzymes, and thus changes in histone acetylation, are believed to play a crucial role in the unbalanced pro-inflammatory/anti-inflammatory gene expression profiles observed.[97] Finally, steroid-induced suppression of inflammation, as well as beneficial effects from treatment with naturally occurring compounds, might be influenced by the presence of chromatin modifiers (Figure 6.1).

Figure 6.1 **(Opposite)** (*A color version of this figure follows page 20.*) Regulation of chromatin structure influences the expression of pro-inflammatory genes. The recruitment of cofactors with HAT activity, stimulated by pro-oxidants, increases NFκB transcriptional activity and pro-inflammatory gene expression. In contrast, glucocorticoids and natural chromatin-modifying agents trigger HDAC recruitment and HAT inhibition, which results in NFκB inactivation, histone deacetylation, and blockade of the inflammatory process.

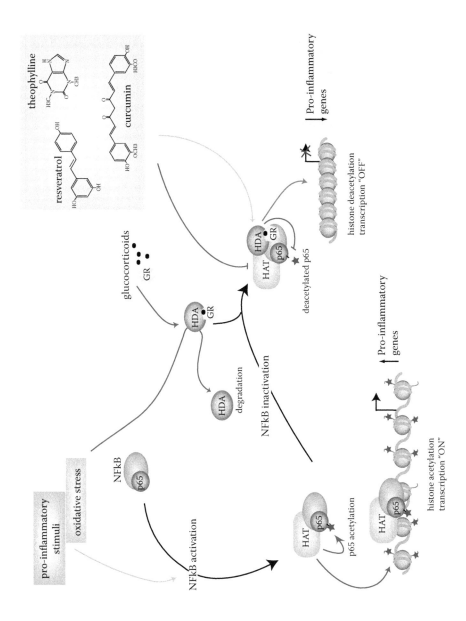

Figure 6.1.

6.3.2 Targeting HAT and HDAC enzymes with dietary and other natural compounds

See Table 6.1. Glucocorticoids are highly efficient at inhibiting inflammation in a number of chronic inflammatory disorders, such as asthma, rheumatoid arthritis, and inflammatory bowel diseases. This anti-inflammatory action is mediated by glucocorticoid receptors (GR) in the cytoplasm that dimerize and translocate to the nucleus, where they bind to the consensus glucocorticoid response element (GRE) on target gene promoters. The increased expression of anti-inflammatory factors, including IL-10, IκBα (inhibitor of NFκB), and MAP kinase phosphatase 1 (MKP1), inactivates MAP kinases and downstream transcription factors, like AP-1.[98] Glucocorticoids may also block the transcription of genes that encode pro-inflammatory proteins such as cytokines, enzymes, receptors, and adhesion molecules. This appears to be mediated by

Table 6.1 Examples of dietary compounds able to modulate HAT or HDAC activities and exhibiting anti-inflammatory potentials

Plant sources	Dietary components	References
Modulators of classic HDAC		
Allium sativum L. (garlic)		160, 161
	Diallyl disulfide (DADS)	
	S-allylmercaptocysteine	
	Allyl mercaptan	
Dietary fiber fermentation	Butyrate	156
Brassicaceae family		159, 162, 163
Broccoli sprouts	Sulforaphane	
Japanese horseradish (wasabi)	6-methylsulfinylhexyl-isothiocyanate	
Modulators of SIRT		164
Vitis vinifera (red grapes, wines)	Resveratrol	120, 165
Rhus verniciflua (stems)	Butein	166, 167
Rhus toxicodendron (leaves)	Fisetin	168, 169
Apple, tea, onion, nuts, berries,	Quercetin	170, 171, 172
Blueberries	Piceatannol	173
Sweet red pepper, celery, parsley	Luteolin	174
Modulators of HAT		
Curcuma longa (tumeric roots)	Curcumin	125
Garcina indica (fruit)	Garcinol	175, 176
Camellia sinensis (black and green tea)	Theophylline	110, 112

GRE-independent mechanisms. Glucocorticoid receptors suppress iNOS expression, and thus NO generation, by blocking AP-1- and NFκB-activated transcription.[99,100] It is also possible for GR to promote NFκB sequestration in the cytosolic compartment or alter the DNA-binding activity of NFκB.[101] Interestingly, naturally occurring HDACi, such as TSA (isolated from bacteria *Streptomyces*) and apicidin (isolated from fungi *Fusarium*), also suppress the inhibitory effects of glucocorticoids on LPS-induced iNOS mRNA expression in macrophages.[102] Similarly, HDAC1 was able to interact with GR and to potentiate GR-mediated repression of IL5 gene transcription in human T-helper 2 lymphocytes (Th2).[103] This strongly suggested that histone deacetylation was required for glucocorticoid mediated-transcriptional suppression. Moreover, Th2-driven epithelium activation in asthma, efficiently repressed by inhaled corticosteroids,[104] has been associated with altered HAT and HDAC activities in the alveolar macrophages of untreated asthmatic patients.[105] The reduction in HDAC activity, together with the increased HAT activity, detected in bronchial biopsies of asthmatic patients,[106] is thought to promote NFκB proinflammatory function[107] (Figure 6.1).

A natural compound extracted from tea leaves (*Camellia sinensis*), theophylline (also called dimethylxanthine), was first recognized as a phosphodiesterase inhibitor and has long been used in the treatment of respiratory diseases like asthma.[108,109] Recently, theophylline has been reported to enhance HDAC activity.[110,111] Theophyllin was able to potentiate the glucocorticoid-induced increase in HDAC activity and the decrease of IL-8 production in LPS-challenged bronchoalveolar macrophages isolated from asthmatic patients.[110] Moreover, the decrease in histone H4 acetylation within the NFκB-responsive GM-CSF promoter[110] suggested the recruitment and activation of class I HDACs[107,110] by combined treatment in human lung cells. It is, however, not known if theophylline stimulated HDAC2-induced GR deacetylation, which may be required for the suppression of NFκB function by GR.[112]

The correlation between HDAC activity and the inhibitory effect of glucocorticoids on anti-inflammatory gene expression has been further supported by the reduction in HDAC (especially HDAC2) expression and activity found in patients with chronic obstructive pulmonary disease (COPD).[101,113] Loss of HDAC2 was indeed associated with unresponsiveness to glucocorticoids.[114,115] Recognized as an important factor triggering COPD, cigarette smoke induces oxidative stress and affects the anti-inflammatory effect of corticosteroids,[116] at least in part, through H_2O_2- and peroxynitrite-induced alterations in HAT and HDAC activities.[101] Thus, HDACs are clearly necessary for glucocorticoid-activated anti-inflammatory processes. Accordingly, increased HDAC activity by theophylline may be an interesting therapeutic approach to overcome the glucocorticoid resistance in COPD[111] and in steroid-resistant asthma.[117]

Clinical investigations combining theophylline with glucocorticoid treatment may be informative.

Other possible natural therapies for inflammatory conditions are resveratrol and structurally related plant polyphenols (e.g., butein, fisetin, and quercetin). Resveratrol, found in the skin of red grapes (*Vitis vinifera*) and in red wine, is an antioxidant with potential anticancer, anti-inflammatory, and antiaging properties. The therapeutic interest in resveratrol has been mainly attributed to its ability to control oxidative stress[118] and to activate the NAD+-dependent sirtuins.[119] A recent study revealed that SIRT1 and SIRT2 were dramatically decreased in monocyte-macrophage cells in vitro and rat lungs exposed to cigarette smoke.[120] A similar reduction of SIRT1 was reported in lungs of smokers and COPD patients.[121] This was associated with increased acetylation of the NFκB subunit, p65, which promotes NFκB-induced cytokine expression and release. This also suggested the possibility for p65 to be deacetylated and inactivated in the presence of the deacetylase SIRT1. Resveratrol increased SIRT1 deacetylase activity and inhibited the release of cigarette smoke-induced pro-inflammatory mediators in vitro.[120] However, it is not known whether resveratrol could prevent SIRT nitration and degradation, which is associated with oxidative stress.[121] It will also be of interest to investigate the capacity of resveratrol to improve corticosteroid sensitivity in asthmatic and COPD patients.

Curcumin (diferuloymethane) is another polyphenolic plant compound, found in the rhizome of the Indian curry spice, turmeric (*Curcuma longa L.*). Curcumin is used worldwide as a flavoring and coloring agent. In addition to growing evidence for cancer preventative and therapeutic properties,[122–124] curcumin might be a useful dietary tool to treat inflammation. Indeed, curcumin was shown to interfere with NFκB activation and activity in a significant number of inflammatory diseases[125,126] and may potentially increase the efficacy of glucocorticoids. Curcumin could impair NFκB translocation to the nucleus through inhibition of IKKα phosphorylation and IkBα degradation.[127]

It is also conceivable that curcumin-induced reductions in histone acetylation participate in the inhibition of NFκB-induced inflammation. The capacity of curcumin to specifically inhibit HAT p300 enzymatic activity and upregulate its proteasome-dependent degradation has been highlighted recently.[128,129] Therefore, through inhibiting NFκB,[127,130] curcumin may alter the recruitment of HAT in coactivator complexes and the chromatin remodeling required for NFκB-induced transcription of pro-inflammatory mediators[131] in lung cells challenged by cigarette smoke. This may also explain the inhibition of TNFα-induced p65 acetylation by curcumin, which was recently observed in human myeloid leukemia cells.[132] In a rat model of bleomycin-induced pulmonary fibrosis, Xu et al.[133] have shown that hydrocortisone and curcumin separately decreased lung inflammation and collagen content by targeting similar proteins (i.e., Col-1, iNOS, and TGF-β1). Examination of a combined treatment could be of great interest in order to evaluate potential synergistic effects. Other natural compounds like anacardic acid (*Anacardium occidentale*)[134] and garcinol (*Garcinia indica*)[135] may also be of interest, because both are HAT inhibitors.

Although the use of HDAC inhibitors may possibly worsen the aforementioned inflammatory diseases,[136] a great deal of interest has developed in their use for blocking inflammation at other sites, as illustrated by inflammatory bowel diseases (IBD: ulcerative colitis and Crohn disease), systemic lupus erythematosus, and rheumatoid arthritis.[137] Reductions in disease severity have been associated with increased histone acetylation at inflammatory sites in dextran sodium sulfate (DSS)-induced colitis in mice treated with the synthetic HDACi valproic acid (VPA).[138] Anti-inflammatory effects of HDACi have been described mainly for the hydroxamic acids, TSA and SAHA. Nevertheless, butyrate, a short-chain fatty acid identified 50 years ago, appears to be efficient at blocking inflammation in certain digestive tract-related diseases. Butyrate is the main end product of the intestinal microbial fermentation of dietary fibers. Low consumption of soluble fibers (along with "unhealthy" nutritional habits, i.e., high consumption of saturated fat, simple sugars, or well-done meat) has been associated with ulcerative colitis[139] and heightened risk of developing colorectal cancers.[140,141] Among possible mechanisms, butyrate could decrease TNFα-induced IκBα proteosome-dependent degradation by downregulating the mRNA expression of proteasome subunits[142] and by blocking TNFα-induced cyclooxygenase 2 (COX2),[143] a known NFκB target in colon cancer cells. COX2, which converts arachidonic acid into prostaglandins, is deregulated in ulcerative colitis,[144] as well as in colorectal tumors.[145] COX2 regulation by butyrate is unclear, but it may involve chromatin remodeling. Butyrate may also interfere with the recruitment and migration of circulating leukocytes to the areas of inflammation; this may play a critical role in IBD.[146] Specifically, the expression of vascular cell adhesion molecules (VCAM) and intracellular adhesion molecules (ICAM) by endothelial cells, correlated with leukocyte adhesion, was blocked by butyrate through an NFκB-dependent mechanism.[147,148] Butyrate prevented p65 translocation and blocked NFκB activation by TNFα but no change in NFκB acetylation status was detected.

Butyrate also might offer some benefit in neuroinflammation-associated diseases. Activation of microglial cells (brain macrophages) is required for protection from microorganism invasion. It also facilitates communication between neurons, astrocytes and microglia with cytokines, trophic factors and neuromodulators. However, it is believed that the pathological activation of microglia may be toxic to neurons, leading to neurodegeneration, as observed in multiple sclerosis, Alzheimer, Parkinson and Huntington diseases, as well as in cerebral ischemia (stroke).[149] In these pathologies, microglial hyperactivation has been associated with neuroinflammation.[150] Specifically, brain excitotoxicity has been related to the release of pro-inflammatory cytokines (TNFα, IL1, IL6, IL12) as well as nitric oxide (NO) and reactive oxygen species (ROS). LPS, a gram-negative cell wall component, and the pro-inflammatory interferon-γ (IFN-γ) are well known to activate, through distinct pathways, the microglia. Butyrate pretreatment suppressed LPS-mediated inflammation in primary cultures of astrocytes, microglia, and cerebellar granule cells,[151] but not in transformed microglial cells.[151,152] However, butyrate also suppressed IFN-γ-induced iNOS mRNA expression, NO generation, and altered NFκB DNA-binding activity in mouse transformed BV-2 microglial cell line.[152] VPA, commonly used as a mood stabilizer, also exhibited neuroprotective activity[153] and anti-inflammatory effects through the inhibition of LPS-induced microglia activation.[154] Specifically, VPA pretreatment prevented the production of TNF-α and, to a lesser extent, ROS and NO induced by LPS.[155] However, the mechanisms underlying the modulation of inflammation by VPA and butyrate have not yet been investigated. Therefore, the possibility that inhibition of HDAC by VPA and butyrate interferes with LPS- and TNF-α-activated gene expression still needs to be considered. Interestingly, histone deacetylation, observed in the brain hemisphere affected by a permanent middle cerebral artery occlusion-inducing stroke (pMCAO rodent model), was blocked by butyrate, TSA, and VPA postischemic injections.[156] Neuroprotection provided by these HDACi was mediated by the downregulation of neuroinflammation-promoting enzymes (i.e., inducible NO synthase and COX2) and the regulation of apoptotic mediators (i.e., increase in HSP70 and Bcl2 levels, decrease in Bak and Bid levels).[157,158] If neuroinflammation is, at least in part, related to a HAT/HDAC imbalance, the use of HDACi may be considered for the treatment of other inflammatory diseases affecting the central nervous system, such as multiple sclerosis.[157] Other dietary approaches with chromatin modifying agents, such as the isothiocyanate sulforaphane (*Brassica* family members, such as broccoli) or organosulfur compounds diallyl disulfide and its derivative allyl mercaptan from garlic (*Allium sativum* L.), may also alter NFκB function and markedly attenuate aberrant activation of inflammatory processes.[159]

However, HDAC inhibitors differentially impact inflammatory pathways depending on the nature of the compound used, which may affect other biological targets (e.g., oxidants and regulators of cell cycle).[151] In addition, although dietary HAT and HDAC modulators can affect NFκB pro-inflammatory function in several inflammatory diseases, the mechanisms of action still need to be examined more carefully.[125]

6.4   Conclusions

There continues to be a great deal of interest in the role of epigenetics in normal physiology and in various pathological conditions, including several diseases with an underlying inflammatory component. There is a delicate balance here, in that low-level inflammation is considered beneficial and important for surveillance purposes, in rapidly responding to exogenous insults such as bacterial infection, but too much inflammation can provoke an oxidative stress scenario. The general paradigm of an HDAC inhibitor working in the cancer therapeutic setting via "de-repression" of aberrantly silenced genes is appealing but, in some cases, the toxic insult, such as cigarette smoke, can attenuate absolute expression levels of HDACs. In the latter case, treatment regimens may seek to increase, rather than decrease HDAC activity, reestablishing homeostatic norms, and repressing certain gene expression pathways related to inflammation and cytokine signaling.[95] This aspect reemphasizes the possible "double-edged sword" of epigenetic interventions, discussed elsewhere in the context of the different HDAC classes and their downstream pathways.[64] One approach may be to adopt a cocktail of agents, in which several different mechanisms are targeted simultaneously, such as an HDAC inhibitor and one or more agents that block the activity of DNA methyltransferases. The growing list of natural dietary compounds with an epigenetic mechanism of action (Table 6.1) is adding an interesting new angle to this story, and one that is likely to develop in exciting new directions in the future.

References

1. Shogren-Knaak, M., Ishii, H., Sun, J. M., Pazin, M. J., Davie, J. R., and Peterson, C. L. (2006). Histone H4-K16 acetylation controls chromatin structure and protein interactions. *Science* 311, 844–847.
2. Jacobson, R. H., Ladurner, A. G., King, D. S., and Tjian, R. (2000). Structure and function of a human TAFII250 double bromodomain module. *Science* 288, 1422–1425.
3. Bannister, A. J., Zegerman, P., Partridge, J. F., Miska, E. A., Thomas, J. O., Allshire, R. C., and Kouzarides, T. (2001). Selective recognition of methylated lysine 9 on histone H3 by the HP1 chromo domain. *Nature* 410, 120–124.
4. Pray-Grant, M. G., Daniel, J. A., Schieltz, D., Yates, J. R. III, and Grant, P. A. (2005). Chd1 chromodomain links histone H3 methylation with SAGA- and SLIK-dependent acetylation. *Nature* 433, 434–438.
5. Huyen, Y., Zgheib, O., Ditullio, R. A., Jr., Gorgoulis, V. G., Zacharatos, P., Petty, T. J., Sheston, E. A., Mellert, H. S., Stavridi, E. S., and Halazonetis, T. D. (2004). Methylated lysine 79 of histone H3 targets 53BP1 to DNA double-strand breaks. *Nature* 432, 406–411.
6. Rea, S., Eisenhaber, F., O'Carroll, D., Strahl, B. D., Sun, Z. W., Schmid, M., Opravil, S., Mechtler, K., Ponting, C. P., Allis, C. D., and Jenuwein, T. (2000). Regulation of chromatin structure by site-specific histone H3 methyltransferases. *Nature* 406, 593–599.

7. Wysocka, J., Swigut, T., Milne, T. A., Dou, Y., Zhang, X., Burlingame, A. L., Roeder, R. G., Brivanlou, A. H., and Allis, C. D. (2005). WDR5 associates with histone H3 methylated at K4 and is essential for H3 K4 methylation and vertebrate development. *Cell* 121, 859–872.

8. Berger, S. L. (2002). Histone modifications in transcriptional regulation. *Curr Opin Genet Dev* 12, 142–148.

9. Ozsolak, F., Song, J. S., Liu, X. S., and Fisher, D. E. (2007). High-throughput mapping of the chromatin structure of human promoters. *Nat Biotechnol* 25, 244–248.

10. Heintzman, N. D., Stuart, R. K., Hon, G., Fu, Y., Ching, C. W., Hawkins, R. D., Barrera, L. O., Van Calcar, S., Qu, C., Ching, K. A., Wang, W., Weng, Z., Green, R. D., Crawford, G. E., and Ren, B. (2007). Distinct and predictive chromatin signatures of transcriptional promoters and enhancers in the human genome. *Nat Genet* 39, 311–318.

11. Li, B., Carey, M., and Workman, J. L. (2007). The role of chromatin during transcription. *Cell* 128, 707–719.

12. Allfrey, V. G., Faulkner, R., and Mirsky, A. E. (1964). Acetylation and methylation of histones and their possible role in the regulation of RNA synthesis. *Proc Natl Acad Sci USA* 51, 786–794.

13. Feinberg, A. P., and Vogelstein, B. (1983). Hypomethylation distinguishes genes of some human cancers from their normal counterparts. *Nature* 301, 89–92.

14. Esteller, M., and Herman, J. G. (2002). Cancer as an epigenetic disease: DNA methylation and chromatin alterations in human tumours. *J Pathol* 196, 1–7.

15. Turner, B. M. (1993). Decoding the nucleosome. *Cell* 75, 5–8.

16. Dion, M. F., Altschuler, S. J., Wu, L. F., and Rando, O. J. (2005). Genomic characterization reveals a simple histone H4 acetylation code. *Proc Natl Acad Sci USA* 102, 5501–5506.

17. Henikoff, S. (2005). Histone modifications: Combinatorial complexity or cumulative simplicity? *Proc Natl Acad Sci USA* 102, 5308–5309.

18. Liu, C. L., Kaplan, T., Kim, M., Buratowski, S., Schreiber, S. L., Friedman, N., and Rando, O. J. (2005). Single-nucleosome mapping of histone modifications in *S. cerevisiae*. *PLoS Biol* 3, e328.

19. Vakoc, C. R., Sachdeva, M. M., Wang, H., and Blobel, G. A. (2006). Profile of histone lysine methylation across transcribed mammalian chromatin. *Mol Cell Biol* 26, 9185–9195.

20. Ooi, S. K., Qiu, C., Bernstein, E., Li, K., Jia, D., Yang, Z., Erdjument-Bromage, H., Tempst, P., Lin, S. P., Allis, C. D., Cheng, X., and Bestor, T. H. (2007). DNMT3L connects unmethylated lysine 4 of histone H3 to de novo methylation of DNA. *Nature* 448, 714–717.

21. Jia, D., Jurkowska, R. Z., Zhang, X., Jeltsch, A., and Cheng, X. (2007). Structure of Dnmt3a bound to Dnmt3L suggests a model for de novo DNA methylation. *Nature* 449, 248–251.

22. Deplus, R., Brenner, C., Burgers, W. A., Putmans, P., Kouzarides, T., de Launoit, Y., and Fuks, F. (2002). Dnmt3L is a transcriptional repressor that recruits histone deacetylase. *Nucleic Acids Res* 30, 3831–3838.

23. Zhu, P., Zhou, W., Wang, J., Puc, J., Ohgi, K. A., Erdjument-Bromage, H., Tempst, P., Glass, C. K., and Rosenfeld, M. G. (2007). A histone H2A deubiquitinase complex coordinating histone acetylation and H1 dissociation in transcriptional regulation. *Mol Cell* 27, 609–621.

24. Nakagawa, T., Kajitani, T., Togo, S., Masuko, N., Ohdan, H., Hishikawa, Y., Koji, T., Matsuyama, T., Ikura, T., Muramatsu, M., and Ito, T. (2008). Deubiquitylation of histone H2A activates transcriptional initiation via trans-histone cross-talk with H3K4 di- and trimethylation. *Genes Dev* 22, 37–49.

25. Lee, M. G., Villa, R., Trojer, P., Norman, J., Yan, K. P., Reinberg, D., Di Croce, L., and Shiekhattar, R. (2007). Demethylation of H3K27 regulates polycomb recruitment and H2A ubiquitination. *Science* 318, 447–450.

26. Hernandez-Munoz, I., Taghavi, P., Kuijl, C., Neefjes, J., and van Lohuizen, M. (2005). Association of BMI1 with polycomb bodies is dynamic and requires PRC2/EZH2 and the maintenance DNA methyltransferase DNMT1. *Mol Cell Biol* 25, 11047–11058.

27. Cao, R., Tsukada, Y., and Zhang, Y. (2005). Role of BMI-1 and RING1A in H2A ubiquitylation and Hox gene silencing. *Mol Cell* 20, 845–854.

28. de la Cruz, C. C., Kirmizis, A., Simon, M. D., Isono, K., Koseki, H., and Panning, B. (2007). The polycomb group protein SUZ12 regulates histone H3 lysine 9 methylation and HP1 alpha distribution. *Chromosome Res* 15, 299–314.

29. Tachibana, M., Sugimoto, K., Nozaki, M., Ueda, J., Ohta, T., Ohki, M., Fukuda, M., Takeda, N., Niida, H., Kato, H., and Shinkai, Y. (2002). G9a histone methyltransferase plays a dominant role in euchromatic histone H3 lysine 9 methylation and is essential for early embryogenesis. *Genes Dev* 16, 1779–1791.

30. Lehnertz, B., Ueda, Y., Derijck, A. A., Braunschweig, U., Perez-Burgos, L., Kubicek, S., Chen, T., Li, E., Jenuwein, T., and Peters, A. H. (2003). Suv39h-mediated histone H3 lysine 9 methylation directs DNA methylation to major satellite repeats at pericentric heterochromatin. *Curr Biol* 13, 1192–1200.

31. Stewart, M. D., Li, J., and Wong, J. (2005). Relationship between histone H3 lysine 9 methylation, transcription repression, and heterochromatin protein 1 recruitment. *Mol Cell Biol* 25, 2525–2538.

32. Eskeland, R., Eberharter, A., and Imhof, A. (2007). HP1 binding to chromatin methylated at H3K9 is enhanced by auxiliary factors. *Mol Cell Biol* 27, 453–465.

33. Mateos-Langerak, J., Brink, M. C., Luijsterburg, M. S., van der Kraan, I., van Driel, R., and Verschure, P. J. (2007). Pericentromeric heterochromatin domains are maintained without accumulation of HP1. *Mol Biol Cell* 18, 1464–1471.

34. Peters, A. H., O'Carroll, D., Scherthan, H., Mechtler, K., Sauer, S., Schofer, C., Weipoltshammer, K., Pagani, M., Lachner, M., Kohlmaier, A., Opravil, S., Doyle, M., Sibilia, M., and Jenuwein, T. (2001). Loss of the Suv39h histone methyltransferases impairs mammalian heterochromatin and genome stability. *Cell* 107, 323–337.

35. Rhee, I., Bachman, K. E., Park, B. H., Jair, K. W., Yen, R. W., Schuebel, K. E., Cui, H., Feinberg, A. P., Lengauer, C., Kinzler, K. W., Baylin, S. B., and Vogelstein, B. (2002). DNMT1 and DNMT3b cooperate to silence genes in human cancer cells. *Nature* 416, 552–556.

36. Dodge, J. E., Okano, M., Dick, F., Tsujimoto, N., Chen, T., Wang, S., Ueda, Y., Dyson, N., and Li, E. (2005). Inactivation of DNMT3b in mouse embryonic fibroblasts results in DNA hypomethylation, chromosomal instability, and spontaneous immortalization. *J Biol Chem* 280, 17986–17991.

37. Gonzalo, S., Jaco, I., Fraga, M. F., Chen, T., Li, E., Esteller, M., and Blasco, M. A. (2006). DNA methyltransferases control telomere length and telomere recombination in mammalian cells. *Nat Cell Biol* 8, 416–424.

38. Fuks, F., Hurd, P. J., Deplus, R., and Kouzarides, T. (2003). The DNA methyltransferases associate with HP1 and the SUV39H1 histone methyltransferase. *Nucleic Acids Res* 31, 2305–2312.

39. Knudson, A. G., Jr. (1971). Mutation and cancer: Statistical study of retinoblastoma. *Proc Natl Acad Sci USA* 68, 820–823.

40. Mastrangelo, D., De Francesco, S., Di Leonardo, A., Lentini, L., and Hadjistilianou, T. (2007). Does the evidence matter in medicine? The retinoblastoma paradigm. *Int J Cancer* 121, 2501–2505.

41. Jones, P. A., and Baylin, S. B. (2002). The fundamental role of epigenetic events in cancer. *Nat Rev Genet* 3, 415–428.

42. Ushijima, T. (2005). Detection and interpretation of altered methylation patterns in cancer cells. *Nat Rev Cancer* 5, 223–231.

43. Kanai, Y., and Hirohashi, S. (2007). Alterations of DNA methylation associated with abnormalities of DNA methyltransferases in human cancers during transition from a precancerous to a malignant state. *Carcinogenesis* 28, 2434–2442.

44. Hao, C. Y., Moore, D. H., Wong, P., Bennington, J. L., Lee, N. M., and Chen, L. C. (2005). Alteration of gene expression in macroscopically normal colonic mucosa from individuals with a family history of sporadic colon cancer. *Clin Cancer Res* 11, 1400–1407.

45. Cravo, M., Pinto, R., Fidalgo, P., Chaves, P., Gloria, L., Nobre-Leitao, C., and Costa Mira, F. (1996). Global DNA hypomethylation occurs in the early stages of intestinal type gastric carcinoma. *Gut* 39, 434–438.

46. Rodriguez, J., Frigola, J., Vendrell, E., Risques, R. A., Fraga, M. F., Morales, C., Moreno, V., Esteller, M., Capella, G., Ribas, M., and Peinado, M. A. (2006). Chromosomal instability correlates with genome-wide DNA demethylation in human primary colorectal cancers. *Cancer Res* 66, 8462–9468.

47. Rhee, I., Jair, K. W., Yen, R. W., Lengauer, C., Herman, J. G., Kinzler, K. W., Vogelstein, B., Baylin, S. B., and Schuebel, K. E. (2000). CpG methylation is maintained in human cancer cells lacking DNMT1. *Nature* 404, 1003–1007.

48. Girault, I., Tozlu, S., Lidereau, R., and Bieche, I. (2003). Expression analysis of DNA methyltransferases 1, 3A, and 3B in sporadic breast carcinomas. *Clin Cancer Res* 9, 4415–4422.

49. Kn, H., Bassal, S., Tikellis, C., and El-Osta, A. (2004). Expression analysis of the epigenetic methyltransferases and methyl-CpG binding protein families in the normal B-cell and B-cell chronic lymphocytic leukemia (CLL). *Cancer Biol Ther* 3, 989–994.

50. Lin, R. K., Hsu, H. S., Chang, J. W., Chen, C. Y., Chen, J. T., and Wang, Y. C. (2007). Alteration of DNA methyltransferases contributes to 5'CpG methylation and poor prognosis in lung cancer. *Lung Cancer* 55, 205–213.

51. Vertino, P. M., Yen, R. W., Gao, J., and Baylin, S. B. (1996). De novo methylation of CpG island sequences in human fibroblasts overexpressing DNA (cytosine-5-)-methyltransferase. *Mol Cell Biol* 16, 4555–4565.

52. Ehrlich, M. (2002). DNA hypomethylation, cancer, the immunodeficiency, centromeric region instability, facial anomalies syndrome and chromosomal rearrangements. *J Nutr* 132, 2424S–2429S.

53. Reynolds, P. A., Sigaroudinia, M., Zardo, G., Wilson, M. B., Benton, G. M., Miller, C. J., Hong, C., Fridlyand, J., Costello, J. F., and Tlsty, T. D. (2006). Tumor suppressor p16INK4A regulates polycomb-mediated DNA hypermethylation in human mammary epithelial cells. *J Biol Chem* 281, 24790–24802.

54. Vire, E., Brenner, C., Deplus, R., Blanchon, L., Fraga, M., Didelot, C., Morey, L., Van Eynde, A., Bernard, D., Vanderwinden, J. M., Bollen, M., Esteller, M., Di Croce, L., de Launoit, Y., and Fuks, F. (2006). The Polycomb group protein EZH2 directly controls DNA methylation. *Nature* 439, 871–874.

55. Ikegami, K., Iwatani, M., Suzuki, M., Tachibana, M., Shinkai, Y., Tanaka, S., Greally, J. M., Yagi, S., Hattori, N., and Shiota, K. (2007). Genome-wide and locus-specific DNA hypomethylation in G9a deficient mouse embryonic stem cells. *Genes Cells* 12, 1–11.

56. Smallwood, A., Esteve, P. O., Pradhan, S., and Carey, M. (2007). Functional cooperation between HP1 and DNMT1 mediates gene silencing. *Genes Dev* 21, 1169–1178.

57. van der Vlag, J., and Otte, A. P. (1999). Transcriptional repression mediated by the human polycomb-group protein EED involves histone deacetylation. *Nat Genet* 23, 474–478.

58. Seligson, D. B., Horvath, S., Shi, T., Yu, H., Tze, S., Grunstein, M., and Kurdistani, S. K. (2005). Global histone modification patterns predict risk of prostate cancer recurrence. *Nature* 435, 1262–1266.

59. Feng, W., Lu, Z., Luo, R. Z., Zhang, X., Seto, E., Liao, W. S., and Yu, Y. (2007). Multiple histone deacetylases repress tumor suppressor gene ARHI in breast cancer. *Int J Cancer* 120, 1664–1668.

60. Wilson, A. J., Byun, D. S., Popova, N., Murray, L. B., L'Italien, K., Sowa, Y., Arango, D., Velcich, A., Augenlicht, L. H., and Mariadason, J. M. (2006). Histone deacetylase 3 (HDAC3) and other class I HDACs regulate colon cell maturation and p21 expression and are deregulated in human colon cancer. *J Biol Chem* 281, 13548–13558.

61. Huang, W., Tan, D., Wang, X., Han, S., Tan, J., Zhao, Y., Lu, J., and Huang, B. (2006). Histone deacetylase 3 represses p15(INK4b) and p21(WAF1/cip1) transcription by interacting with Sp1. *Biochem Biophys Res Commun* 339, 165–171.

62. Nakagawa, M., Oda, Y., Eguchi, T., Aishima, S., Yao, T., Hosoi, F., Basaki, Y., Ono, M., Kuwano, M., Tanaka, M., and Tsuneyoshi, M. (2007). Expression profile of class I histone deacetylases in human cancer tissues. *Oncol Rep* 18, 769–774.

63. Zimmermann, S., Kiefer, F., Prudenziati, M., Spiller, C., Hansen, J., Floss, T., Wurst, W., Minucci, S., and Gottlicher, M. (2007). Reduced body size and decreased intestinal tumor rates in HDAC2-mutant mice. *Cancer Res* 67, 9047–9054.

64. Dashwood, R. H., Myzak, M. C., and Ho, E. (2006). Dietary HDAC inhibitors: Time to rethink weak ligands in cancer chemoprevention? *Carcinogenesis* 27, 344–349.

65. Atsumi, A., Tomita, A., Kiyoi, H., and Naoe, T. (2006). Histone deacetylase 3 (HDAC3) is recruited to target promoters by PML-RARalpha as a component of the N-CoR co-repressor complex to repress transcription in vivo. *Biochem Biophys Res Commun* 345, 1471–1480.

66. Carbone, R., Botrugno, O. A., Ronzoni, S., Insinga, A., Di Croce, L., Pelicci, P. G., and Minucci, S. (2006). Recruitment of the histone methyltransferase SUV39H1 and its role in the oncogenic properties of the leukemia-associated PML-retinoic acid receptor fusion protein. *Mol Cell Biol* 26, 1288–1296.

67. Villa, R., Pasini, D., Gutierrez, A., Morey, L., Occhionorelli, M., Vire, E., Nomdedeu, J. F., Jenuwein, T., Pelicci, P. G., Minucci, S., Fuks, F., Helin, K., and Di Croce, L. (2007). Role of the polycomb repressive complex 2 in acute promyelocytic leukemia. *Cancer Cell* 11, 513–525.

68. Di Croce, L., Raker, V. A., Corsaro, M., Fazi, F., Fanelli, M., Faretta, M., Fuks, F., Lo Coco, F., Kouzarides, T., Nervi, C., Minucci, S., and Pelicci, P. G. (2002). Methyltransferase recruitment and DNA hypermethylation of target promoters by an oncogenic transcription factor. *Science* 295, 1079–1082.

69. Gelmetti, V., Zhang, J., Fanelli, M., Minucci, S., Pelicci, P. G., and Lazar, M. A. (1998). Aberrant recruitment of the nuclear receptor corepressor-histone deacetylase complex by the acute myeloid leukemia fusion partner ETO. *Mol Cell Biol* 18, 7185–7191.

70. Liu, X., Wang, L., Zhao, K., Thompson, P. R., Hwang, Y., Marmorstein, R., and Cole, P. A. (2008). The structural basis of protein acetylation by the p300/CBP transcriptional coactivator. *Nature* 451, 846–850.

71. Miller, R. W., and Rubinstein, J. H. (1995). Tumors in Rubinstein-Taybi syndrome. *Am J Med Genet* 56, 112–115.

72. Murata, T., Kurokawa, R., Krones, A., Tatsumi, K., Ishii, M., Taki, T., Masuno, M., Ohashi, H., Yanagisawa, M., Rosenfeld, M. G., Glass, C. K., and Hayashi, Y. (2001). Defect of histone acetyltransferase activity of the nuclear transcriptional coactivator CBP in Rubinstein-Taybi syndrome. *Hum Mol Genet* 10, 1071–1076.

73. Zimmermann, N., Acosta, A. M., Kohlhase, J., and Bartsch, O. (2007). Confirmation of EP300 gene mutations as a rare cause of Rubinstein-Taybi syndrome. *Eur J Hum Genet* 15, 837–842.

74. Gayther, S. A., Batley, S. J., Linger, L., Bannister, A., Thorpe, K., Chin, S. F., Daigo, Y., Russell, P., Wilson, A., Sowter, H. M., Delhanty, J. D., Ponder, B. A., Kouzarides, T., and Caldas, C. (2000). Mutations truncating the EP300 acetylase in human cancers. *Nat Genet* 24, 300–303.

75. Zhang, C., Li, K., Wei, L., Li, Z., Yu, P., Teng, L., Wu, K., and Zhu, J. (2007). p300 expression repression by hypermethylation associated with tumour invasion and metastasis in oesophageal squamous cell carcinoma. *J Clin Pathol* 60, 1249–1253.

76. Ionov, Y., Matsui, S., and Cowell, J. K. (2004). A role for p300/CREB binding protein genes in promoting cancer progression in colon cancer cell lines with microsatellite instability. *Proc Natl Acad Sci USA* 101, 1273–1278.

77. Ishihama, K., Yamakawa, M., Semba, S., Takeda, H., Kawata, S., Kimura, S., and Kimura, W. (2007). Expression of HDAC1 and CBP/p300 in human colorectal carcinomas. *J Clin Pathol* 60, 1205–1210.

78. Panagopoulos, I., Fioretos, T., Isaksson, M., Samuelsson, U., Billstrom, R., Strombeck, B., Mitelman, F., and Johansson, B. (2001). Fusion of the MORF and CBP genes in acute myeloid leukemia with the t(10;16)(q22;p13). *Hum Mol Genet* 10, 395–404.

79. Taki, T., Sako, M., Tsuchida, M., and Hayashi, Y. (1997). The t(11;16)(q23;p13) translocation in myelodysplastic syndrome fuses the MLL gene to the CBP gene. *Blood* 89, 3945–3950.
80. Ida, K., Kitabayashi, I., Taki, T., Taniwaki, M., Noro, K., Yamamoto, M., Ohki, M., and Hayashi, Y. (1997). Adenoviral E1A-associated protein p300 is involved in acute myeloid leukemia with t(11;22)(q23;q13). *Blood* 90, 4699–4704.
81. Chaffanet, M., Gressin, L., Preudhomme, C., Soenen-Cornu, V., Birnbaum, D., and Pebusque, M. J. (2000). MOZ is fused to p300 in an acute monocytic leukemia with t(8;22). *Genes Chromosomes Cancer* 28, 138–144.
82. Deguchi, K., Ayton, P. M., Carapeti, M., Kutok, J. L., Snyder, C. S., Williams, I. R., Cross, N. C., Glass, C. K., Cleary, M. L., and Gilliland, D. G. (2003). MOZ-TIF2-induced acute myeloid leukemia requires the MOZ nucleosome binding motif and TIF2-mediated recruitment of CBP. *Cancer Cell* 3, 259–271.
83. Wang, L., Grossman, S. R., and Kieff, E. (2000). Epstein-Barr virus nuclear protein 2 interacts with p300, CBP, and PCAF histone acetyltransferases in activation of the LMP1 promoter. *Proc Natl Acad Sci USA* 97, 430–435.
84. Valls, E., de la Cruz, X., and Martinez-Balbas, M. A. (2003). The SV40 T antigen modulates CBP histone acetyltransferase activity. *Nucleic Acids Res* 31, 3114–3122.
85. Turnell, A. S., and Mymryk, J. S. (2006). Roles for the coactivators CBP and p300 and the APC/C E3 ubiquitin ligase in E1A-dependent cell transformation. *Br J Cancer* 95, 555–560.
86. Ramirez, J. A., and Nyborg, J. K. (2007). Molecular characterization of HTLV-1 Tax interaction with the KIX domain of CBP/p300. *J Mol Biol* 372, 958–969.
87. Germaniuk-Kurowska, A., Nag, A., Zhao, X., Dimri, M., Band, H., and Band, V. (2007). Ada3 requirement for HAT recruitment to estrogen receptors and estrogen-dependent breast cancer cell proliferation. *Cancer Res* 67, 11789–11797.
88. Wang, T., Kobayashi, T., Takimoto, R., Denes, A. E., Snyder, E. L., el-Deiry, W. S., and Brachmann, R. K. (2001). hADA3 is required for p53 activity. *EMBO J* 20, 6404–6413.
89. Galbiati, L., Mendoza-Maldonado, R., Gutierrez, M. I., and Giacca, M. (2005). Regulation of E2F-1 after DNA damage by p300-mediated acetylation and ubiquitination. *Cell Cycle* 4, 930–939.
90. Pediconi, N., Ianari, A., Costanzo, A., Belloni, L., Gallo, R., Cimino, L., Porcellini, A., Screpanti, I., Balsano, C., Alesse, E., Gulino, A., and Levrero, M. (2003). Differential regulation of E2F1 apoptotic target genes in response to DNA damage. *Nat Cell Biol* 5, 552–558.
91. Zhao, Y., Tan, J., Zhuang, L., Jiang, X., Liu, E. T., and Yu, Q. (2005). Inhibitors of histone deacetylases target the Rb-E2F1 pathway for apoptosis induction through activation of proapoptotic protein Bim. *Proc Natl Acad Sci USA* 102, 16090–16095.
92. Ogura, K., Hirata, Y., Yanai, A., Shibata, W., Ohmae, T., Mitsuno, Y., Maeda, S., Watabe, H., Yamaji, Y., Okamoto, M., Yoshida, H., Kawabe, T., and Omata, M. (2008). The effect of *Helicobacter pylori* eradication on reducing the incidence of gastric cancer. *J Clin Gastroenterol* 42, 279–283.
93. Karin, M., and Greten, F. R. (2005). NF-kappaB: Linking inflammation and immunity to cancer development and progression. *Nat Rev Immunol* 5, 749–759.

94. Aggarwal, B. B., Shishodia, S., Sandur, S. K., Pandey, M. K., and Sethi, G. (2006). Inflammation and cancer: How hot is the link? *Biochem Pharmacol* 72, 1605–1621.

95. Rahman, I., Marwick, J., and Kirkham, P. (2004). Redox modulation of chromatin remodeling: Impact on histone acetylation and deacetylation, NF-kappaB and pro-inflammatory gene expression. *Biochem Pharmacol* 68, 1255–1267.

96. Yamaguchi, K., Lantowski, A., Dannenberg, A. J., and Subbaramaiah, K. (2005). Histone deacetylase inhibitors suppress the induction of c-Jun and its target genes including COX-2. *J Biol Chem* 280, 32569–32577.

97. Bhavsar, P., Ahmad, T., and Adcock, I. M. (2008). The role of histone deacetylases in asthma and allergic diseases. *J Allergy Clin Immunol* 121, 171–178.

98. Kassel, O., and Herrlich, P. (2007). Crosstalk between the glucocorticoid receptor and other transcription factors: molecular aspects. *Mol Cell Endocrinol* 275, 13–29.

99. Smith, P. J., Cousins, D. J., Jee, Y. K., Staynov, D. Z., Lee, T. H., and Lavender, P. (2001). Suppression of granulocyte-macrophage colony-stimulating factor expression by glucocorticoids involves inhibition of enhancer function by the glucocorticoid receptor binding to composite NF-AT/activator protein-1 elements. *J Immunol* 167, 2502–2510.

100. McKay, L. I., and Cidlowski, J. A. (1999). Molecular control of immune/inflammatory responses: Interactions between nuclear factor-kappa B and steroid receptor-signaling pathways. *Endocr Rev* 20, 435–459.

101. Moodie, F. M., Marwick, J. A., Anderson, C. S., Szulakowski, P., Biswas, S. K., Bauter, M. R., Kilty, I., and Rahman, I. (2004). Oxidative stress and cigarette smoke alter chromatin remodeling but differentially regulate NF-kappaB activation and proinflammatory cytokine release in alveolar epithelial cells. *FASEB J* 18, 1897–1899.

102. Hamalainen, M., Lilja, R., Kankaanranta, H., and Moilanen, E. (2008). Inhibition of iNOS expression and NO production by anti-inflammatory steroids: Reversal by histone deacetylase inhibitors. *Pulm Pharmacol Ther* 21, 331–339.

103. Jee, Y. K., Gilmour, J., Kelly, A., Bowen, H., Richards, D., Soh, C., Smith, P., Hawrylowicz, C., Cousins, D., Lee, T., and Lavender, P. (2005). Repression of interleukin-5 transcription by the glucocorticoid receptor targets GATA3 signaling and involves histone deacetylase recruitment. *J Biol Chem* 280, 23243–23250.

104. John, M., Lim, S., Seybold, J., Jose, P., Robichaud, A., O'Connor, B., Barnes, P. J., and Chung, K. F. (1998). Inhaled corticosteroids increase interleukin-10 but reduce macrophage inflammatory protein-1alpha, granulocyte-macrophage colony-stimulating factor, and interferon-gamma release from alveolar macrophages in asthma. *Am J Respir Crit Care Med* 157, 256–262.

105. Cosio, B. G., Mann, B., Ito, K., Jazrawi, E., Barnes, P. J., Chung, K. F., and Adcock, I. M. (2004). Histone acetylase and deacetylase activity in alveolar macrophages and blood monocytes in asthma. *Am J Respir Crit Care Med* 170, 141–147.

106. Ito, K., Caramori, G., Lim, S., Oates, T., Chung, K. F., Barnes, P. J., and Adcock, I. M. (2002). Expression and activity of histone deacetylases in human asthmatic airways. *Am J Respir Crit Care Med* 166, 392–396.

107. Ito, K., Barnes, P. J., and Adcock, I. M. (2000). Glucocorticoid receptor recruitment of histone deacetylase 2 inhibits interleukin-1beta-induced histone H4 acetylation on lysines 8 and 12. *Mol Cell Biol* 20, 6891–6903.

108. Kosmas, E. N., Michaelides, S. A., Polychronaki, A., Roussou, T., Toukmatzi, S., Polychronopoulos, V., and Baxevanis, C. N. (1999). Theophylline induces a reduction in circulating interleukin-4 and interleukin-5 in atopic asthmatics. *Eur Respir J* 13, 53–58.

109. Makino, S., Adachi, M., Ohta, K., Kihara, N., Nakajima, S., Nishima, S., Fukuda, T., and Miyamoto, T. (2006). A prospective survey on safety of sustained-release theophylline in treatment of asthma and COPD. *Allergol Int* 55, 395–402.

110. Ito, K., Lim, S., Caramori, G., Cosio, B., Chung, K. F., Adcock, I. M., and Barnes, P. J. (2002). A molecular mechanism of action of theophylline: Induction of histone deacetylase activity to decrease inflammatory gene expression. *Proc Natl Acad Sci USA* 99, 8921–8926.

111. Cosio, B. G., Tsaprouni, L., Ito, K., Jazrawi, E., Adcock, I. M., and Barnes, P. J. (2004). Theophylline restores histone deacetylase activity and steroid responses in COPD macrophages. *J Exp Med* 200, 689–695.

112. Ito, K., Yamamura, S., Essilfie-Quaye, S., Cosio, B., Ito, M., Barnes, P. J., and Adcock, I. M. (2006). Histone deacetylase 2-mediated deacetylation of the glucocorticoid receptor enables NF-kappaB suppression. *J Exp Med* 203, 7–13.

113. Ito, K., Ito, M., Elliott, W. M., Cosio, B., Caramori, G., Kon, O. M., Barczyk, A., Hayashi, S., Adcock, I. M., Hogg, J. C., and Barnes, P. J. (2005). Decreased histone deacetylase activity in chronic obstructive pulmonary disease. *N Engl J Med* 352, 1967–1976.

114. Postma, D. S., and Kerstjens, H. A. (1999). Are inhaled glucocorticosteroids effective in chronic obstructive pulmonary disease? *Am J Respir Crit Care Med* 160, S66–S71.

115. Barnes, P. J. (2000). Inhaled corticosteroids are not beneficial in chronic obstructive pulmonary disease. *Am J Respir Crit Care Med* 161, 342–344.

116. Marwick, J. A., Kirkham, P. A., Stevenson, C. S., Danahay, H., Giddings, J., Butler, K., Donaldson, K., Macnee, W., and Rahman, I. (2004). Cigarette smoke alters chromatin remodeling and induces proinflammatory genes in rat lungs. *Am J Respir Cell Mol Biol* 31, 633–642.

117. Goleva, E., Hauk, P. J., Boguniewicz, J., Martin, R. J., and Leung, D. Y. (2007). Airway remodeling and lack of bronchodilator response in steroid-resistant asthma. *J Allergy Clin Immunol* 120, 1065–1072.

118. Kode, A., Rajendrasozhan, S., Caito, S., Yang, S. R., Megson, I. L., and Rahman, I. (2008). Resveratrol induces glutathione synthesis by activation of NRF2 and protects against cigarette smoke-mediated oxidative stress in human lung epithelial cells. *Am J Physiol Lung Cell Mol Physiol* 294, L478–L488.

119. Howitz, K. T., Bitterman, K. J., Cohen, H. Y., Lamming, D. W., Lavu, S., Wood, J. G., Zipkin, R. E., Chung, P., Kisielewski, A., Zhang, L. L., Scherer, B., and Sinclair, D. A. (2003). Small molecule activators of sirtuins extend *Saccharomyces cerevisiae* lifespan. *Nature* 425, 191–196.

120. Yang, S. R., Wright, J., Bauter, M., Seweryniak, K., Kode, A., and Rahman, I. (2007). Sirtuin regulates cigarette smoke-induced proinflammatory mediator release via RelA/p65 NF-kappaB in macrophages in vitro and in rat lungs in vivo: Implications for chronic inflammation and aging. *Am J Physiol Lung Cell Mol Physiol* 292, L567–L576.

121. Rajendrasozhan, S., Yang, S. R., Kinnula, V. L., and Rahman, I. (2008). SIRT1, an anti-inflammatory and anti-aging protein, is decreased in lungs of patients with chronic obstructive pulmonary disease. *Am J Respir Crit Care Med* 177, 861–870.

122. Singh, S. V., Hu, X., Srivastava, S. K., Singh, M., Xia, H., Orchard, J. L., and Zaren, H. A. (1998). Mechanism of inhibition of benzo[a]pyrene-induced forestomach cancer in mice by dietary curcumin. *Carcinogenesis* 19, 1357–1360.

123. Arbiser, J. L., Klauber, N., Rohan, R., van Leeuwen, R., Huang, M. T., Fisher, C., Flynn, E., and Byers, H. R. (1998). Curcumin is an in vivo inhibitor of angiogenesis. *Mol Med* 4, 376–383.

124. Duvoix, A., Blasius, R., Delhalle, S., Schnekenburger, M., Morceau, F., Henry, E., Dicato, M., and Diederich, M. (2005). Chemopreventive and therapeutic effects of curcumin. *Cancer Lett* 223, 181–190.

125. Jagetia, G. C., and Aggarwal, B. B. (2007). "Spicing up" of the immune system by curcumin. *J Clin Immunol* 27, 19–35.

126. Khanna, D., Sethi, G., Ahn, K. S., Pandey, M. K., Kunnumakkara, A. B., Sung, B., Aggarwal, A., and Aggarwal, B. B. (2007). Natural products as a gold mine for arthritis treatment. *Curr Opin Pharmacol* 7, 344–351.

127. Shishodia, S., Potdar, P., Gairola, C. G., and Aggarwal, B. B. (2003). Curcumin (diferuloylmethane) down-regulates cigarette smoke-induced NF-kappaB activation through inhibition of IkappaBalpha kinase in human lung epithelial cells: Correlation with suppression of COX-2, MMP-9 and cyclin D1. *Carcinogenesis* 24, 1269–1279.

128. Marcu, M. G., Jung, Y. J., Lee, S., Chung, E. J., Lee, M. J., Trepel, J., and Neckers, L. (2006). Curcumin is an inhibitor of p300 histone acetyltransferase. *Med Chem* 2, 169–174.

129. Kang, J., Chen, J., Shi, Y., Jia, J., and Zhang, Y. (2005). Curcumin-induced histone hypoacetylation: The role of reactive oxygen species. *Biochem Pharmacol* 69, 1205–1213.

130. Biswas, S. K., McClure, D., Jimenez, L. A., Megson, I. L., and Rahman, I. (2005). Curcumin induces glutathione biosynthesis and inhibits NF-kappaB activation and interleukin-8 release in alveolar epithelial cells: Mechanism of free radical scavenging activity. *Antioxid Redox Signal* 7, 32–41.

131. Kiernan, R., Bres, V., Ng, R. W., Coudart, M. P., El Messaoudi, S., Sardet, C., Jin, D. Y., Emiliani, S., and Benkirane, M. (2003). Post-activation turn-off of NF-kappa B-dependent transcription is regulated by acetylation of p65. *J Biol Chem* 278, 2758–2766.

132. Aggarwal, S., Ichikawa, H., Takada, Y., Sandur, S. K., Shishodia, S., and Aggarwal, B. B. (2006). Curcumin (diferuloylmethane) down-regulates expression of cell proliferation and antiapoptotic and metastatic gene products through suppression of IkappaBalpha kinase and AKT activation. *Mol Pharmacol* 69, 195–206.

133. Xu, M., Deng, B., Chow, Y. L., Zhao, Z. Z., and Hu, B. (2007). Effects of curcumin in treatment of experimental pulmonary fibrosis: A comparison with hydrocortisone. *J Ethnopharmacol* 112, 292–299.

134. Balasubramanyam, K., Swaminathan, V., Ranganathan, A., and Kundu, T. K. (2003). Small molecule modulators of histone acetyltransferase p300. *J Biol Chem* 278, 19134–19140.

135. Balasubramanyam, K., Altaf, M., Varier, R. A., Swaminathan, V., Ravindran, A., Sadhale, P. P., and Kundu, T. K. (2004). Polyisoprenylated benzophenone, garcinol, a natural histone acetyltransferase inhibitor, represses chromatin transcription and alters global gene expression. *J Biol Chem* 279, 33716–33726.

136. Keslacy, S., Tliba, O., Baidouri, H., and Amrani, Y. (2007). Inhibition of tumor necrosis factor-alpha-inducible inflammatory genes by interferon-gamma is associated with altered nuclear factor-kappaB transactivation and enhanced histone deacetylase activity. *Mol Pharmacol* 71, 609–618.

137. Huang, L. (2006). Targeting histone deacetylases for the treatment of cancer and inflammatory diseases. *J Cell Physiol* 209, 611–616.

138. Glauben, R., Batra, A., Fedke, I., Zeitz, M., Lehr, H. A., Leoni, F., Mascagni, P., Fantuzzi, G., Dinarello, C. A., and Siegmund, B. (2006). Histone hyperacetylation is associated with amelioration of experimental colitis in mice. *J Immunol* 176, 5015–5022.

139. Rosman-Urbach, M., Niv, Y., Birk, Y., Morgenstern, S., and Schwartz, B. (2006). Relationship between nutritional habits adopted by ulcerative colitis relevant to cancer development patients at clinical remission stages and molecular-genetic parameters. *Br J Nutr* 95, 188–195.

140. Bingham, S. A., Day, N. E., Luben, R., Ferrari, P., Slimani, N., Norat, T., Clavel-Chapelon, F., Kesse, E., Nieters, A., Boeing, H., Tjonneland, A., Overvad, K., Martinez, C., Dorronsoro, M., Gonzalez, C. A., Key, T. J., Trichopoulou, A., Naska, A., Vineis, P., Tumino, R., Krogh, V., Bueno-de-Mesquita, H. B., Peeters, P. H., Berglund, G., Hallmans, G., Lund, E., Skeie, G., Kaaks, R., and Riboli, E. (2003). Dietary fibre in food and protection against colorectal cancer in the European Prospective Investigation into Cancer and Nutrition (EPIC): An observational study. *Lancet* 361, 1496–1501.

141. Potter, J. D., Slattery, M. L., Bostick, R. M., and Gapstur, S. M. (1993). Colon cancer: A review of the epidemiology. *Epidemiol Rev* 15, 499–545.

142. Place, R. F., Noonan, E. J., and Giardina, C. (2005). HDAC inhibition prevents NF-kappa B activation by suppressing proteasome activity: Downregulation of proteasome subunit expression stabilizes I kappa B alpha. *Biochem Pharmacol* 70, 394–406.

143. Tong, X., Yin, L., and Giardina, C. (2004). Butyrate suppresses Cox-2 activation in colon cancer cells through HDAC inhibition. *Biochem Biophys Res Commun* 317, 463–471.

144. Paiotti, A. P., Artigiani Neto, R., Forones, N. M., Oshima, C. T., Miszputen, S. J., and Franco, M. (2007). Immunoexpression of cyclooxygenase-1 and -2 in ulcerative colitis. *Braz J Med Biol Res* 40, 911–918.

145. Kutchera, W., Jones, D. A., Matsunami, N., Groden, J., McIntyre, T. M., Zimmerman, G. A., White, R. L., and Prescott, S. M. (1996). Prostaglandin H synthase 2 is expressed abnormally in human colon cancer: Evidence for a transcriptional effect. *Proc Natl Acad Sci USA* 93, 4816–4820.

146. Burns, R. C., Rivera-Nieves, J., Moskaluk, C. A., Matsumoto, S., Cominelli, F., and Ley, K. (2001). Antibody blockade of ICAM-1 and VCAM-1 ameliorates inflammation in the SAMP-1/Yit adoptive transfer model of Crohn's disease in mice. *Gastroenterology* 121, 1428–1436.

147. Menzel, T., Luhrs, H., Zirlik, S., Schauber, J., Kudlich, T., Gerke, T., Gostner, A., Neumann, M., Melcher, R., and Scheppach, W. (2004). Butyrate inhibits leukocyte adhesion to endothelial cells via modulation of VCAM-1. *Inflamm Bowel Dis* 10, 122–128.

148. Sans, M., Panes, J., Ardite, E., Elizalde, J. I., Arce, Y., Elena, M., Palacin, A., Fernandez-Checa, J. C., Anderson, D. C., Lobb, R., and Pique, J. M. (1999). VCAM-1 and ICAM-1 mediate leukocyte-endothelial cell adhesion in rat experimental colitis. *Gastroenterology* 116, 874–883.

149. McGeer, P. L., Itagaki, S., Boyes, B. E., and McGeer, E. G. (1988). Reactive microglia are positive for HLA-DR in the substantia nigra of Parkinson's and Alzheimer's disease brains. *Neurology* 38, 1285–1291.

150. Minghetti, L. (2005). Role of inflammation in neurodegenerative diseases. *Curr Opin Neurol* 18, 315–321.

151. Huuskonen, J., Suuronen, T., Nuutinen, T., Kyrylenko, S., and Salminen, A. (2004). Regulation of microglial inflammatory response by sodium butyrate and short-chain fatty acids. *Br J Pharmacol* 141, 874–880.

152. Kim, H. S., Whang, S. Y., Woo, M. S., Park, J. S., Kim, W. K., and Han, I. O. (2004). Sodium butyrate suppresses interferon-gamma-, but not lipopolysaccharide-mediated induction of nitric oxide and tumor necrosis factor-alpha in microglia. *J Neuroimmunol* 151, 85–93.

153. Chen, P. S., Peng, G. S., Li, G., Yang, S., Wu, X., Wang, C. C., Wilson, B., Lu, R. B., Gean, P. W., Chuang, D. M., and Hong, J. S. (2006). Valproate protects dopaminergic neurons in midbrain neuron/glia cultures by stimulating the release of neurotrophic factors from astrocytes. *Mol Psychiatry* 11, 1116–1125.

154. Peng, G. S., Li, G., Tzeng, N. S., Chen, P. S., Chuang, D. M., Hsu, Y. D., Yang, S., and Hong, J. S. (2005). Valproate pretreatment protects dopaminergic neurons from LPS-induced neurotoxicity in rat primary midbrain cultures: Role of microglia. *Brain Res Mol Brain Res* 134, 162–169.

155. Gao, H. M., Jiang, J., Wilson, B., Zhang, W., Hong, J. S., and Liu, B. (2002). Microglial activation-mediated delayed and progressive degeneration of rat nigral dopaminergic neurons: Relevance to Parkinson's disease. *J Neurochem* 81, 1285–1297.

156. Kim, H. J., Rowe, M., Ren, M., Hong, J. S., Chen, P. S., and Chuang, D. M. (2007). Histone deacetylase inhibitors exhibit anti-inflammatory and neuroprotective effects in a rat permanent ischemic model of stroke: Multiple mechanisms of action. *J Pharmacol Exp Ther* 321, 892–901.

157. Camelo, S., Iglesias, A. H., Hwang, D., Due, B., Ryu, H., Smith, K., Gray, S. G., Imitola, J., Duran, G., Assaf, B., Langley, B., Khoury, S. J., Stephanopoulos, G., De Girolami, U., Ratan, R. R., Ferrante, R. J., and Dangond, F. (2005). Transcriptional therapy with the histone deacetylase inhibitor trichostatin A ameliorates experimental autoimmune encephalomyelitis. *J Neuroimmunol* 164, 10–21.

158. Sinn, D. I., Kim, S. J., Chu, K., Jung, K. H., Lee, S. T., Song, E. C., Kim, J. M., Park, D. K., Kun Lee, S., Kim, M., and Roh, J. K. (2007). Valproic acid-mediated neuroprotection in intracerebral hemorrhage via histone deacetylase inhibition and transcriptional activation. *Neurobiol Dis* 26, 464–472.

159. Noyan-Ashraf, M. H., Sadeghinejad, Z., and Juurlink, B. H. (2005). Dietary approach to decrease aging-related CNS inflammation. *Nutr Neurosci* 8, 101–110.

160. Rassoul, F., Salvetter, J., Reissig, D., Schneider, W., Thiery, J., and Richter, V. (2006). The influence of garlic (*Allium sativum*) extract on interleukin 1alpha-induced expression of endothelial intercellular adhesion molecule-1 and vascular cell adhesion molecule-1. *Phytomedicine* 13, 230–235.

161. Lang, A., Lahav, M., Sakhnini, E., Barshack, I., Fidder, H. H., Avidan, B., Bardan, E., Hershkoviz, R., Bar-Meir, S., and Chowers, Y. (2004). Allicin inhibits spontaneous and TNF-alpha induced secretion of proinflammatory cytokines and chemokines from intestinal epithelial cells. *Clin Nutr* 23, 1199–1208.

162. Woo, K. J., and Kwon, T. K. (2007). Sulforaphane suppresses lipopolysaccharide-induced cyclooxygenase-2 (COX-2) expression through the modulation of multiple targets in COX-2 gene promoter. *Int Immunopharmacol* 7, 1776–1783.

163. Wu, L., Noyan Ashraf, M. H., Facci, M., Wang, R., Paterson, P. G., Ferrie, A., and Juurlink, B. H. (2004). Dietary approach to attenuate oxidative stress, hypertension, and inflammation in the cardiovascular system. *Proc Natl Acad Sci USA* 101, 7094–7099.

164. Hamalainen, M., Nieminen, R., Vuorela, P., Heinonen, M., and Moilanen, E. (2007). Anti-inflammatory effects of flavonoids: Genistein, kaempferol, quercetin, and daidzein inhibit STAT-1 and NF-kappaB activations, whereas flavone, isorhamnetin, naringenin, and pelargonidin inhibit only NF-kappaB activation along with their inhibitory effect on iNOS expression and NO production in activated macrophages. *Mediators Inflamm* 2007, 45673.

165. Yoshida, Y., Shioi, T., and Izumi, T. (2007). Resveratrol ameliorates experimental autoimmune myocarditis. *Circ J* 71, 397–404.

166. Lee, S. H., Seo, G. S., Jin, X. Y., Ko, G., and Sohn, D. H. (2007). Butein blocks tumor necrosis factor alpha-induced interleukin 8 and matrix metalloproteinase 7 production by inhibiting p38 kinase and osteopontin mediated signaling events in HT-29 cells. *Life Sci* 81, 1535–1543.

167. Lee, S. H., Seo, G. S., and Sohn, D. H. (2004). Inhibition of lipopolysaccharide-induced expression of inducible nitric oxide synthase by butein in RAW 264.7 cells. *Biochem Biophys Res Commun* 323, 125–132.

168. Higa, S., Hirano, T., Kotani, M., Matsumoto, M., Fujita, A., Suemura, M., Kawase, I., and Tanaka, T. (2003). Fisetin, a flavonol, inhibits TH2-type cytokine production by activated human basophils. *J Allergy Clin Immunol* 111, 1299–1306.

169. Sung, B., Pandey, M. K., and Aggarwal, B. B. (2007). Fisetin, an inhibitor of cyclin-dependent kinase 6, down-regulates nuclear factor-kappaB-regulated cell proliferation, antiapoptotic and metastatic gene products through the suppression of TAK-1 and receptor-interacting protein-regulated IkappaBalpha kinase activation. *Mol Pharmacol* 71, 1703–1714.

170. Ruiz, P. A., Braune, A., Holzlwimmer, G., Quintanilla-Fend, L., and Haller, D. (2007). Quercetin inhibits TNF-induced NF-kappaB transcription factor recruitment to proinflammatory gene promoters in murine intestinal epithelial cells. *J Nutr* 137, 1208–1215.

171. Min, Y. D., Choi, C. H., Bark, H., Son, H. Y., Park, H. H., Lee, S., Park, J. W., Park, E. K., Shin, H. I., and Kim, S. H. (2007). Quercetin inhibits expression of inflammatory cytokines through attenuation of NF-kappaB and p38 MAPK in HMC-1 human mast cell line. *Inflamm Res* 56, 210–215.

172. Rogerio, A. P., Kanashiro, A., Fontanari, C., da Silva, E. V., Lucisano-Valim, Y. M., Soares, E. G., and Faccioli, L. H. (2007). Anti-inflammatory activity of quercetin and isoquercitrin in experimental murine allergic asthma. *Inflamm Res* 56, 402–408.
173. Jin, C. Y., Moon, D. O., Lee, K. J., Kim, M. O., Lee, J. D., Choi, Y. H., Park, Y. M., and Kim, G. Y. (2006). Piceatannol attenuates lipopolysaccharide-induced NF-kappaB activation and NF-kappaB-related proinflammatory mediators in BV2 microglia. *Pharmacol Res* 54, 461–467.
174. Chen, C. Y., Peng, W. H., Tsai, K. D., and Hsu, S. L. (2007). Luteolin suppresses inflammation-associated gene expression by blocking NF-kappaB and AP-1 activation pathway in mouse alveolar macrophages. *Life Sci* 81, 1602–1614.
175. Liao, C. H., Sang, S., Liang, Y. C., Ho, C. T., and Lin, J. K. (2004). Suppression of inducible nitric oxide synthase and cyclooxygenase-2 in downregulating nuclear factor-kappa B pathway by Garcinol. *Mol Carcinog* 41, 140–149.
176. Hong, J., Sang, S., Park, H. J., Kwon, S. J., Suh, N., Huang, M. T., Ho, C. T., and Yang, C. S. (2006). Modulation of arachidonic acid metabolism and nitric oxide synthesis by garcinol and its derivatives. *Carcinogenesis* 27, 278–286.

chapter seven

Nutrients, epigenetics, and embryonic development

Craig A. Cooney

Contents

Maternal nutrition can affect a wide variety of characteristics in offspring, including health, appearance, memory and morphology. Many of these effects are life long but can be achieved with just a brief treatment—during part or all of gestation. In most cases the most effective treatments to achieve these maternal effects have not been determined. In other cases, effective treatments have not been chemically defined. Only a minute fraction of potential treatments and putative toxic agents have been tested for epigenetic effects. The strong effects of maternal diet on offspring make it imperative that the role of maternal nutrition and exposure to various environmental agents in offspring and multigenerational health be a research and public health priority.

7.1   Introduction

Most cells of an organism are of one genotype and yet this same genotype produces a huge number of cell types. For example, it is estimated that there are over 400 cell types in humans.[1] Many cell types are stable for the lifetime of the organism, which can range from weeks (e.g., *Caenorhabditis elegans*) to decades (e.g., humans) to millennia (e.g., bristle cone pine trees). Stability of the differentiated state occurs in dividing cells (e.g., hematopoietic and liver cells) as well as nondividing cells (e.g., neurons). Most of the initial cell differentiation occurs during embryonic and fetal development. The establishment and maintenance of the differentiated state requires epigenetic mechanisms to define patterns of gene expression characteristic of each state. Accumulating evidence shows that exposure of the embryo and fetus to nutrients and various other compounds can affect epigenetics. In mammals, the nutrients and other environmental variables during this time are maternally derived.

7.2   Epigenetic mechanisms

The genome contains thousands of genes as well as thousands of other functional sequences, such as replication origins, centromeres and endogenous retroviruses. In a particular cell type only a fraction of these may be active. At any given time in that cell type even fewer of these sequences may be active. The control of this activity is dependent on local chromatin structure and accessibility to factors that promote and cause expression. Inaccessibility of chromatin is not merely the absence of factors for activity but is a "conspiracy of silence" where specific proteins and specific covalent modifications see to the maintenance of the inactive state.[2] In addition to constitutively active and "constitutively silenced" sequences, there are probably cell type-specific sequences that are maintained in a poised chromatin state ready to become active, when appropriately signaled.[3] Factors involved in gene activity include histone acetylation, site-specific histone methylation, histone acetyltransferases, certain histone methyltransferases, transcription factors, transcription coactivators and RNA polymerases. Factors involved in gene silencing include site-specific histone methylation (at different sites than those used to signal activity), DNA methylation, interfering

RNAs, histone deacetylases, certain histone methyltransferases, DNA methyltransferases, and methylated DNA binding proteins. Many, if not all, of these factors work together to perpetuate the active or silent state.[2–5]

This chromatin structure of the genome is called the epigenome. The epigenome varies between different cell types and may differ even between cells of the same type. The epigenome is duplicated through cell growth and division. In this way the activities of the genome are duplicated in daughter cells. Changes in the local environment of cells— signaling, hormones, drugs and nutrients—may lead to changes in the epigenome and establish a new pattern of gene expression. Most of the epigenome appears to be established in embryonic and fetal development although some normal epigenetic changes do occur in postnatal development[6,7] and epigenomic changes with aging and cancer are extensive (reviewed in Reference 8).

Some of the most extensively studied epigenetic mechanisms are DNA methylation, histone acetylation and histone methylation. DNA methylation usually promotes silencing of chromatin and associated genes, whereas histone acetylation usually promotes gene activation. In contrast, histone methylation either activates or silences chromatin depending on the specific site. Metabolic control of gene expression may most likely be effected by influences on DNA methylation or histone acetylation because of their largely unidirectional responses to silence or activate, respectively.[3]

Mammals, higher plants, birds, reptiles, fish, some fungi and some insects use DNA methylation as a means of genome control to silence genes, including many showing genomic imprinting and epigenetic inheritance.[7,9–11] DNA methyltransferases Dnmt1, Dnmt3a and Dnmt3b are essential for mammalian development as is at least one methylated DNA binding protein, MeCP2.[12–15] There is some evidence for active DNA demethylation.[16,17]

Histone modifications include enzymatic methylation and acetylation of specific sites mainly on the N-terminal tails. Both histone acetyltransferase and deacetylase enzymes are well studied and each acts on multiple sites. In contrast, nearly all methylated sites on histones H3 and H4 have their own histone MTase. Methylation of some histone sites promotes active chromatin, while methylation of other histone sites promotes inactive chromatin. Methylation and acetylation can be in competition. For example, methylation of lysine 9 on histone H3 promotes gene silencing, whereas acetylation of this lysine is found in transcriptionally active chromatin.[18] Acetyl and methyl groups for these reactions come from metabolism and can therefore be influenced by metabolic state and diet.

7.3   Methyl and acetyl metabolism provide donors for epigenetic modifications

Methylation of DNA and histones requires the methyl donor S-adenosylmethionine (AdoMet, SAM), which is a product of methyl metabolism. Dnmts and HMTs use AdoMet to methylate cytosines in DNA and some lysines and arginines of histones. Dnmt1 is inhibited by the reaction product S-adenosylhomocysteine (AdoHcy, SAH).[19] HMTs are also likely inhibited by AdoHcy.[20] The methyl groups for AdoMet are newly synthesized in one-carbon metabolism or are from preformed methyl groups from the diet. Zinc is a cofactor for Dnmt1 and for the betaine homocysteine MTase.[21–23]

Methyl metabolism, and the broader one-carbon metabolism, use dietary folates (or folic acid), dietary methionine and dietary or endogenous betaine and choline. Folate, methionine, zinc and vitamin B12 are intermediates and enzymatic cofactors to transport and transfer methyl groups (Figure 7.1).[23–26] Except for betaine, all of these components are dietary essentials. Choline and betaine are found in many foods and are important dietary sources of preformed methyl groups.[27]

For histone acetylation the donor is acetyl-coenzyme A (AcCoA) which is an intermediate in fat and carbohydrate catabolism feeding

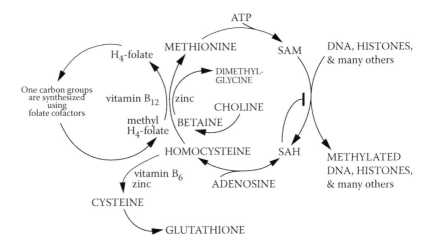

Figure 7.1 Methyl metabolism. S-adenosylmethionine (AdoMet, SAM) is the methyl donor used for enzymatic methylation of DNA, histone and other molecules. Production of AdoMet and recycling of S-adenosylhomocysteine (AdoHcy, SAH) are dependent on methyl metabolism. Many components of this metabolism are essential nutrients or provide alternative metabolic pathways to make AdoMet and recycle AdoHcy. (Adapted from Cooney, C.A. (2008). Cancer and aging: The epigenetic connection. In *Cancer Epigenetics*, Trygve Tollefsbol, ed., 303–316. Boca Raton, FL: CRC Press.)

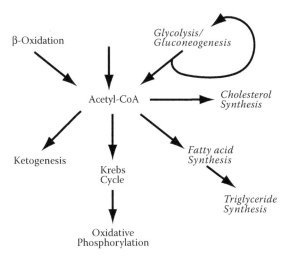

Figure 7.2 Acetate metabolism. Acetyl-CoA is the acetyl donor for enzymatic acetylation of histones and other molecules. Glucose and fats can be completely metabolized via acetyl-CoA, the TCA cycle and oxidative phosphorylation. However, when glucose is abundant or mitochondrial function is compromised, cells can rely on glycolysis and avoid production of acetyl-CoA. (From Cooney, C.A. (2008). Cancer and aging: The epigenetic connection. In *Cancer Epigenetics*, Trygve Tollefsbol, ed., 303–316. Boca Raton, FL: CRC Press.)

acetyl groups to the citric acid cycle (Figure 7.2). Acetyl groups are a source of available energy and could signal the potential for growth. The production and transport of acetyl groups involves many regulatory molecules, cofactors and vitamins, including insulin, epinephrine, carnitine and pantothenate. Acetate availability and subcellular compartmentalization may also depend on macronutrient levels and balance (carbohydrate, protein, and fat) and on physiological factors, including fasting and exercise.[28] In addition to histones, acetylation of some transcription factors can increase their activity.[29,30]

It has been proposed that gene regulation by methylation of DNA,[24] methylation of histones[31] and acetylation of chromatin proteins[32] respond to levels of dietary and metabolic precursors and cofactors for methylation and acetylation. Interactions of epigenetics and gene regulation with diet and metabolism may be evolved responses to environmental variation.

The availability of acetyl groups may vary greatly with many aspects of metabolism. Low oxygen concentrations, as might occur with intrauterine growth restriction (IUGR), may limit oxidative phosphorylation, forcing cells to rely on glycolysis and not produce acetate. A recent study describes neonatal changes in histone modification of the glucose transporter 4 (GLUT4) receptor after IUGR in rats.[33] Acetate levels or acetate compartmentalization may be affected by high glucose levels that promote glycolysis but not acetate production and oxidative phosphorylation. Likewise, the exposure to alcohol, especially at high doses or repeatedly, may affect the concentration of its metabolite acetate.

7.4   Yellow agouti mouse models provide visible readouts of epigenetic effects

Some of the most useful models in epigenetics are *agouti* alleles in mice that lead to a spectrum of yellow and agouti coat colors in the mouse population. These "yellow" alleles include A^{vy} and A^{iapy}, both of which produce a spectrum of coats that vary between entirely yellow to entirely agouti with a variety of mottled patterns in between (Figure 7.3).

In this model, mice carry a null *agouti* gene (*a* allele) that produces black mice in homozygotes (*a/a*). An epigenetically controlled *agouti* allele (e.g., A^{vy} or A^{iapy} alleles) produces a yellow coat when overexpressed and an agouti coat (brownish) when expressed at normal, wild-type levels.

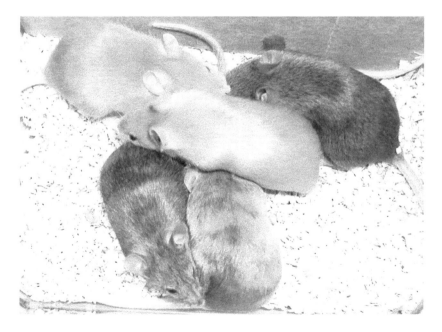

*Figure 7.3 (**A color version of this figure follows page 20.**)* Examples of mice from the yellow agouti mouse model. Strain VY mice showing A^{vy}/a mice, top left, a clear yellow, Y5 mouse; top right, a pseudoagouti, Y0 mouse; middle, a slightly mottled, Y4 mouse; bottom left, a heavily mottled, Y2, mouse; and bottom right, a mottled, Y3 mouse. These five mice are genetically identical. Coat color patterns are due to the degree of A^{vy} expression.

(The wild type, *A* allele, of *agouti* would also produce mice with an agouti or brownish coat but the *A* allele is not always part of this model.) Epigenetic modification of the A^{vy} or A^{iapy} alleles regulates *agouti* expression and coat color. This silencing provides A^{vy}/a and A^{iapy}/a mice with an agouti (brownish) coat and with many health characteristics similar to mice homozygous for a null *agouti* allele (*a/a* genotype, black coat). The majority of A^{vy}/a and A^{iapy}/a mice are part of a continuous spectrum of variegated agouti patterns (mottling) on yellow backgrounds (Figure 7.2). In A^{vy} and related alleles, the extent of agouti mottling and the degree of *agouti* allele DNA methylation are correlated.[9,10,34] The coat color of these mice provides a readout of their genetics and epigenetics at the *agouti locus* (reviewed in References 35 and 36).

The intermediate steps between ectopic *agouti* overexpression and many gross biological endpoints have been studied in some detail.[37] The agouti protein antagonizes melanocortin receptors. Normally (e.g., mice with the *A* allele) agouti acts on hair follicles and effects cyclic yellow pigment deposition in the hair (which combined with black pigment produces the agouti or brownish coat). In A^{vy}/a and A^{iapy}/a mice, agouti is overexpressed and ectopically expressed and interferes with melanocortin signaling multiple cell types. For example, in adipocytes, agouti promotes pathways associated with adipocyte differentiation.[37] Ectopic *agouti* expression causes obesity and type 2 diabetes mellitus (T2DM).[38] Yellow mice (with ectopic *agouti* overexpression) convert food calories to fat stores more efficiently (they are more metabolically efficient) compared to agouti mice (*A/a* genotype).[39] These alleles and caloric intake also affect expression of hepatic genes likely to be important in T2DM.[40] *Agouti* overexpression increases cancer susceptibility[41,42] and can lower 2-year survival.[39,42] In addition to a readout of their genetics and epigenetics, the coat color of these mice provides a readout of their long-term health prospects (reviewed in References 35 and 36).

7.5   Maternal diet affects the epigenetics of yellow agouti offspring

Compared to a maternal control diet, the proportion of epigenetic phenotypes in offspring is changed when dams are fed before and during pregnancy with a methyl-supplemented diet.[10,43] These diets are supplemented with substantial amounts of betaine, choline, folic acid and vitamin B12 or with these plus methionine and zinc (3SZM). The proportion of agouti in the offspring population increases as increasing levels of methyl supplement are added to the maternal diet. The proportion of mice with majority agouti coat was 43% for mice from mothers fed control diet and increased to 66% for mice from mothers on the high methyl 3SZM diet.

We observed a new phenotype, Y1, *only* in litters from dams fed the 3SZM diet.[10,43] These Y1 mice had a high degree of DNA methylation on their *agouti* allele commensurate with their high degree of agouti coat color. We did not observe any adverse effects on litter size, neonatal mortality, health, etc. even with the highest supplement levels.[10] Subsequent studies have shown that maternal dietary genistein, an estrogen-like compound from soybeans, has a similar effect as methyl supplements on offspring epigenetics.[44,45] The above studies supplemented mothers throughout pregnancy and did not determine the timing during pregnancy of nutritional influence in epigenetics.

The lowest levels of agouti coat in this system have been achieved by knocking down *Dnmt1* expression to a fraction of normal.[46] In these experiments the average percent of agouti coat was reduced from 71% for controls (*Dnmt1* wild type) to 29% for low *Dnmt1* mice. No purely nutritional studies have reported lowering agouti coat proportion. However, bisphenol A, which is an estrogen-like contaminant in food and water,[47] has been shown to lower agouti coat levels compared to controls, and methyl or genistein dietary supplementation was shown to substantially reverse this effect.[45] Bisphenol A may also have multigenerational effects.[48]

Even highly methyl supplemented maternal diets[10,43,49] still produce a small proportion of mostly yellow mice. Genetic studies that knock down the expression of *Dnmt1* still produce some mainly agouti mice.[46] The span of percent agouti in populations can be estimated to be between about 30%[46] and about 70%.[10,43] In theory at least, it should be possible to push epigenetic phenotype such that nearly all offspring are fully agouti or nearly all offspring are entirely yellow. However, no treatment has been devised that achieves this.

Mice bearing the A^{vy} allele have also been used to study the effect of methyl-supplemented diet on a subsequent generation and to study the time during pregnancy when the methyl supplement is effective.

7.6   Maternal nutrition can affect at least two generations

The epigenetic phenotype of yellow agouti mice is partially maternally inherited. This is based on the observation that agouti dams are more likely to produce agouti offspring than are yellow dams.[43,50] Later, Morgan et al.[9] showed that when mother and grandmother are fully agouti, a higher proportion of offspring have fully agouti coats than when grandmother has a mottled or yellow phenotype. Cropley et al.[49] studied the effects of a highly methyl-supplemented *grandmaternal diet* on offspring epigenetics.

They mated *a/a* dams with A^{vy}/a sires (P1), supplemented the pregnant dams and then without further supplementation, mated their pseudoagouti female offspring (F1) to *a/a* sires. The proportion of agouti coat was higher in offspring (F2) from supplemented grandmothers than from grandmothers on control diet. This demonstrates a transgenerational effect of maternal diet on the F2 generation. The extent of epigenetic change in the offspring phenotype was similar in the F1 and F2 generations.

Cropley et al. suggested that highly supplemented maternal (P1) diet results in modification of the F1 germline. These effects would then carry through and appear in the postnatal F2 offspring. This indicates that germline A^{vy} silencing is well maintained through gametogenesis, fertilization and development.

In a much different experimental design, Waterland et al.[51] did not find a second-generation effect of maternal diets. However, among other differences, they used a much lower dose diet than did Cropley et al.[49,52] Cropley et al. used a diet supplementing betaine, choline, folic acid, vitamin B12, methionine and zinc.[10,43] Human diets span a huge range for these same nutrients. These nutrient levels can be very low in refined foods and high, if not therapeutic, in some whole foods.[35]

7.7 Nutrition in mid-pregnancy can change epigenetics of yellow agouti offspring

In early mammalian development, the genome is substantially demethylated between fertilization and preimplantation. After implantation there is a wave of new methylation.[53] A substantial amount of A^{vy} silencing is epigenetically inherited from previous generations,[9,43] although some is newly established in gestation. A^{vy} silencing is often attributed to DNA methylation because there is a high correlation between A^{vy} LTR methylation and the silent state (agouti coat color).[10] As with many other genes it is likely that histone modifications and other aspects of the silenced chromatin repertoire are also involved. Some data indicates that both maternally and paternally inherited A^{vy} alleles are substantially or completely hypomethylated by the blastocyst stage and that DNA methylation reappears at approximately postnatal levels by 12.5 days gestation.[54] However, it is quite possible that cells in the inner cell mass that produce the fetus retain DNA methylated A^{vy} alleles continuously. Nevertheless as is the case with many other sequences, it is likely that some A^{vy} silencing occurs between 4.5 and 12.5 days gestation in mice. This does not exclude silencing later in development.

DNA methylation is established and maintained by Dnmts. An oocyte-specific form of Dnmt1, called Dnmt1o, is found in the cleavage embryo but disappears after implantation. The somatic form of Dnmt1 appears necessary for maintenance of DNA methylation after implantation and mouse embryos null for the *Dnmt1* gene do not develop past mid-gestation.[12] Substantial reductions in either the oocyte or somatic Dnmt1 forms during gestation resulted in significant decreases in the agouti coat color in mouse offspring carrying the A^{iapy} allele.[46] This indicates that most times of gestation (early and mid to late gestation) may be important for silencing A^{iapy}.

Cropley et al.[49] used gestational timing of maternal methyl supplementation to determine if A^{vy} silencing could be influenced mid-gestation. They treated pregnant dams with a high-level methyl supplement (3SZM) between gestational days 8.5 and 15.5. Full gestation is 21 days in mice. The proportion of agouti coat was higher in offspring from mid-gestation-supplemented dams than from control diet dams but very similar to that from dams supplemented throughout pregnancy. These results show that a significant amount, if not a majority, of A^{vy} silencing can occur after gestational day 8.5. It may be that epigenetics can be influenced at most times in gestation.

7.8   Maternal choline intake affects epigenetics, memory, and aging

Another long-term effect of maternal nutrition and metabolism is on long-term memory and mental function. Although choline is produced in mammalian metabolism, we evolved while getting substantial choline in our food and dietary choline is essential to maintain normal choline levels.[55] Choline is important for mobilizing fats, for the fluidity of cell membranes (e.g., as phosphatidylcholine) and as a precursor of the neurotransmitter acetylcholine. Choline is also a source of methyl groups in methyl metabolism after its enzymatic oxidation to betaine. Choline can be important for the control of blood plasma homocysteine levels.[56] Choline is transported against a concentration gradient to the fetus and to breast milk to help assure the fetus and neonate an adequate supply of choline. This can deplete maternal choline stores (reviewed in Reference 55).

In studies where pregnant rats are fed a normal, control diet plus a choline supplement from middle to late pregnancy (embryonic days 11 to 17), their offspring have better memory than do offspring of pregnant control rats fed only the control diet. This improved memory in the offspring is life long. Unlike control rats and many humans, the memory of rats from supplemented mothers did not decline with age[57–59] (reviewed in References 55 and 60).

Supplemental maternal choline may improve offspring memory by a number of mechanisms. Increased fetal acetylcholine levels could foster synapse formation and communication between neurons. Increased methyl donor availability could affect any of numerous *S*-adenosylmethionine-dependent methylation reactions, including DNA and histone methylation.

Choline could increase neuron membrane fluidity and fat transport to the brain. Any or all of these factors could affect fetal brain growth.

Several effects on brain development are associated with maternal choline supplementation. There is increased proliferation and decreased apoptosis of hippocampal progenitor cells in fetuses. In adult offspring of supplemented mothers the hippocampus shows increased sensitivity to long-term potentiation (long-lasting enhancement of communication between neurons). Generally the opposite effects are seen with maternal choline deficiency (reviewed by Reference 55). Meck and Williams[61] describe an organizational change in brain function in response to choline, possibly at the cholinergic synapse, which they call "metabolic imprinting."

Improved memory by maternal choline supplements appears to have an epigenetic component, at least during fetal development. Kovacheva and coworkers studied three levels of maternal choline (deficient, control and supplemented) during embryonic days 11 to 17 in rats.[62] Control and deficient embryos at day 17 had lower *Dnmt1* gene methylation in the cerebral cortex and higher expression of the *Dnmt1*, *Dnmt3a* and *Mdb2* genes in the frontal cortex. In liver, they showed some similar results, as well as altered methylation and expression of the imprinted *Igf2* gene. In the brain, the expression patterns for control and deficient groups were similar and the supplemented group was the exception. They discuss how choline deficiency may induce a compensatory response in the expression levels of Dnmt1 and other machinery of epigenetic regulation. This compensatory response may not be enough to bring memory or other characteristics up to normal levels. Overall, their results suggest that epigenetics is probably involved in brain development, and possibly memory, in response to choline. These results, as well as previous studies of offspring memory, suggest that "normal" choline levels may be too low and that supplemented levels are closer to the optimum. Additional studies are needed to determine what maternal choline consumption levels will produce optimum memory in offspring.

7.9   *Maternal effects on the development of T2DM*

The incidence of T2DM is increasing in many developed nations and worldwide. This increase is substantially due to lifestyle and other environmental factors. This increase is not due mainly to an aging population, because many children are developing T2DM—a disease once called "adult onset diabetes." Although genetics plays a role in diabetes it is probably not responsible for the *increased incidence* of diabetes. This is because there are no large demographic shifts in population or other changes that could affect the average genetics of the affected populations to account for such substantial increases in T2DM. There is the unlikely possibility that maternal effects are leading to genetic selection in utero but there are few, if any, data to argue for this and it would require that the maternal effect (e.g., high glucose) be lethal to a substantial number of early embryos. Instead the available evidence points to lifestyle factors, especially diet and sedentary behavior, of children and adults as the likely causes. For pregnant mothers their behavior prior to and during pregnancy, may be especially important because maternal effects likely affect the risk of offspring developing T2DM. Further, these maternal effects may compound and accumulate over generations (reviewed in References 63 and 36).

As early as 1975 Dörner et al. reported a possible epigenetic role in the transmission of T2DM between generations in humans.[64] Diabetes with an age of onset greater than 10 years was much more likely to be associated with a family history of diabetes on the maternal side than on the paternal side. Such differences were not found in juvenile (type 1) diabetes.[64,65]

Women with gestational diabetes were also more likely to have mothers with diabetes than were pregnant controls.[66] In a follow up report, women with gestational diabetes were eight times more likely to have mothers with diabetes than were controls. No difference was found for the incidence of diabetes in the fathers of the two groups.[67] Harder et al.[68] showed that women with gestational diabetes are more likely to have grandmothers with T2DM than to have grandfathers with T2DM.

Rat and mouse strains without known genetic susceptibilities to diabetes can be induced to develop diabetes with drugs or glucose loading. Diabetes or related disorders are then often passed on to subsequent generations. Treatment of rats with the drugs alloxan or streptozotocin induces diabetes. The F1, or subsequent generation offspring of treated female rats, have hallmarks of diabetes that can include hyperinsulinemia, hypoinsulinemia, pancreatic islet hyperplasia and beta cell degranulation.[69–72] In some cases these effects worsen with subsequent generations. These effects were not found in F1 or subsequent generations from normal, untreated, mothers (P1). Although both male and female offspring would be diabetic, in most cases, paternal transmission of diabetes was not observed.

Transgenerational diabetes can also be induced by continuously infusing pregnant rats with glucose during the last week of pregnancy.[73,74] The adult offspring from hyperglycemic mothers had mild glucose intolerance and impaired insulin secretion that worsened with age. F2 newborns of F1 hyperglycemic dams were also hyperglycemic, hyperinsulinemic and macrosomic. They later developed basal hyperglycemia and defective glucose tolerance and insulin secretion. These results demonstrate that maternal glucose intake in pregnancy can produce heritable diabetes in offspring.

Chronically high levels of insulin signaling and/or glucose metabolism may lead to epigenetic modifications in genes of various pathways for metabolism and signaling. This may be similar to the glucose hysteresis proposed by Mobbs et al.[75] Any alteration of macronutrient levels such as protein restriction will necessitate an overall change in nutrient balance that will affect the content of fat, carbohydrates and/or calories in the diet. Lillycrop et al.[76] showed that maternal protein restriction in rats lowered DNA methylation levels of several CpGs in the PPARα promoter of rat pups (34 days postnatal). These effects persisted to adulthood (80 days postnatal). In another study they showed lower hepatic glucocorticoid receptor promoter methylation and lower *Dnmt1* expression in offspring due to maternal protein restriction.[77]

The molecular mechanism for multigenerational inheritance and progression of diabetes has not been determined in rats, mice or humans. It appears that some epigenetic effect is involved, such as metabolic imprinting by each mother on her offspring during pregnancy. It seems likely that some effects will be found at the level of gene-specific expression or epigenetic modification. The mechanisms of diabetes, especially multigenerational diabetes, are of great interest because of the current rise in childhood and adult diabetes in the United States and many other countries.

7.10   Honey bee phenotypes are determined epigenetically

In honey bees (*Apis mellifera*) dramatically different phenotypes are obtained from the same genotype depending on what is fed to the larvae. Feeding larvae royal jelly results in their development into queen bees. Queen bees and worker bees have dramatically different phenotypes, including marked morphological, physiological, behavioral and reproductive differences. Their life spans differ, with queens outliving workers 10–fold.[78,79] Unlike some other insects, *Apis* has DNA methylation globally and in at least several genes and has homologs of mammalian DNA methyltransferases and methylated DNA binding proteins.[80]

A study by Kucharski et al.[81] shows that inhibition of *Dnmt3* expression in *Apis* larvae by siRNA leads to the development of most larvae into queen bees. Controls were injected with siRNA to a nonlarval gene resulting in development into mainly worker bees. They also studied DNA methylation of CpG sites in the exons of the *dynactin p62* gene. (Most *Apis* gene methylation is in CpGs of exons.) The *dynactin p62* gene is differentially methylated during development. In both hive-reared queen larvae and in Dnmt3 RNAi-treated, in vitro-reared larvae, the *dynactin p62* CpG methylation was lower than in corresponding controls. This difference was most pronounced in larval heads that have higher levels of *dynactin p62* gene DNA methylation than whole body larvae.

Certainly, insect development is substantially different from mammalian development, which makes the relevance of this insect model to mouse and human epigenetics debatable. However, *Apis* is an attractive model on several scores. Most notably is the clear and dramatic difference in phenotype and life span between queen and worker bees. Unlike some other animal models of extended longevity[82–84] the increased fecundity of the queen is accompanied by greatly *increased* longevity. Thus, the long-term health and the ability of the queen to perform evolutionary essential functions go hand in hand in this model. The epigenetics of this model is particularly clear—queens and workers each maintain their phenotypes and, for experimental purposes, subjects can be chosen at will for one treatment or another from a population that is a large group of genetically clonal larvae. Although a specialty, bee breeding, maintenance and experimentation are far less costly than similar studies with mice.

The identification of active components of royal jelly[85] and the pathways controlling bee development that connect feeding of royal jelly to epigenetics have yet to be elucidated. Likewise, much work remains to connect nutrition, metabolism, signaling, development and epigenetics in mammals.[3,86–88]

7.11   Conclusions

If we assume that epigenetics of the fetus is more malleable than that of the adult, then the fetal response to high glucose, high or low choline or methyl supplements may be greater and longer lasting than similar exposure of the adult. A few months of exposure to the fetus may have lifelong effects, whereas a few months exposure in the adult may have little or no lasting effect.

Most successful interventions so far are mixtures or not fully chemically defined. The methyl supplements used in yellow agouti studies, while chemically defined, are a combination, and presumably there are simpler combinations or single compound treatments to produce similar results. The interventions of bisphenol A and genistein, while chemically defined, are not normal constituents of mouse metabolism, leaving their mechanism of action uncertain. In honey bees, royal jelly produces a dramatic shift in phenotype and some experiments shed light on a mechanism;[81] however, the active ingredient in royal jelly is not known. Interventions using choline provide an example of a chemically defined normal metabolite and dietary constituent with a strong phenotypic effect.

Most interventions thus far show only a moderate effect on epigenetics. If the modifications of DNA, histones, transcription factors, signaling proteins and others were better understood, and interventions were designed to effectively target them, it should be possible to dramatically shift epigenetics such that a highly variable phenotype would be pushed to one extreme or the other. For example, in the yellow agouti mouse model it should be possible to produce a population of offspring that are nearly all agouti (e.g., nearly all pseudoagouti) or, by another intervention, to produce a population of offspring that are nearly all yellow.

There are thousands of nutrients and other compounds in food and only a handful of compounds and nutrient combinations have been tested for maternal effects on offspring epigenetics. Increased testing to screen compounds and nutrient balances is essential if we are to protect public health and set sensible public policy. What we do now is important not just for mothers and their offspring but for future generations as well.

Acknowledgments

I thank Tonya Rafferty for mouse photographs and Kimberly Cooney for drawing most of the figures. This work is supported by grants P01AG20641 from the NIA/NIH and R01AA016676 from the NIAAA/NIH.

References

1. Vickaryous, M.K. and Hall, B.K. (2006). Human cell type diversity, evolution, development, and classification with special reference to cells derived from the neural crest. *Biol Rev Camb Philos Soc* 81, 425–455.
2. Laird, P. (2005). Cancer epigenetics. *Human Molecular Genetics* 14, R65–R76.
3. Meaney, M.J. and Szyf, M. (2005). Maternal care as a model for experience-dependent chromatin plasticity? *Trends Neurosci* 28, 456–463.
4. Taverna, S. D., Ilin, S., Rogers, R.S., Tanny, J.C., Lavender, H., Li, H., Baker, L., Boyle, J., Blair, L.P., Chait, B.T., Patel, D.J., Aitchison, J.D., Tackett, A.J., and Allis, C.D. (2006). Yng1 PHD finger binding to H3 trimethylated at K4 promotes NuA3 HAT activity at K14 of H3 and transcription at a subset of targeted ORFs. *Mol Cell* 24, 785–796.
5. Kouzarides, T. (2007). Chromatin modifications and their function. *Cell* 128, 693–705.
6. Hershko, A.Y., Kafri, T., Fainsod, A., and Razin, A. (2003). Methylation of HoxA5 and HoxB5 and its relevance to expression during mouse development. *Gene* 302, 65–72.
7. Weaver, I.C., Cervoni, N., Champagne, F.A., D'Alessio, A.C., Sharma, S., Seckl, J.R., Dymov, S., Szyf, M., and Meaney, M.J. (2004). Epigenetic programming by maternal behavior. *Nat Neurosci* 7, 847–854.
8. Cooney, C.A. (2008). Cancer and aging: The epigenetic connection. In *Cancer Epigenetics*, Trygve Tollefsbol, ed., 303–316. Boca Raton, FL: CRC Press.
9. Morgan, H.D., Sutherland, H.G., Martin, D.I., and Whitelaw, E. (1999). Epigenetic inheritance at the agouti locus in the mouse. *Nat Genet* 23, 314–318.
10. Cooney, C.A., Dave, A.A., and Wolff, G.L. (2002). Maternal methyl supplements in mice affect epigenetic variation and DNA methylation of offspring. *J Nutr* 132, 2393S–2400S.

11. Rakyan, V.K., Chong, S., Champ, M.E., Cuthbert, P.C., Morgan, H.D., Luu, K.V., and Whitelaw, E. (2003). Transgenerational inheritance of epigenetic states at the murine Axin(Fu) allele occurs after maternal and paternal transmission. *Proc Natl Acad Sci USA* 100, 2538–2543.

12. Li, E., Bestor, T.H., and Jaenisch, R. (1992). Targeted mutation of the DNA methyltransferase gene results in embryonic lethality. *Cell* 69, 915–926.

13. Tate, P., Skarnes, W., and Bird, A. (1996). The methyl-CpG binding protein MeCP2 is essential for embryonic development in the mouse. *Nat Genet* 12, 205–208.

14. Okano, M., Bell, D.W., Haber, D.A., and Li, E. (1999). DNA methyltransferases Dnmt3a and Dnmt3b are essential for de novo methylation and mammalian development. *Cell* 99, 247–257.

15. Goll, M.G. and Bestor, T.H. (2005). Eukaryotic cytosine methyltransferases. *Annu Rev Biochem* 74, 481–514.

16. D'Alessio, A.C., Weaver, I.C., and Szyf, M. (2007). Acetylation-induced transcription is required for active DNA demethylation in methylation-silenced genes. *Mol Cell Biol* 27, 7462–7474.

17. Métivier, R., Gallais, R., Tiffoche, C., Le Péron, C., Jurkowska, R.Z., Carmouche, R.P., Ibberson, D., Barath, P., Demay, F., Reid, G., Benes, V., Jeltsch, A., Gannon, F., and Salbert, G. (2008). Cyclical DNA methylation of a transcriptionally active promoter. *Nature* 452, 45–50.

18. Kondo, Y., Shen, L., Yan, P.S., Huang, T.H., and Issa, J.P. (2004). Chromatin immunoprecipitation microarrays for identification of genes silenced by histone H3 lysine 9 methylation. *Proc Natl Acad Sci USA* 101, 7398–7403.

19. Adams, R. and Burdon, R. (1985). *Molecular Biology of DNA Methylation*. New York: Springer-Verlag.

20. Jacobs, S.A., Harp, J.M., Devarakonda, S., Kim, Y., Rastinejad, F., and Khorasanizadeh, S. (2002). The active site of the SET domain is constructed on a knot. *Nat Struct Biol* 9, 833–838.

21. Bestor, T.H. (1992). Activation of mammalian DNA methyltransferase by cleavage of a Zn binding regulatory domain. *EMBO J* 11, 2611–2617.

22. Chuang, L.S., Ng, H.H., Chia, J.N., and Li, B.F. (1996). Characterisation of independent DNA and multiple Zn-binding domains at the N terminus of human DNA-(cytosine-5) methyltransferase: Modulating the property of a DNA-binding domain by contiguous Zn-binding motifs. *J Mol Biol* 257, 935–948.

23. Millian, N.S. and Garrow, T.A. (1998). Human betaine-homocysteine methyltransferase is a zinc metalloenzyme. *Arch Biochem Biophys* 356, 93–98.

24. Cooney, C.A. (1993). Are somatic cells inherently deficient in methylation metabolism? A proposed mechanism for DNA methylation loss, senescence and aging. *Growth Dev Aging* 57, 261–273.

25. Mosharov, E., Cranford, M.R., and Banerjee, R. (2000). The quantitatively important relationship between homocysteine metabolism and glutathione synthesis by the transsulfuration pathway and its regulation by redox changes. *Biochemistry* 39, 13005–13011.

26. Uthus, E.O. and Brown-Borg, H.M. (2003). Altered methionine metabolism in long living Ames dwarf mice. *Exp Gerontol* 38, 491–498.

27. Zeisel, S.H., Mar, M.H., Howe, J.C., and Holden, J.M. (2003). Concentrations of choline-containing compounds and betaine in common foods. *J Nutr* 133, 1302–1307.

28. Jeukendrup, A.E. (2002). Regulation of fat metabolism in skeletal muscle. *Ann NY Acad Sci* 967, 217–235.
29. Choi, C.H., Hiromura, M., and Usheva, A. (2003). Transcription factor IIB acetylates itself to regulate transcription. *Nature* 424, 965–969.
30. Imhof, A., Yang, X.J., Ogryzko, V.V., Nakatani, Y., Wolffe, A.P., and Ge, H. (1997). Acetylation of general transcription factors by histone acetyltransferases. *Curr Biol* 7, 689–692.
31. Huang, S. (2002). Histone methyltransferases, diet nutrients and tumour suppressors. *Nat Rev Cancer* 2, 469–476.
32. Choi, C.H., Zimon, A., and Usheva, A. (2005). Metabolic stress regulates basic transcription through acetyl-coenzyme A. *Cell Mol Life Sci* 62, 625–628.
33. Raychaudhuri, N., Raychaudhuri, S., Thamotharan, M., and Devaskar, S.U. (2008). Histone code modifications repress glucose transporter 4 expression in the intra-uterine growth restricted offspring. *J Biol Chem* 283, 13611–13626.
34. Waterland, R.A. and Jirtle, R.L. (2003). Transposable elements: Targets for early nutritional effects on epigenetic gene regulation. *Mol Cell Biol* 23, 5293–5300.
35. Cooney, C.A. (2006). Maternal nutrition: Nutrients and control of expression. In *Nutrigenomics: Concepts and Technologies*, James Kaput and Raymond L. Rodriguez, ed., 219–254. Hoboken, NJ: John Wiley & Sons.
36. Cooney, C.A. (2007). Epigenetics: DNA-based mirror of our environment. *Disease Markers* 23, 121–137.
37. Mynatt, R.L. and Stephens, J.M. (2001). Agouti regulates adipocyte transcription factors, *Am J Physiol Cell Physiol* 280, C954–C961.
38. Wolff, G.L., Roberts, D.W., and Mountjoy, K.G. (1999). Physiological consequences of ectopic agouti gene expression: The yellow obese mouse syndrome. *Physiol Genomics* 1, 151–163.
39. Wolff, G.L., Kodell, R.L., Kaput, J.A., and Visek, W.J. (1999). Caloric restriction abolishes enhanced metabolic efficiency induced by ectopic agouti protein in yellow mice. *Proc Soc Exp Biol Med* 221, 99–104.
40. Kaput, J., Klein, K.G., Reyes, E.J., Kibbe, W.A., Cooney, C.A., Jovanovic, B., Visek, W.J., and Wolff, G.L. (2004). Identification of genes contributing to the obese yellow Avy phenotype: Caloric restriction, genotype, diet × genotype interactions. *Physiol Genomics* 18, 316–324.
41. Wolff, G.L., Kodell, R.L., Cameron, A.M., and Medina, D. (1982). Accelerated appearance of chemically induced mammary carcinomas in obese yellow (Avy/A) (BALB/c X VY) F1 hybrid mice. *J Toxicol Environ Health* 10, 131–142.
42. Wolff, G.L., Morrissey, R.L., and Chen, J.J. (1986). Susceptible and resistant subgroups in genetically identical populations: Response of mouse liver neoplasia and body weight to Phenobarbital. *Carcinogenesis* 7, 1935–1937.
43. Wolff, G.L., Kodell, R.L., Moore, S.R., and Cooney, C.A. (1998). Maternal epigenetics and methyl supplements affect agouti gene expression in Avy/a mice, *FASEB J* 12, 949–957.
44. Dolinoy, D.C., Weidman, J.R., Waterland, R.A., and Jirtle, R.L. (2006). Maternal genistein alters coat color and protects Avy mouse offspring from obesity by modifying the fetal epigenome. *Environ Health Perspect* 114, 567–572.
45. Dolinoy, D.C., Huang, D., and Jirtle, R.L. (2007). Maternal nutrient supplementation counteracts bisphenol A-induced DNA hypomethylation in early development. *Proc Natl Acad Sci USA* 104, 13056–13061.

46. Gaudet, F., Rideout, W. M. III, Meissner, A., Dausman, J., Leonhardt, H., and Jaenisch, R. (2004). Dnmt1 expression in pre- and postimplantation embryogenesis and the maintenance of IAP silencing. *Mol Cell Biol* 24, 1640–1648.

47. Vandenberg, L.N., Hauser, R., Marcus, M., Olea, N., and Welshons, W.V. (2007). Human exposure to bisphenol A (BPA). *Reprod Toxicol* 24,139–177.

48. Susiarjo, M. and Hunt, P. (2008). Bisphenol A exposure disrupts egg development in the mouse. *Fertil Steril* 89 (2 Suppl), e97.

49. Cropley, J.E., Suter, C.M., Beckman, K.B., and Martin, D.I.K. (2006). Germline epigenetic modification of the murine A vy allele by nutritional supplementation. *Proc Natl Acad Sci USA* 103, 17308–17312.

50. Wolff, G.L. (1978). Influence of maternal phenotype on metabolic differentiation of agouti locus mutants in the mouse. *Genetics* 88, 529–539.

51. Waterland, R.A., Travisano, M., and Tahiliani, K.G. (2007). Diet-induced hypermethylation at agouti viable yellow is not inherited transgenerationally through the female. *FASEB J* 21, 3380–3385.

52. Cropley, J.E., Suter, C.M., and Martin, D.I. (2007). Methyl donors change the germline epigenetic state of the A(vy) allele. *FASEB J* 21, 3021.

53. Li, E. (2002). Chromatin modification and epigenetic reprogramming in mammalian development. *Nat Rev Genet* 3, 662–673.

54. Blewitt, M.E., Vickaryous, N.K., Paldi, A., Koseki, H., and Whitelaw, E. (2006). Dynamic reprogramming of DNA methylation at an epigenetically sensitive allele in mice. *PLoS Genet* 2, e49.

55. Zeisel, S.H. (2007). Gene response elements, genetic polymorphisms and epigenetics influence the human dietary requirement for choline. *IUBMB Life* 59, 380–387.

56. da Costa, K.A., Gaffney, C.E., Fischer, L.M., and Zeisel, S.H. (2005). Choline deficiency in mice and humans is associated with increased plasma homocysteine concentration after a methionine load. *Am J Clin Nutr* 81, 440–444.

57. Meck, W.H., Smith, R.A., and Williams, C.L. (1989). Organizational changes in cholinergic activity and enhanced visuospatial memory as a function of choline administered prenatally or postnatally or both. *Behav Neurosci* 103, 1234–1241.

58. Meck, W.H. and Williams, C.L. (1997). Perinatal choline supplementation increases the threshold for chunking in spatial memory. *Neuroreport* 8, 3053–3059.

59. Meck, W.H. and Williams, C.L. (1997). Simultaneous temporal processing is sensitive to prenatal choline availability in mature and aged rats. *Neuroreport* 8, 3045–3051.

60. Blusztajn, J.K. (1998). Choline, a vital amine. *Science* 281, 794–795.

61. Meck, W.H., and Williams, C.L. (2003). Metabolic imprinting of choline by its availability during gestation: Implications for memory and attentional processing across the lifespan. *Neurosci Biobehav Rev* 27, 385–399.

62. Kovacheva, V.P., Mellott, T.J., Davison, J.M., Wagner, N., Lopez-Coviella, I., Schnitzler, A.C., and Blusztajn, J.K. (2007). Gestational choline deficiency causes global and Igf2 gene DNA hypermethylation by up-regulation of Dnmt1 expression. *J Biol Chem* 282, 31777–31788.

63. Fetita, L.S., Sobngwi, E., Serradas, P., Calvo, F., and Gautier, J.F. (2006). Consequences of fetal exposure to maternal diabetes in offspring. *J Clin Endocrinol Metab* 91, 3718–3724.

64. Dörner, G., Mohnike, A., and Steindel, E. (1975). On possible genetic and epigenetic modes of diabetes transmission. *Endokrinologie* 66, 225–227.
65. Dörner, G., and Mohnike, A. (1976). Further evidence for a predominantly maternal transmission of maturity-onset type diabetes. *Endokrinologie* 68, 121–124.
66. Martin, A.O., Simpson J.L., Ober, C., and Freinkel, N. (1985). Frequency of diabetes mellitus in mothers of probands with gestational diabetes: Possible maternal influence on the predisposition to gestational diabetes. *Am J Obstet Gynecol* 151, 471–475.
67. Freinkel, N., Metzger, B.E., Phelps, R.L., Simpson, J.L., Martin, A.O., Radvany, R., Ober, C., Dooley, S.L., Depp, R.O., and Belton, A. (1986). Gestational diabetes mellitus: A syndrome with phenotypic and genotypic heterogeneity. *Horm Metab Res* 18, 427–430.
68. Harder, T., Franke, K., Kohlhoff, R., and Plagemann, A. (2001). Maternal and paternal family history of diabetes in women with gestational diabetes or insulin-dependent diabetes mellitus type I. *Gynecol Obstet Invest* 51, 160–164.
69. Spergel, G., Khan, F., and Goldner, M.G. (1975). Emergence of overt diabetes in offspring of rats with induced latent diabetes. *Metabolism* 24, 1311–1319.
70. van Assche, F.A., and Aerts, L. (1985). Long-term effect of diabetes and pregnancy in the rat. *Diabetes* 34 (Suppl 2), 116–118.
71. Baranov, V.G., Sokoloverova, I.M., Sitnikova, A.M., and Onegova, R.F. (1988). Development of diabetes mellitus in the progeny of 6 generations of female rats with alloxan diabetes. *Biull Eksp Biol Med* 105, 13–15.
72. Dorner, G., Plagemann, A., Ruckert, J., Gotz, F., Rohde, W., Stahl, F., Kurschner, U., Gottschalk, J., Mohnike, A., and Steindel, E. (1988). Teratogenetic maternofoetal transmission and prevention of diabetes susceptibility. *Exp Clin Endocrinol* 91, 247–258.
73. Gauguier, D., Bihoreau, M.T., Ktorza, A., Berthault, M.F., and Picon, L. (1990). Inheritance of diabetes mellitus as consequence of gestational hyperglycemia in rats. *Diabetes* 39, 734–739.
74. Gauguier, D., Bihoreau, M.T., Picon, L., and Ktorza, A. (1991). Insulin secretion in adult rats after intrauterine exposure to mild hyperglycemia during late gestation, *Diabetes* 40 (Suppl 2), 109–114.
75. Mobbs, C.V., Mastaitis, J.W., Zhang, M., Isoda, F., Cheng, H., and Yen, K. (2007). Secrets of the lac operon. Glucose hysteresis as a mechanism in dietary restriction, aging and disease. *Interdiscip Top Gerontol* 35, 39–68.
76. Lillycrop, K.A., Phillips, E.S., Torrens, C., Hanson, M.A., Jackson, A.A., and Burdge, G.C. (2008). Feeding pregnant rats a protein-restricted diet persistently alters the methylation of specific cytosines in the hepatic PPARalpha promoter of the offspring. *Br J Nutr* 100, 278–282.
77. Lillycrop, K.A., Slater-Jefferies, J.L., Hanson, M.A., Godfrey, K.M., Jackson, A.A., and Burdge, G.C. (2007). Induction of altered epigenetic regulation of the hepatic glucocorticoid receptor in the offspring of rats fed a protein-restricted diet during pregnancy suggests that reduced DNA methyltransferase-1 expression is involved in impaired DNA methylation and changes in histone modifications. *Br J Nutr* 97, 1064–1073.
78. Page, R.E., Jr., and Peng, C.Y. (2001). Aging and development in social insects with emphasis on the honey bee, *Apis mellifera* L. *Exp Gerontol* 36, 695–711.

79. Corona, M., Velarde R.A., Remolina, S., Moran-Lauter, A., Wang, Y., Hughes, K.A., and Robinson, G.E. (2007). Vitellogenin, juvenile hormone, insulin signaling, and queen honey bee longevity. *Proc Natl Acad Sci USA* 104, 7128–7133.
80. Wang, Y., Jorda, M., Jones, P.L., Maleszka, R., Ling, X., Robertson, H.M., Mizzen, C.A., Peinado, M.A., and Robinson, G.E. (2006). Functional CpG methylation system in a social insect. *Science* 314, 645–647.
81. Kucharski, R., Maleszka, J., Foret, S., and Maleszka, R. (2008). Nutritional control of reproductive status in honeybees via DNA methylation. *Science* 319, 1827–1830.
82. Ayyadevara, S., Alla, R., Thaden, J.J., and Shmookler Reis, R.J. (2008). Remarkable longevity and stress resistance of nematode PI3K-null mutants. *Aging Cell* 7, 13–22.
83. Yamawaki, T.M., Arantes-Oliveira, N., Berman, J.R., Zhang, P., and Kenyon, C. (2008). Distinct activities of the germline and somatic reproductive tissues in the regulation of *Caenorhabditis elegans'* longevity. *Genetics* 178, 513–526.
84. Bartke, A., and Brown-Borg, H. (2004). Life extension in the dwarf mouse. *Curr Top Dev Biol* 63, 189–225.
85. Schönleben, S., Sickmann, A., Mueller, M.J., and Reinders, J. (2007). Proteome analysis of *Apis mellifera* royal jelly. *Anal Bioanal Chem* 389, 1087–1093.
86. Slack, A., Cervoni, N., Pinard, M., and Szyf, M. (1999). Feedback regulation of DNA methyltransferase gene expression by methylation. *Eur J Biochem* 264, 191–199.
87. Slack, A., Pinard, M., Araujo, F.D., and Szyf, M. (2001). A novel regulatory element in the dnmt1 gene that responds to co-activation by Rb and c-Jun. *Gene* 268, 87–96.
88. Xie, C.H., Naito, A., Mizumachi, T., Evans, T.T., Douglas, M.G., Cooney, C.A., Fan, C.Y., and Higuchi, M. (2007). Mitochondrial regulation of cancer associated nuclear DNA methylation. *Biochem Biophys Res Commun* 364, 656–661.

chapter eight

Nutrition, epigenetics, and aging

John C. Mathers and Dianne Ford

Contents

8.1 Epidemiology and biology of aging

Over the past two centuries, one of the most remarkable human achievements has been the apparently inexorable increase in life expectancy observed in most countries. Apparently authoritative predictions of limits to human longevity have been confounded consistently for the last 80 years.[1] Before 1950 most of this gain in years of life was due to reductions in deaths in childhood but there is now a clear increase in survival after age 65 years. For example, life expectancy of Japanese women has increased by 3 months per annum throughout the last 160 years and one in four Japanese girls born in the millennium year 2000 can expect to celebrate their 100th birthday. Until recently, population aging has been associated with the more developed regions of the world but the number of older people (defined as those aged 65 years or more) living in less developed regions is expected to increase from ~400 million people in 2002 to ~840 million in 2025.[2] Globally, people over the age of 80 are the fastest growing segment of the population.[2]

In most cases the increase in longevity has brought with it more years of chronic morbidity so that much of humankind's experience of ill health and expenditure on medical and social care (especially in Western countries) are concentrated in the later years of life. Indeed, for a large proportion of common chronic medical conditions, age is the single greatest risk factor. Among older people in America, 50% have chronic diseases or some other form of disability,[3] including hypertension (49.2%), arthritic symptoms (36.1%), heart disease (31.4%), sinusitis (15%) and diabetes (15%).[4] In the United Kingdom, although older people make up only 16% of the population, they account for more than a third of hospital and community health service spending[5] and, in England, almost two-thirds of general and acute hospital beds are used by older people.[6]

This worldwide increase in life span is evidence of considerable malleability in the aging process and argues against the idea that humans are genetically programmed to die.[7] The challenge is to understand the factors influencing aging so that strategies that facilitate healthy aging, that is, maintenance of the healthy aging phenotype, can be maximized. At its most fundamental, aging appears to be due to damage to macromolecules that results in loss of, or aberrant, function,[7] including changes in chromatin structure,[8] which may contribute to altered gene expression.[9] Such damage affects (probably) all cells in the body and includes damage to the nuclear genome (somatic mutations and telomere shortening[10]) and accumulation of both mitochondrial mutations[11] and altered cellular proteins.[7] It seems likely that damage to stem cells may be particularly important in limiting capacity for regeneration with age.[12] Emerging evidence suggests that nutrition and lifestyle may be key environmental determinants of aging because they have profound effects on the genomic and cellular damage which appears to be the fundamental cause of reduced function and increasing frailty that characterize physiological aging.

8.2   *Nutritional modulation of aging*

Food restriction is the only proven nongenetic experimental paradigm for increasing life span in many animal species[13] but its effects on longevity in humans remain uncertain.[14] A recent review of the literature since 1966 concluded that experimental restriction of dietary intake in adult men and women elicited metabolic adaptations similar to those seen in energy restricted rodents and monkeys but the authors warned that "even moderate calorie restriction may be harmful in … lean persons who have minimal amounts of body fat."[14] Nevertheless, there is observational evidence that diet quality affects both length of life[15] and risk of a wide range of age-related diseases and conditions, including cognitive decline.[16] While there is encouraging epidemiological evidence that dietary choices influence aging, there is a paucity of intervention studies in humans that have tested the impact of particular nutrients, foods or dietary patterns on aging in general or aging of particular body systems. An exception is vitamin D supplementation, which seems to be associated with decreased total mortality although it is important to note that death was not the primary endpoint in the studies considered in this review.[17]

8.3   Epigenetic changes associated with aging

A quarter of a century ago, Wilson and Jones[18] observed that the methyl-cytosine content of DNA of mammalian cells decreased with time in culture. These authors could not distinguish between effects of time in culture and age per se but favored the latter explanation and went on to speculate that this alteration in DNA methylation might explain reported changes in gene expression with age. Much of this loss of genomic methyl groups occurs in repeated sequences within DNA[19] especially within Alu sequences,[20] which are short (~300 bp) interspersed nuclear elements (SINEs) making up about 10% of the mass of the human genome. Loss of DNA methylation may contribute to genomic instability[21,22] and so contribute to an aging cellular phenotype through this process. Age-related demethylation appears to be a passive process associated with reduced expression and activity of the DNA methyltransferase DNMT1.[23,24] At the same time, a number of normally unmethylated domains, especially CpG islands within the promoters of housekeeping genes, become methylated during aging. For example, Issa et al. report CpG island methylation within the estrogen receptor (*ESR1*) gene with age in the human colon.[25] Such hypermethylation was observed also in *ESR1, MYOD* and *p16* exon 1 in the macroscopically normal epithelium from ulcerative colitis (UC) patients, indicating that UC may be a disease of premature aging of the colorectal mucosa.[26] Passage-dependent increase in *ESR2* methylation was observed when human aortic endothelial and smooth muscle cells were cultured in vitro.[27] In addition, coronary atherosclerotic tissues had higher *ESR2* methylation than apparently normal femoral artery tissue, suggesting that epigenetic dysregulation of *ESR2* may occur in atherosclerosis and vascular aging.[27] In normal prostate tissue, there is a significant increase with age in promoter methylation for *ESR1, RARβ2, RASSF1A, GSTP1* and *NKX2-5*.[28] The mechanism for the greater gene-specific methylation with age is not well understood but may be related to enhanced activity of the de novo DNA methyltransferase DNMT3b.[24]

The limited evidence available to date supports the view that several genes in many (if not all) tissue types are susceptible to age-dependent hypermethylation and this epigenetic change would be expected to result in loss of function of these genes in the affected cells. It is important to note that age-related aberrant methylation does not occur

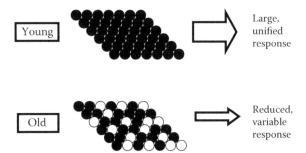

Figure 8.1 Conceptual functional consequences of increased intercellular hetero-geneity in promoter methylation and subsequent silencing of a gene with age in a given tissue. • = unmethylated gene, expression; ○ = methylated gene, no expression.

in all cells in a tissue but that aging increases the degree of epigenetic mosaicism within a tissue. In other words, in a single cell at a given CpG site in a specific gene, methylation is a binary phenomenon, that is, the cytosine in question is either methylated or unmethylated. Since DNA methylation patterns across cell generations are much less well policed than is the primary sequence, it would be anticipated that methylation patterns would drift over time leading to greater intercellular diver-gence in methylation patterns within a tissue with age. By expanding HMEC cells from 1 to 10^6 followed by bisulfite sequencing, Ushijima et al. quantified epigenetic error rates for a panel of six genes and reported a mean of 0.1% "errors" per site per cell generation.[29] This growing heterogeneity in epigenetic markings may explain, to some extent, the greater cell-to-cell variation in gene expression observed with age in mouse cardiomyocytes.[30] The greater cell-to-cell variation appeared to be random (i.e., differed between genes within a cell[30]), which would be consistent with epigenetic drift occurring over time. These observations suggest that the increased cell-to-cell diversity in epigenetic marking with age may have important functional conse-quences and, at a tissue level, may explain some of the reduction in speed and magnitude of response to stimuli which characterizes aging and the development of frailty (Figure 8.1).

8.4   Impact of nutrition on DNA methylation

The observation that the susceptibility of rat liver chromatin to digestion by micrococcal nuclease was altered as a function of diet was an early indication of the potential of diet to modify gross chromatin structure.[31] The more recent observation that DNA methylation and histone acetyla-tion patterns are less similar in older than in younger homozygous twins is indicative of an environmental influence, likely to include diet, on epigenomic status.[32] Evidence for specific effects of dietary components on DNA methylation and histone modification will be summarized in the following sections, with particular consideration of the potential relevance to aging.

A number of specific nutrients and micronutrients or other bioactive dietary constituents influence DNA methylation, both globally and at specific loci. These dietary components include intermediates involved in one-carbon (methyl) metabolism (folate, methionine, choline, and betaine), bioactive polyphenols and isothiocyanates, zinc, selenium, arsenic, vitamin A and alcohol. In addition to specific dietary components, broader nutritional strategies or interventions, specifically dietary restriction and (in utero) a low protein diet, might have epigenetic effects. These effects might be one of the mechanisms through which the very well-established effect of dietary restriction to increase life span is mediated. Obesity, which may be considered a consequence of nutrition, might have epigenetic effects that are independent of the influences of the causal nutritional status.

Much of the research on the epigenetic effects of dietary components, in particular methyl donors and bioactive polyphenols, has focused on exposure in utero. This focus has been driven largely by the now-compelling evidence that nutritional stresses during gestation result in lifelong consequences for health,[33] coupled with the apparent feasibility of epigenetic modification as a mechanism through which these in utero challenges might be recorded in a manner that will allow functional consequences to persist throughout the life course. It remains to be established directly if epigenetic marking in utero, or indeed epigenetic effects of diet later in the life course, has an effect on aging per se, but studies on epigenetic effects of nutrition in utero, and also on epigenetic effects of diet in a more general context (unrelated specifically to aging), deserve consideration here for three reasons. First, such studies provide proof of the principle that nutrition can have profound effects on epigenetic marking and identify individual dietary components with such activity. Second, the risk of disease states linked with nutritional challenge in utero—specifically cancer and type 2 diabetes—increases with aging. There is also debate about the possibility that cancer and aging may share common etiology, particularly with respect to epigenetic changes.[19,34] Thus, there is strong argument for an influence of epigenetic marking in utero on at least some parameters of aging. Third, mechanisms through which specific dietary components may affect epigenetic marking are likely to be conserved between the developing embryo and the adult, albeit that embryonic development is likely to represent a particular stage in the life course at which the epigenome is particularly labile and, therefore, susceptible to dietary modification. Table 8.1 summarizes some of the evidence for epigenetic effects

Table 8.1 A summary of selected evidence for effects of specific dietary components on DNA methylation based on studies in cell culture models, rodents and humans

Dietary component/intervention	Model	Observations	Refs
Methyl donors	Cell culture	Global and *p53*-specific DNA hypomethylation induced by folate-free medium in the colon adenocarcinoma cell line SW620; reversed by folic acid addition	83
		Global DNA hypomethylation induced by folate-depleted medium in immortalized human colonocytes	84
		Hypermethylation of *H-cadherin* gene in nasopharyngeal carcinoma cells	85
		Global DNA hypomethylation induced by folate deficiency in NIH/3T3 and CHO-K1 (nontransformed) cell lines, but not in HCT116 and Caco-2 colon cancer (transformed) cell lines	86
	Rodent	Increased proportion of pseudoagouti over yellow pups (indicative of increased methylation at A^{vy} allele) in agouti mice fed methyl-supplemented diet	87
		DNA hypermethylation at A^{vy} allele, accompanied by shift in coat color towards pseudoagouti, in pups of agouti mice fed methyl-supplemented diet	88, 89
		Reversal of bisphenol A-induced DNA hypomethylation at A^{vy} allele in pups, and shift towards yellow coat color, reversed by folate supplementation of agouti mice	90
		Hypomethylation of *p53* locus in liver in male weanling rats induced by folate-deficient diet	91
		Gobal and Cdkn3-specific DNA hypomethylation in fetal brain induced by choline-deficient diet in mice	92
		Transient global DNA hypermethylation induced by folate-deficient diet in weanling male rats	93

		No effect of folate deficiency on global DNA methylation at *Hpa*II and *Msp*I sites in maternal or fetal liver in rats, despite measured indicators of perturbation in methyl group supply	94
		No effect of folate deficiency on global DNA methylation in rat liver or colon, despite measured indicators of perturbation in methyl group supply	95
		Global and *IgF2* DNA hypermethylation induced in liver and brain of E17 embryos by choline-deficient diet in rats	96
	Human	Weak, significant association between serum and cervical folate concentration and DNA hypomethylation in cervical tissue	97
		Global colonic DNA hypomethylation and reduced folate status in patients with colorectal neoplasia compared with controls; DNA hypomethylation correlated negatively with folate status and positively with plasma homocysteine concentration	98
		Inverse correlation between DNA hypomethylation in colonic mucosa and erythrocyte/serum folate concentration in healthy subjects	98, 99
		Global lymphocyte DNA hypomethylation induced in postmenopausal women by low folate diet; reversed by folate-supplemented diet	100, 101
		Increased global DNA methylation in lymphocytes and colonic mucosa induced by folate supplement in patients with colorectal adenoma	102
		Arsenic exposure in Bangladeshi adults correlated positively with leukocyte DNA methylation only in individuals with high folate intake	70
Bioactive polyphenols	Cell culture	Reversal of gene-specific DNA hypermethylation (*p16^INK4a*, *RARβ*, *MGMT*, *hMLH1*) and increased expression of the corresponding mRNA transcripts in KYSE 501 (human esophageal carcinoma) and HT-29 (human adenocarcinoma) cell lines on treatment with epigallocatechin-3-gallate	49
		Demethylation of *RARβ* locus by epigallocatechin-3-gallate in MCF-7 and MDA-MB-231 breast cancer cell lines	51
		No substantial effects of epigallocatechin-3-gallate on gene-specific DNA methylation	50, 52

(Continued)

Table 8.1 (*Continued*)

Dietary component/ intervention	Model	Observations	Refs
		Reversal of gene-specific DNA hypermethylation (*p16^INK4a*, *RARβ*, *MGMT*) in KYSE 510 cells by genistein; reversal of *RARβ* methylation and induction of corresponding mRNA expression by genistein in PC3 and LNCaP prostate cancer cell lines and by biochanin A and daidzein in KYSE 510 cells	103
		Demethylation of GSTP1 promoter and restoration of corresponding mRNA expression induced by phenethyl isothiocyanate in LNCaP cells	104
	Rodent	No effect of green or black tea extract (rich in epigallocatechin-3-gallate) on transfer to lung or liver DNA of tritiated methyl groups from tobacco carcinogen 4-(methylnitrosamino)-1-(3-pyridyl)-1-buanone administered IP to mice	105
		Three of 900 CpG island clones screened hypermethylated in mice fed genistein-supplemented diet	106
		Shift towards pseudoagouti coat color, and corresponding increase in methylation at the *A^vy* locus, in agouti mice pups from dams fed genistein supplemented diet	36
		Reversal of bisphenol A-induced DNA hypomethylation at *A^vy* locus in agouti mouse pups by co-administration of dietary genistein in utero	90
	Human	Increased plasma homocysteine concentration and reduced folate concentration in subjects consuming coffee polyphenol chlorogenic acid (no direct measure of DNA methylation)	107
Zinc	Rodent	Depressed immune function induced by gestational zinc deficiency in mice persisted for two generations, after zinc repletion, indicating epigenetic effect	108
		Global DNA hypomethylation measured in liver of rats in response to zinc-deficient diet	109

Selenium	Cell culture	Global DNA hypomethylation in Caco-2 and HT-29 (colon adenocarcinoma) cells induced by removal of selenium from culture medium, along with demethylation of *p53* promoter in Caco-2 cells	55, 110
	Rodent	Global DNA hypomethylation in rat liver and colon in response to selenium-deficient diet	111
Vitamin A	Cell culture	Demethylation of *RARβ2* promoter in NB4 (promyelocytic leukaemia) cells, but not in T47D or MCF7 (breast cancer) cells, induced by all-*trans* retinoic acid	112, 113
	Rodent	Global hepatic DNA hypomethylation in rats in response to dietary all-trans retinoic acid, but not in response to retinyl-palmitate or 13-*cis*-retinoic acid	114
	Rodent	No effect of dietary beta-carotene or retinyl-palmitate on gene-specific methylation (hydroxmethylglutaryl coenzyme A reductase, *c-myc, c-Ha-ras*) in rat model of hepatocarcinogenesis	115
Arsenic	Cell culture	Global DNA hypermethylation in Caco-2 cells on addition of arsenite to culture medium	110
	Cell culture	Global DNA hypomethylation in human prostate cancer cells on addition of arsenite to culture medium	116
	Rodent	Global and *ER-α* DNA hypomethylation in mice in response to sodium arsenite in drinking water	117
	Rodent	Global DNA hypomethylation in rat liver in response to sodium arsenite in drinking water	118
	Human	Arsenic exposure positively correlated with DNA methylation in peripheral blood leukocytes in Bangladeshi adults	70
Alcohol	Rodent	Global DNA hypomethylation, with no effect on methylation of *p53* and β-*actin* genes in rat colonic mucosa induced by alcohol consumption	119
	Rodent	Global and *c-myc* DNA hypomethylation in rat model of early-stage, ethanol-induced liver injury	120

(Continued)

Table 8.1 (*Continued*)

Dietary Component/ Intervention	Model	Observations	Refs
	Human	Demethylation of *NR2B* (NMDA receptor) gene in mouse cortical neurons induced by chronic alcohol exposure	121
		Global DNA hypermethylation in peripheral blood mononuclear cells of patients with alcoholism	122
		Positive correlation between methylation of panel of genes and alcohol consumption in oral squamous cell carcinomas	123
		Increased methylation of *p15* (cyclin-dependent kinase inhibitor) gene in regular smokers/ alcohol consumers	124
Dietary restriction	Rodent	Transient global DNA hypomethylation in liver and suppression of age-dependent changes in methylation of *c-myc* in response to dietary restriction in mice	125
		Hypermethylation of *c-Hα-ras* oncogene in rat pancreatic acinar cells in response to dietary restriction.	126
Protein restriction	Rodent	Hypomethylation of *PPARα* and $GR1_{10}$ (glucocorticoid receptor) promoters in rat liver in response to protein-restricted diet in utero	127, 128, 129

of each of the above dietary components or interventions based, where available, on cell culture, animal and human studies.

A number of the studies cited in Table 8.1 are based on the variable yellow agouti (*Avy*) mouse, which provides a particularly convenient and tractable model for the study of dietary effects on DNA methylation during gestational exposure. In this model a long terminal repeat (LTR) retrotransposon insertion, the intracisternal A particle (IAP), at the 5′ end of the agouti gene, provides a cryptic promoter and also confers stochastic, variable CpG methylation on the *Avy* allele. In the wild-type mouse, expression of the agouti A gene product, which signals yellow hair pigmentation, is restricted to the hair follicle over a specific stage of hair growth, resulting in yellow banding of the hair and giving the agouti coat color. Constitutive expression of the agouti A gene product, driven by a hypomethylated IAP cryptic promoter, results in a yellow coat color (and also associated predisposition to obesity, diabetes and cancer). Methylation of the IAP LTR represses constitutive expression of the agouti A gene product, resulting in a brown, or pseudoagouti, coat color. Mice can be scored visually according to coat color to generate a visual readout of the level of DNA methylation at this locus. Hence, effects of dietary interventions during development on DNA methylation can be measured easily. The epigenetic lability conferred by the IAP LTR may be a general property of transposable elements in the genome, which are stabilized by methylation,[35] so data based on the agouti mouse model have possible implications for an influence of nutrition in utero on genome stability, and therefore on aging.

Intermediates in one-carbon metabolism, specifically folate, choline, betaine and methionine, are compelling candidates as dietary agents likely to affect DNA methylation through effects on the supply of methyl groups (ultimately as *S*-adenosylmethionine [AdoMet], the methyl donor to cytosine in the reaction catalyzed by the DNMTs). As such, these compounds have been a focus for much of the research on effects of nutrition on DNA methylation, albeit outside of the specific context of aging.

The potential role of bioactive dietary phytochemicals, principally polyphenols and isothiocyanates, in moderating DNA methylation received less attention initially than that of methyl donors, probably because mechanistic links are not as immediately obvious, but the literature in this area is now expanding rapidly. An observation on epigenetic effects of dietary phytoestrogens of particular relevance to aging was that an increase in DNA methylation at the *Avy* locus in the agouti mouse model in the offspring of mice fed a genistein-supplemented diet throughout gestation and weaning manifest phenotypically as a shift in coat color towards pseudoagouti, persisted into adulthood and afforded protection against obesity.[36]

The mechanistic involvement of zinc in epigenetic processes, particularly in histone deacetylase (HDAC) inhibition,[37,38] highlights this essential dietary micronutrient as a prime candidate for affecting the epigenome, yet the literature on effects of zinc on DNA methylation is not extensive. This lack of published data on epigenetic effects of zinc may be indicative that zinc has minimal effects on DNA methylation or, alternatively, may indicate that the area has not yet been studied extensively.

As already noted, it has been known for several decades that food restriction in laboratory rodents increases life span and, more recently, it has been shown that reduced energy intake can delay or even prevent late-onset diseases in animal models.[39] To date, however, the effect of dietary restriction on DNA methylation appears to be a little-studied phenomenon, highlighting this topic as one for future research effort to elucidate causal links between epigenetic effects of nutrition and aging.

Direct links between obesity and DNA methylation patterns have not been established, yet it is likely that DNA methylation may be influenced by adiposity, particularly in view of the opinion that obesity is a low-grade inflammatory condition,[40] coupled with the strong association between inflammation and cancer,[41,42] a condition in which substantial changes to the DNA methylation profile are observed. Potential mechanisms through which obesity may influence DNA methylation include the secretion by adipose tissue of adipokines and/or pro-inflammatory cytokines such as TNFα and IL6.[40,43,44]

It should be noted that results of individual studies cited in Table 8.1 are not always in apparent concordance with specific nutrients or interventions having apparently opposing effects on DNA methylation. These apparent differences in DNA methylation in response to individual interventions might reflect responses that are cell line/tissue-specific or might be indicative of complex effects of specific dietary agents on DNA methylation that are dependent on experimental model, dose, exposure time and/or interactions with dietary and other factors. As a specific example, the apparent discrepancy between effects of genistein in vitro (site-specific DNA hypomethylation) and in vivo (site-specific hypermethylation) might reflect two different potential mechanisms for the effect of genistein on the epigenome: effects on DNMT activity and effects on histone acetylation (see the following sections). Alternatively, discrepancy between effects observed in vivo and in vitro may be the result of different activities of the aglycone (studied in vitro) and the major circulating forms observed in vivo, which are the glucuronide and sulfate conjugates.[45–48] Given that the loci studied in vivo and in vitro are distinct, an alternative explanation is differential effects of genistein at specific loci. Similarly, the apparent lack of concordance in the literature concerning whether or not the green tea polyphenol epigallocatechin-3-gallate affects DNA methylation[49–52] may be due to gene- or cell-line-specific effects. Furthermore, the reader should be aware that all inferences from studies reporting no effect of changes in nutrient supply on DNA methylation must be with the caveat that effects on site-specific DNA methylation at loci other than those examined or on global DNA methylation at sites not interrogated by the specific assay employed cannot be excluded.

8.5   Impact of nutrition on histone modification

It is evident that, in addition to effects on DNA methylation, diet can affect histone modification. Such observations are not surprising, given the interrelationship between these two levels of epigenetic modification, but direct evidence for effects of diet on histone modification deserves specific consideration. The dietary agents best studied in this context are the short chain fatty acid butyrate, generated in the large bowel as a result of bacterial fermentation of dietary fiber, and organosulfur compounds, including the isothiocyanates. For these compounds an apparently clear mechanistic basis for their histone-modifying activity underpins observations concerning their effects on histone decoration. Examples of other dietary agents or nutritional modifications that appear to or have the potential to influence histone modification include methyl donors, retinoic acid (the active metabolite of vitamin A), ethanol, dietary restriction and protein restriction in utero. Table 8.2 summarizes some of the evidence for effects of these dietary agents or modifications on histone modification. It should be noted that, while all of these agents or modifications might have the potential to influence the aging process through changes in histone decoration, only in the case of dietary restriction is an effect of the dietary strategy on aging in any way established. Even in this case, accompanying changes in histone modification status remain to be identified, in spite of the fact that an epigenetic mechanism through which the beneficial effects of dietary restriction on aging are mediated is compelling, given the strong evidence for the pivotal role of the histone deacetylase Sirt1.[39] This area should be a priority for future research on the links between epigenetics, nutrition and aging.

8.6   Mechanisms through which diet influences epigenetic markings

Conceivable, and known, mechanisms through which diet may influence epigenetic marking include effects on the supply of methyl groups for DNA methylation and effects on the activity and/or expression of enzymes involved in epigenetic modification. These enzymes potentially include DNMTs, DNA demethylases, histone acetyltransferases, histone deacetylases, histone methyltransferases and histone demethylases. The interrelationship between DNA methylation and histone modification renders it very likely that dietary agents acting primarily at one epigenetic level may produce effects at the other. For example, recruitment of

Table 8.2 A summary of selected evidence for effects of specific dietary components on histone modification based on studies in cell culture models, rodents and humans

Dietary component/ intervention	Model	Observations	Refs
Butyrate	Cell culture	Increased histone H4 acetylation induced by butyrate in human A375 and mouse S91 melanoma cells	130
		Increased overall histone H3 and H4 acetylation induced by butyrate in HepG2 human hepatocarcinoma cells, but H3 and H4 deacetylation close to transcription start sites of multiple genes in HepG2 and HT29 (human colon adenocarcinoma) cells	131
		Increased histone H3 and H4 acetylation associated with promoter of cathelicidin (antibacterial peptide) gene induced by butyrate in EBC-1 (human lung epithelial) cell line	132
Organosulfur compounds	Cell culture	Transient increase in acetylation of H3K14, H3K9, H4K12 and H4K16, but not H4K9, in Caco-2 (human intestinal) cells in response to diallyl sulfide	133
		Increased histone H3 acetylation, increased H3K4 methylation and reduced H3K9 methylation (consistent with active chromatin configuration) induced by phenyl isothiocyanate in LNCaP human prostate cancer cells	104
Methyl donors	Rodent	Reduced H3K9 trimethylation and acetylation, reduced H4K20 trimethylation, increased H3S10 phosphorylation in rats fed methyl-deficient diet	134
Vitamin A	Cell culture	Increased histone H3 and H4 acetylation at silenced retinoic acid receptor β P2 promoter induced by treatment of T47D breast cancer cell line with all-*trans* retinoic acid	113

Alcohol	Cell culture	Increased H3K9 acetylation, with no effect on H3K14 acetylation, in cultured rat hepatocytes in response to ethanol	135
		Reduced H3K9 methylation and increased H3K4 methylation in primary rat hepatocytes in response to ethanol	136
	Rodent	Increased hepatic chromatin condensation in rats given ethanol orally	137
		Increased H3K9 acetylation in rat liver, lung and spleen, but not kidney brain and heart, induced by intragastric administration of ethanol	138
Dietary restriction	Rodent	Observed reduction in histone H1 and H3/H2B/H2A carbonylation in rat liver with aging reversed by caloric restriction	139
Protein restriction	Rodent	Increased H3K9 acetylation, H4K9 acetylation, H3K9 methylation (associated with more active chromatin configuration) and reduced H3K9 dimethylation (associated with repressed chromatin configuration) induced at glucocorticoid *GR110* promoter in rat liver in response to protein-restricted diet in utero	129

histone deacetylases to sites methylated as a result of dietary influences may lead to histone deacetylation secondary to an effect on DNA methylation. Conversely, changes to histone acetylation status may drive changes in the methylation state of the associated DNA, although the mechanisms underlying this second interrelationship are less clear. Similarly, it is somewhat artificial to categorize dietary agents on the basis of effects on only one of the above variables that modulate epigenetic marking. For example, as outlined below, a restriction to the methyl group supply can reduce both DNA and histone methylation "directly," through limited availability of substrate for methyltransferase enzymes, and through effects of the accumulation of the product AdoHcy, which cannot be efficiently converted back to AdoMet in the absence of an adequate methyl supply and which binds to and inhibits the methyltransferases.

Table 8.3 summarizes some of the evidence that specific dietary components or nutritional interventions act on each of these potential mediators of epigenetic marking. In some instances, identified effects of specific nutrients on modifiers of epigenetic marking appear to be inconsistent with the effect of these nutrients on epigenetic marking per se. For example, the result of selenium deficiency is generally DNA hypomethylation (see preceding sections), indicating that adequate selenium is required to maintain DNA methylation. Selenite itself, however, has been shown in vitro to be a noncompetitive inhibitor of DNA methyltransferase activity[53,54] and also, compared with selenium-free conditions, to reduce DNMT1 protein expression in HT29 cells.[55] Such apparent inconsistencies might be due to there being multiple, opposing points at which specific nutrients influence the activity of the epigenetic machinery. In the specific case of selenium, for example, effects to reduce methyl group supply might predominate. In contrast, there is particularly convincing evidence that the HDAC-inhibitory activity of butyrate is primarily responsible for its gene-regulatory effects. Treatment of HT-29 cells with butyrate induced an identical panel of 23 genes as did the well-characterized pharmacological HDAC inhibitor trichostatin A (TSA) out of a total of 588 investigated by hybridization of cDNA to a low-density, nylon array.[56] The fold induction of each gene by butyrate compared with TSA also showed remarkable concordance.

8.7   Aging-related changes in intake and metabolism of dietary components with epigenetic effects

From a different perspective, it is perhaps relevant to consider here how the intake of dietary components established to have the potential to influence patterns of epigenetic marking changes with aging, since such changes may be a mechanism through which aging influences epigenetic modification.

Table 8.3 A summary of selected evidence for effects of dietary agents on epigenetic modification mediated through specific mechanisms

Mechanism	Dietary agent	Evidence	Refs
Effect on methyl group supply	Vitamin A	Increased expression of glycine *N*-methyltransferase in rat liver in response to dietary supplementation with retinyl palmitate, 13-*cis* retinoic acid or all-*trans* retinoic acid	114
	Selenium	Increased *N*-methyltransferase activity in rat liver in response to diet containing supranutritional selenium	140
Generation of DNMT inhibitor SAH by catechol-o-methyltransferase (COMT)-catalyzed methylation of SAM (in presence of catechol compounds)	Polyphenols	Concentration- and COMT-dependent inhibition of transfer of methyl groups to synthetic DNA substrate by recombinant human DNMT1 and/or prokaryotic methylase *SssI* by catechin, epicatechin, quercetin, fisetin, myricetin, genistein, daidzein, biochanin A, chlorogenic acid	49, 51, 103
Direct, competitive inhibition of DNMT activity	Epigallocatechin-3-gallate	High-affinity, COMT-independent inhibition of transfer of methyl groups to synthetic DNA substrate by recombinant human DNMT1 and prokaryotic methylase *SssI*	49, 51, 103
Non-competitive inhibition of DNMT activity	Selenium	Inhibition of HDAC activity by sodium selenite demonstrated in vitro	53, 54
Reduced DNMT expression	Selenium	DNMT protein expression reduced in HT29 cells in presence of selenium	55
Modification of DNA demethylase activity	Methyl donors	Methyl domain binding protein 2 (MBD2) (putative DNA demethylase) increased at protein and mRNA levels in rat liver in response to folate- and methyl-deficient diet	141, 142

(*Continued*)

Table 8.3 (*Continued*)

Mechanism	Dietary agent	Evidence	Refs
Histone deacetylase inhibition	Butyrate	Inhibition of HDAC activity demonstrated in vitro	143
	S-allylmercaptocysteine (garlic)	Inhibition of HDAC activity demonstrated in vitro	37, 38
	Cysteine conjugates of isothiocyanates	Inhibition of HDAC activity demonstrated in vitro	37, 38
	Genistein	Weak inhibition at high concentrations demonstrated in vitro	103
	Zinc	Structural studies demonstrate importance of buried zinc atom in HDAC pocket for interaction with other dietary HDAC inhibitors	37, 38
Repression of histone methyltransferase activity	Methyl donors	Reduced expression of histone methyltransferases Suv4-20h2, Suv39h1, PRDM2/RIZ1, hPR-SET7 in rat liver in hepatocarcinogenesis induced by methyl-deficient diet	134

A reduction in the ratio of AdoMet to AdoHcy in serum has been observed with age in rats.[57] Aging in human subjects was associated with higher concentrations of SAdoHcy and homocysteine and reduced folate concentration in the cerebrospinal fluid and with an increased concentration of homocysteine in serum[58] and plasma,[59] all indicative of a disturbed methylation status. In view of the abovementioned studies showing effects of methyl supply to influence DNA methylation, these changes may contribute to the global hypomethylation of DNA and site-specific hypermethylation observed with aging. Mean daily folate intake increased significantly with age in adults aged 19 to 64 captured in the UK National Diet and Nutrition Survey,[60] however, so the more negative apparent effects on methyl group supply in older subjects may reflect variability between the different samples and/or inclusion of more elderly subjects in the studies demonstrating reduced folate/methylation status with aging.

Changes in the intake of fruit and vegetables in more elderly cohorts and the consequent exposure to lower levels of bioactive phytochemicals might be a mechanism through which epigenetic marking is affected. However, there is no overall apparent consistent pattern of fruit and vegetable intake with age. Studies in U.S. cohorts reveal an apparent reduction in fruit and vegetable consumption with aging,[61–64] while consumption of these foods increased with age, between the ages of 19 and 64 years, in respondents to the UK National Diet and Nutrition Survey.[60]

With regard to aging-related changes in micronutrient intake, zinc intake in the elderly is reduced and aging-associated changes in zinc homeostasis, including endogenous secretion and absorptive efficiency, may affect epigenetic marking (reviewed in Reference 65). Inspection of the literature suggests that knowledge about the effect of aging on either selenium intake or selenium status is poor, but a study based on a small sample of 105 subjects in Northern Italy found a progressive decrease in selenium status with aging.[66] Similarly, there is an apparent paucity of knowledge about the relationship between vitamin A intake or status and aging, although in this case the evidence available does not support the view that intake and/or status changes substantially with age. Serum vitamin A levels declined only slightly with age in men and women over 50 years of age living in California in the 1950s[67] and plasma concentrations increased in women with age, but not in men, in a cohort aged 20 to 95 years who participated in the Baltimore Longitudinal Study of Aging.[68] The UK National Diet and Nutrition Survey revealed significantly lower vitamin A intakes in the youngest groups of both men and women (19 to 24 years) than in older groups (35 to 49 years for men and 50 to 64 years for women).[60] Vitamin A stored in the liver was reduced in old mice compared with younger adult mice, but was still sufficient to meet nutritional requirements.[69]

Data relating to arsenic exposure, including urinary and plasma concentrations, was apparently not analyzed with respect to effect of age in a sample of Bangladeshi adults taken from a larger cohort aged 18 to 65 years,[70] but might indicate if this environmental and dietary contaminant accumulates with aging and so contributes to aging-associated changes in DNA methylation in exposed populations.

Aging may alter histone modification through effects on the generation of the diet-derived HDAC inhibitor butyrate as indicated by the observation that consumption of an oat-based diet increased the proportion of butyrate to other short chain fatty acids in the rat cecum, but that this response was attenuated in elderly rats, compared with younger animals.[71]

Current data on differences in the intake of dietary components with age are severely limited by the constraint that there is a lack of longitudinal studies to indicate how dietary intake changes with aging in a single cohort. Rather, most existing data relate only to sampling cohorts of different ages, so it is likely that differences in dietary intake between younger and older groups reflect dietary habits long established in the older groups rather than changes in preferences and habits that accompany aging.

8.8   The influence of aging-associated epigenetic modification on nutrient requirements

Another potential link between nutrition, epigenetics and aging is that changes in the methylation status of the genome that accompany aging may have an impact on specific nutrient requirements. It is not difficult to imagine mechanisms through which aging-associated changes in epigenetic marking of key genes might affect the optimum requirement for specific nutrients. For example, the expression of specific intestinal nutrient transporters is responsive to fluctuations in their substrate supply, often contributing to optimum absorption under conditions of a variable nutrient supply (reviewed in Reference 72). Dysregulation of the sensitivity of specific nutrient transporter genes to the availability of their substrate through aging-associated epigenetic modification could, hypothetically, impair this homeostatic response and so invoke the need for tighter regulation of the dietary intake of the affected nutrients to maintain an optimum supply. Currently, such links remain speculative and the topic is one for future research on the links between nutrition, epigenetics and aging.

8.9   Priorities of future research

We coined the term the four "Rs" of epigenomics to encapsulate the key processes through which environmental exposures connect with health via epigenetic mechanisms.[73] These include the processes involved in (1) receiving environmental signals, (2) recording those signals through altered patterns of epigenomic marks, (3) remembering the resulting epigenomic pattern through subsequent cell divisions and (4) revealing the consequences of the altered epigenomic markings in the cell's unique transcriptome. The process by which DNA methylation marks are copied during mitosis (remembering) has been clarified[74] but there is limited understanding of the other three "Rs." In particular, little is known about the epigenetic targets of environmental exposures that lead to differential gene expression and that may be important during aging. Potential targets include (1) the promoter regions of housekeeping genes, (2) genes with metastable epialleles and (3) imprinted genes.[75] One whole genome approach to discovery of potentially epigenetically regulated genes is through examination of outcomes of microarray studies. Transcriptomic analysis of rodent tissues has demonstrated that aging results in differential patterns of gene expression that are specific to each tissue and that dietary restriction partially, or completely, reverses these changes.[9] While individual studies are helpful in identifying potentially interesting genes, combining data from several studies minimizes the risk of false positives and comparative studies of transcriptomic outcomes from different experimental protocols may reveal the key genes that facilitate greater life span. Using the latter approach with microarray data sets from studies with long-lived dwarf strains of mice and mice exposed to energy restriction, low-fat diets and other treatments, Swindell identified 43 longevity-associated genes of which 30 had similar differential expression patterns in several long-lived dwarf strains and following energy restriction.[76] Given the hypothesis that epigenetic processes, which are causal in modulating aging, do so via altered gene expression, the genes identified by Swindell represent an important starting point for further analysis and experimentation.

It remains to be proven that epigenomics or gene expression measurements made in accessible cells such as peripheral blood lymphocytes provide a useful reflection of processes occurring in other target tissues, such as muscle, brain, or bone, which might be of particular interest in studies of human aging. Limited evidence to date suggests that patterns of DNA methylation may be distinctly different between tissues[77] but conclusions about this must await larger-scale epigenomic mapping (such as that described by Eckhardt et al.[78]) carried out systematically on different tissues from the same individual. There appear to be tissue-specific changes in gene expression during aging[9] but, when investigating mechanisms of aging, it may be more useful to look for commonality in differentially expressed genes because these genes would be those expected to be fundamental to aging if the disposable soma theory of aging[7] holds true. As a consequence, these would be prima facie targets for epigenetically regulated genes causal for the aging process. Further, if the damaging events which result in the aging phenotype are modifiable by nutritional means (some of which may be mediated epigenetically), then there is a strong rationale for focusing on cellular repair processes.

At this early stage in research on the mechanisms responsible for nutritional modulation of the aging process, there is merit in considering nutritional interventions at all stages of the life course. Clearly, factors acting in utero that result in slower than normal fetal growth (including inadequate energy and nutrient supply) lead to greater risks of several age-related diseases and to premature mortality.[79,80] In addition, maternal obesity, which is increasingly common worldwide and is associated with adverse effects on the health of the offspring,[81] may contribute to faster aging trajectories. Since epigenetic markings may be more plastic in early life,[82] it will be important to characterize the differential epigenetic markings of newborns associated with adverse intrauterine environments and to determine (1) the extent to which these differential marks are permanent, (2) how the marks are modified by postnatal exposures and (3) the consequences for the aging phenotype.

References

1. Oeppen, J., and Vaupel, J.W. (2002). Demography. Broken limits to life expectancy. *Science* 296, 1029–1031.
2. World Health Organization (2002). *Active Ageing. A Policy Framework*. Geneva: World Health Organization.
3. Blanc, S., Schoeller, D., Bauer, D., Danielson, M., Tylaysky, F., Simonsick, E., Harris, T., Kritchevsky, S., and Everhart, J. (2004). Energy requirements in the eighth decade of life. *Am J Clin Nutr* 79, 303–310.
4. Administration on Aging (2003). A statistical profile of older Americans aged 65+. Washington, D.C.: Administration on Aging.
5. Wanless, D. (2004). *Securing Good Health for the Whole Population*. London: Her Majesty's Stationery Office.
6. Department of Health (2001). *National Service Framework for Older People*. London: Department of Health.
7. Kirkwood, T.B. (2005). Understanding the odd science of aging. *Cell* 120, 437–447.
8. Oberdoerffer, P., and Sinclair, D.A. (2007). The role of nuclear architecture in genomic instability and ageing. *Nat Rev Mol Cell Biol* 8, 692–702.
9. Park, S.K., and Prolla, T.A. (2005). Lessons learned from gene expression profile studies of aging and caloric restriction. *Ageing Res Rev* 4, 55–65.
10. Blasco, M.A. (2005). Telomeres and human disease: Ageing, cancer and beyond. *Nat Rev Genet* 6, 611–622.
11. Taylor, R.W., Barron, M.J., Borthwick, G.M., Gospel, A., Chinnery, P.F., Samuels, D.C., Taylor, G.A., Plusa, S.M., Needham, S.J., Greaves, L.C., Kirkwood, T.B., and Turnbull, D.M. (2003). Mitochondrial DNA mutations in human colonic crypt stem cells. *J Clin Invest* 112, 1351–1360.
12. Sharpless, N.E., and DePinho, R.A. (2007). How stem cells age and why this makes us grow old. *Nat Rev Mol Cell Biol* 8, 703–713.
13. Speakman, J.R., and Hambly, C. (2007). Starving for life: What animal studies can and cannot tell us about the use of caloric restriction to prolong human lifespan. *J Nutr* 137, 1078–1086.

14. Fontana, L., and Klein, S. (2007). Aging, adiposity, and calorie restriction. *JAMA* 297, 986–994.

15. Trichopoulou, A., Orfanos, P., Norat, T., Bueno-de-Mesquita, B., Ocke, M.C., Peeters, P.H., van der Schouw, Y.T., Boeing, H., Hoffmann, K., Boffetta, P., Nagel, G., Masala, G., Krogh, V., Panico, S., Tumino, R., Vineis, P., Bamia, C., Naska, A., Benetou, V., Ferrari, P., Slimani, N., Pera, G., Martinez-Garcia, C., Navarro, C., Rodriguez-Barranco, M., Dorronsoro, M., Spencer, E.A., Key, T.J., Bingham, S., Khaw, K.T., Kesse, E., Clavel-Chapelon, F., Boutron-Ruault, M.C., Berglund, G., Wirfalt, E., Hallmans, G., Johansson, I., Tjonneland, A., Olsen, A., Overvad, K., Hundborg, H.H., Riboli, E., and Trichopoulos, D. (2005). Modified Mediterranean diet and survival: EPIC-elderly prospective cohort study. *BMJ* 330, 991.

16. Panza, F., Solfrizzi, V., Colacicco, A.M., D'Introno, A., Capurso, C., Torres, F., Del Parigi, A., Capurso, S., and Capurso, A. (2004). Mediterranean diet and cognitive decline. *Public Health Nutr* 7, 959–963.

17. Autier, P., and Gandini, S. (2007). Vitamin D supplementation and total mortality: A meta-analysis of randomized controlled trials. *Arch Intern Med* 167, 1730–1737.

18. Wilson, V.L., and Jones, P.A. (1983). DNA methylation decreases in aging but not in immortal cells. *Science* 220, 1055–1057.

19. Fraga, M.F., Agrelo, R., and Esteller, M. (2007). Cross-talk between aging and cancer: The epigenetic language. *Ann NY Acad Sci* 1100, 60–74.

20. Rodriguez, J., Vives, L., Jorda, M., Morales, C., Munoz, M., Vendrell, E., and Peinado, M.A. (2008). Genome-wide tracking of unmethylated DNA Alu repeats in normal and cancer cells. *Nucleic Acids Res* 36, 770–784.

21. Eden, A., Gaudet, F., Waghmare, A., and Jaenisch, R. (2003). Chromosomal instability and tumors promoted by DNA hypomethylation. *Science* 300, 455.

22. Gaudet, F., Hodgson, J.G., Eden, A., Jackson-Grusby, L., Dausman, J., Gray, J.W., Leonhardt, H., and Jaenisch, R. (2003). Induction of tumors in mice by genomic hypomethylation. *Science* 300, 489–492.

23. Lopatina, N., Haskell, J.F., Andrews, L.G., Poole, J.C., Saldanha, S., and Tollefsbol, T. (2002). Differential maintenance and de novo methylating activity by three DNA methyltransferases in aging and immortalized fibroblasts. *J Cell Biochem* 84, 324–334.

24. Casillas, M.A., Jr., Lopatina, N., Andrews, L.G., and Tollefsbol, T.O. (2003). Transcriptional control of the DNA methyltransferases is altered in aging and neoplastically-transformed human fibroblasts. *Mol Cell Biochem* 252, 33–43.

25. Issa, J.P., Ottaviano, Y.L., Celano, P., Hamilton, S.R., Davidson, N.E., and Baylin, S.B. (1994). Methylation of the oestrogen receptor CpG island links ageing and neoplasia in human colon. *Nat Genet* 7, 536–540.

26. Issa, J.P., Ahuja, N., Toyota, M., Bronner, M.P., and Brentnall, T.A. (2001). Accelerated age-related CpG island methylation in ulcerative colitis. *Cancer Res* 61, 3573–3577.

27. Kim, J., Kim, J.Y., Song, K.S., Lee, Y.H., Seo, J.S., Jelinek, J., Goldschmidt-Clermont, P.J., and Issa, J.P. (2007). Epigenetic changes in estrogen receptor beta gene in atherosclerotic cardiovascular tissues and in-vitro vascular senescence. *Biochim Biophys Acta* 1772, 72–80.

28. Kwabi-Addo, B., Chung, W., Shen, L., Ittmann, M., Wheeler, T., Jelinek, J., and Issa, J.P. (2007). Age-related DNA methylation changes in normal human prostate tissues. *Clin Cancer Res* 13, 3796–3802.

29. Ushijima, T., Watanabe, N., Okochi, E., Kaneda, A., Sugimura, T., and Miyamoto, K. (2003). Fidelity of the methylation pattern and its variation in the genome. *Genome Res* 13, 868–874.

30. Bahar, R., Hartmann, C.H., Rodriguez, K.A., Denny, A.D., Busuttil, R.A., Dolle, M.E., Calder, R.B., Chisholm, G.B., Pollock, B.H., Klein, C.A., and Vijg, J. (2006). Increased cell-to-cell variation in gene expression in ageing mouse heart. *Nature* 441, 1011–1014.

31. Castro, C.E., and Sevall, J.S. (1980). Alteration of higher order structure of rat liver chromatin by dietary composition. *J Nutr* 110, 105–116.

32. Fraga, M.F., Ballestar, E., Paz, M.F., Ropero, S., Setien, F., Ballestar, M.L., Heine-Suner, D., Cigudosa, J.C., Urioste, M., Benitez, J., Boix-Chornet, M., Sanchez-Aguilera, A., Ling, C., Carlsson, E., Poulsen, P., Vaag, A., Stephan, Z., Spector, T.D., Wu, Y.Z., Plass, C., and Esteller, M. (2005). Epigenetic differences arise during the lifetime of monozygotic twins. *Proc Natl Acad Sci USA* 102, 10604–10609.

33. Fernandez-Twinn, D.S., and Ozanne, S.E. (2006). Mechanisms by which poor early growth programs type-2 diabetes, obesity and the metabolic syndrome. *Physiol Behav* 88, 234–243.

34. Dreosti, I.E. (1998). Nutrition, cancer, and aging. *Ann NY Acad Sci* 854, 371–377.

35. Miura, A., Yonebayashi, S., Watanabe, K., Toyama, T., Shimada, H., and Kakutani, T. (2001). Mobilization of transposons by a mutation abolishing full DNA methylation in Arabidopsis. *Nature* 411, 212–214.

36. Dolinoy, D.C., Weidman, J.R., Waterland, R.A., and Jirtle, R.L. (2006). Maternal genistein alters coat color and protects Avy mouse offspring from obesity by modifying the fetal epigenome. *Environ Health Perspect* 114, 567–572.

37. Dashwood, R.H., Myzak, M.C., and Ho, E. (2006). Dietary HDAC inhibitors: Time to rethink weak ligands in cancer chemoprevention? *Carcinogenesis* 27, 344–349.

38. Myzak, M.C., Ho, E., and Dashwood, R.H. (2006). Dietary agents as histone deacetylase inhibitors. *Mol Carcinog* 45, 443–446.

39. Guarente, L., and Picard, F. (2005). Calorie restriction: The SIR2 connection. *Cell* 120, 473–482.

40. Mehta, S., and Farmer, J.A. (2007). Obesity and inflammation: A new look at an old problem. *Curr Atheroscler Rep* 9, 134–138.

41. Aggarwal, B.B., Shishodia, S., Sandur, S.K., Pandey, M.K., and Sethi, G. (2006). Inflammation and cancer: How hot is the link? *Biochem Pharmacol* 72, 1605–1621.

42. Lu, H., Ouyang, W., and Huang, C. (2006). Inflammation, a key event in cancer development. *Mol Cancer Res* 4, 221–233.

43. Trayhurn, P., and Beattie, J.H. (2001). Physiological role of adipose tissue: White adipose tissue as an endocrine and secretory organ. *Proc Nutr Soc* 60, 329–339.

44. Rondinone, C.M. (2006). Adipocyte-derived hormones, cytokines, and mediators. *Endocrine* 29, 81–90.

45. Adlercreutz, H., Fotsis, T., Lampe, J., Wahala, K., Makela, T., Brunow, G., and Hase, T. (1993). Quantitative determination of lignans and isoflavonoids in plasma of omnivorous and vegetarian women by isotope dilution gas chromatography-mass spectrometry. *Scand J Clin Lab Invest Suppl* 215, 5–18.

46. Yasuda, T., Kano, Y., Saito, K., and Ohsawa, K. (1994). Urinary and biliary metabolites of daidzin and daidzein in rats. *Biol Pharm Bull* 17, 1369–1374.
47. Adlercreutz, H., van der Wildt, J., Kinzel, J., Attalla, H., Wahala, K., Makela, T., Hase, T., and Fotsis, T. (1995). Lignan and isoflavonoid conjugates in human urine. *J Steroid Biochem Mol Biol* 52, 97–103.
48. Zhang, Y., Hendrich, S., and Murphy, P.A. (2003). Glucuronides are the main isoflavone metabolites in women. *J Nutr* 133, 399–404.
49. Fang, M.Z., Wang, Y., Ai, N., Hou, Z., Sun, Y., Lu, H., Welsh, W., and Yang, C.S. (2003). Tea polyphenol (-)-epigallocatechin-3-gallate inhibits DNA methyltransferase and reactivates methylation-silenced genes in cancer cell lines. *Cancer Res* 63, 7563–7570.
50. Chuang, J.C., Yoo, C.B., Kwan, J.M., Li, T.W., Liang, G., Yang, A.S., and Jones, P.A. (2005). Comparison of biological effects of non-nucleoside DNA methylation inhibitors versus 5-aza-2′-deoxycytidine. *Mol Cancer Ther* 4, 1515–1520.
51. Lee, W.J., Shim, J.Y., and Zhu, B.T. (2005). Mechanisms for the inhibition of DNA methyltransferases by tea catechins and bioflavonoids. *Mol Pharmacol* 68, 1018–1030.
52. Stresemann, C., Brueckner, B., Musch, T., Stopper, H., and Lyko, F. (2006). Functional diversity of DNA methyltransferase inhibitors in human cancer cell lines. *Cancer Res* 66, 2794–2800.
53. Cox, R., and Goorha, S. (1986). A study of the mechanism of selenite-induced hypomethylated DNA and differentiation of Friend erythroleukemic cells. *Carcinogenesis* 7, 2015–2018.
54. Fiala, E.S., Staretz, M.E., Pandya, G.A., El-Bayoumy, K., and Hamilton, S.R. (1998). Inhibition of DNA cytosine methyltransferase by chemopreventive selenium compounds, determined by an improved assay for DNA cytosine methyltransferase and DNA cytosine methylation. *Carcinogenesis* 19, 597–604.
55. Davis, C.D., and Uthus, E.O. (2002). Dietary selenite and azadeoxycytidine treatments affect dimethylhydrazine-induced aberrant crypt formation in rat colon and DNA methylation in HT-29 cells. *J Nutr* 132, 292–297.
56. Della Ragione, F., Criniti, V., Della Pietra, V., Borriello, A., Oliva, A., Indaco, S., Yamamoto, T., and Zappia, V. (2001). Genes modulated by histone acetylation as new effectors of butyrate activity. *FEBS Lett* 499, 199–204.
57. Varela-Moreiras, G., Perez-Olleros, L., Garcia-Cuevas, M., and Ruiz-Roso, B. (1994). Effects of ageing on folate metabolism in rats fed a long-term folate deficient diet. *Int J Vitam Nutr Res* 64, 294–299.
58. Obeid, R., Kostopoulos, P., Knapp, J.P., Kasoha, M., Becker, G., Fassbender, K., and Herrmann, W. (2007). Biomarkers of folate and vitamin B12 are related in blood and cerebrospinal fluid. *Clin Chem* 53, 326–333.
59. Brattstrom, L., Lindgren, A., Israelsson, B., Andersson, A., and Hultberg, B. (1994). Homocysteine and cysteine: Determinants of plasma levels in middle-aged and elderly subjects. *J Intern Med* 236, 633–641.
60. Henderson, L., Gregory, J., and Swan, G. (2003). The National Diet and Nutrition Survey: Adults Aged 19 to 64 Years. London: Her Majesty's Stationery Office.
61. Posner, B.E., Smigelski, C.G., and Krachenfels, M.M. (1987). Dietary characteristics and nutrient intake in an urban homebound population. *J Am Diet Assoc* 87, 452–456.

62. U.S. Department of Health and Human Services (2000). *Healthy People 2010: Understanding and Improving Health*. Washington, D.C.: U.S. Government Printing Office.

63. Millen, B.E., Silliman, R.A., Cantey-Kiser, J., Copenhafer, D.L., Ewart, C.V., Ritchie, C.S., Quatromoni, P.A., Kirkland, J.L., Chipkin, S.R., Fearon, N.A., Lund, M.E., Garcia, P.I., and Barry, P.P. (2001). Nutritional risk in an urban homebound older population. The Nutrition and Healthy Aging Project. *J Nutr Health Aging* 5, 269–277.

64. Keller, H.H., and Hedley, M.R. (2002). Nutritional risk needs assessment of community-living seniors: Prevalence of nutrition problems and priorities for action. *J Community Health* 27, 121–132.

65. Fairweather-Tait, S., Harvery, L.J., and Ford, D. (2008). Does ageing affect zinc homeostasis and dietary requirements? *Exp Gerontol* 43, 382–388.

66. Olivieri, O., Stanzial, A.M., Girelli, D., Trevisan, M.T., Guarini, P., Terzi, M., Caffi, S., Fontana, F., Casaril, M., Ferrari, S., and Corrocher, R. (1994). Selenium status, fatty acids, vitamins A and E, and aging: The Nove Study. *Am J Clin Nutr* 60, 510–517.

67. Gillum, H.L., Morgan, A.F., and Sailer, F. (1955). Nutritional status of the aging. V. Vitamin A and carotene. *J Nutr* 55, 655–670.

68. Hallfrisch, J., Muller, D.C., and Singh, V.N. (1994). Vitamin A and E intakes and plasma concentrations of retinol, beta-carotene, and alpha-tocopherol in men and women of the Baltimore Longitudinal Study of Aging. *Am J Clin Nutr* 60, 176–182.

69. Sundboom, J., and Olson, J.A. (1984). Effect of aging on the storage and catabolism of vitamin A in mice. *Exp Gerontol* 19, 257–265.

70. Pilsner, J.R., Liu, X., Ahsan, H., Ilievski, V., Slavkovich, V., Levy, D., Factor-Litvak, P., Graziano, J.H., and Gamble, M.V. (2007). Genomic methylation of peripheral blood leukocyte DNA: Influences of arsenic and folate in Bangladeshi adults. *Am J Clin Nutr* 86, 1179–1186.

71. Mathers, J.C., Kennard, J., and James, O.F. (1993). Gastrointestinal responses to oats consumption in young adult and elderly rats: Digestion, large bowel fermentation and crypt cell proliferation rates. *Br J Nutr* 70, 567–584.

72. Thomson, A.B., and Wild, G. (1997). Adaptation of intestinal nutrient transport in health and disease. Part I. *Dig Dis Sci* 42, 453–469.

73. Mathers, J.C., and McKay, J.A. (2009). Epigenetics: Potential contribution to fetal programming. In *Early Nutrition Programming and Health Outcomes in Later Life. Adv Exp Biol Med* [Koletzko, B., Desci, T., Molnar, D., and de la Huntry, A., (Eds.)] pp. 119–123. Springer Science.

74. Bird, A. (2002). DNA methylation patterns and epigenetic memory. *Genes Dev* 16, 6–21.

75. Jirtle, R.L., and Skinner, M.K. (2007). Environmental epigenomics and disease susceptibility. *Nat Rev Genet* 8, 253–262.

76. Swindell, W.R. (2007). Gene expression profiling of long-lived dwarf mice: Longevity-associated genes and relationships with diet, gender and aging. *BMC Genomics* 8, 353.

77. Rakyan, V.K., Hildmann, T., Novik, K.L., Lewin, J., Tost, J., Cox, A.V., Andrews, T.D., Howe, K.L., Otto, T., Olek, A., Fischer, J., Gut, I.G., Berlin, K., and Beck, S. (2004). DNA methylation profiling of the human major histocompatibility complex: A pilot study for the human epigenome project. *PLoS Biol* 2, e405.

78. Eckhardt, F., Lewin, J., Cortese, R., Rakyan, V.K., Attwood, J., Burger, M., Burton, J., Cox, T.V., Davies, R., Down, T.A., Haefliger, C., Horton, R., Howe, K., Jackson, D.K., Kunde, J., Koenig, C., Liddle, J., Niblett, D., Otto, T., Pettett, R., Seemann, S., Thompson, C., West, T., Rogers, J., Olek, A., Berlin, K., and Beck, S. (2006). DNA methylation profiling of human chromosomes 6, 20 and 22. *Nat Genet* 38, 1378–1385.

79. Leon, D.A., Lithell, H.O., Vagero, D., Koupilova, I., Mohsen, R., Berglund, L., Lithell, U.B., and McKeigue, P.M. (1998). Reduced fetal growth rate and increased risk of death from ischaemic heart disease: Cohort study of 15000 Swedish men and women born 1915–29. *BMJ* 317, 241–245.

80. Andersen, A.M., and Osler, M. (2004). Birth dimensions, parental mortality, and mortality in early adult age: A cohort study of Danish men born in 1953. *Int J Epidemiol* 33, 92–99.

81. Catalano, P.M., and Ehrenberg, H.M. (2006). The short- and long-term implications of maternal obesity on the mother and her offspring. *BJOG* 113, 1126–1133.

82. Godfrey, K.M., Lillycrop, K.A., Burdge, G.C., Gluckman, P.D., and Hanson, M.A. (2007). Epigenetic mechanisms and the mismatch concept of the developmental origins of health and disease. *Pediatr Res* 61, 5R–10R.

83. Wasson, G.R., McGlynn, A.P., McNulty, H., O'Reilly, S.L., McKelvey-Martin, V.J., McKerr, G., Strain, J.J., Scott, J., and Downes, C.S. (2006). Global DNA and p53 region-specific hypomethylation in human colonic cells is induced by folate depletion and reversed by folate supplementation. *J Nutr* 136, 2748–2753.

84. Duthie, S.J., Narayanan, S., Blum, S., Pirie, L., and Brand, G.M. (2000). Folate deficiency in vitro induces uracil misincorporation and DNA hypomethylation and inhibits DNA excision repair in immortalized normal human colon epithelial cells. *Nutr Cancer* 37, 245–251.

85. Jhaveri, M.S., Wagner, C., and Trepel, J.B. (2001). Impact of extracellular folate levels on global gene expression. *Mol Pharmacol* 60, 1288–1295.

86. Stempak, J.M., Sohn, K.J., Chiang, E.P., Shane, B., and Kim, Y.I. (2005). Cell and stage of transformation-specific effects of folate deficiency on methionine cycle intermediates and DNA methylation in an in vitro model. *Carcinogenesis* 26, 981–990.

87. Wolff, G.L., Kodell, R.L., Moore, S.R., and Cooney, C.A. (1998). Maternal epigenetics and methyl supplements affect agouti gene expression in Avy/a mice. *FASEB J* 12, 949–957.

88. Waterland, R.A., and Jirtle, R.L. (2003). Transposable elements: Targets for early nutritional effects on epigenetic gene regulation. *Mol Cell Biol* 23, 5293–5300.

89. Waterland, R.A., Travisano, M., and Tahiliani, K.G. (2007). Diet-induced hypermethylation at agouti viable yellow is not inherited transgenerationally through the female. *FASEB J* 21, 3380–3385.

90. Dolinoy, D.C., Huang, D., and Jirtle, R.L. (2007). Maternal nutrient supplementation counteracts bisphenol A-induced DNA hypomethylation in early development. *Proc Natl Acad Sci USA* 104, 13056–13061.

91. Kim, Y.I., Pogribny, I.P., Basnakian, A.G., Miller, J.W., Selhub, J., James, S.J., and Mason, J.B. (1997). Folate deficiency in rats induces DNA strand breaks and hypomethylation within the p53 tumor suppressor gene. *Am J Clin Nutr* 65, 46–52.

92. Niculescu, M.D., Craciunescu, C.N., and Zeisel, S.H. (2006). Dietary choline deficiency alters global and gene-specific DNA methylation in the developing hippocampus of mouse fetal brains. *FASEB J* 20, 43–49.

93. Sohn, K.J., Stempak, J.M., Reid, S., Shirwadkar, S., Mason, J.B., and Kim, Y.I. (2003). The effect of dietary folate on genomic and p53-specific DNA methylation in rat colon. *Carcinogenesis* 24, 81–90.

94. Maloney, C.A., Hay, S.M., and Rees, W.D. (2007). Folate deficiency during pregnancy impacts on methyl metabolism without affecting global DNA methylation in the rat fetus. *Br J Nutr* 97, 1090–1098.

95. Kim, Y.I., Christman, J.K., Fleet, J.C., Cravo, M.L., Salomon, R.N., Smith, D., Ordovas, J., Selhub, J., and Mason, J.B. (1995). Moderate folate deficiency does not cause global hypomethylation of hepatic and colonic DNA or c-myc-specific hypomethylation of colonic DNA in rats. *Am J Clin Nutr* 61, 1083–1090.

96. Kovacheva, V.P., Mellott, T.J., Davison, J.M., Wagner, N., Lopez-Coviella, I., Schnitzler, A.C., and Blusztajn, J.K. (2007). Gestational choline deficiency causes global and Igf2 gene DNA hypermethylation by up-regulation of Dnmt1 expression. *J Biol Chem* 282, 31777–31788.

97. Fowler, B.M., Giuliano, A.R., Piyathilake, C., Nour, M., and Hatch, K. (1998). Hypomethylation in cervical tissue: Is there a correlation with folate status? *Cancer Epidemiol Bio Prevt* 7, 901–906.

98. Pufulete, M., Al-Ghnaniem, R., Leather, A.J., Appleby, P., Gout, S., Terry, C., Emery, P.W., and Sanders, T.A. (2003). Folate status, genomic DNA hypomethylation, and risk of colorectal adenoma and cancer: A case control study. *Gastroenterology* 124, 1240–1248.

99. Pufulete, M., Al-Ghnaniem, R., Khushal, A., Appleby, P., Harris, N., Gout, S., Emery, P.W., and Sanders, TA. (2005). Effect of folic acid supplementation on genomic DNA methylation in patients with colorectal adenoma. *Gut* 54, 648–653.

100. Jacob, R.A., Gretz, D.M., Taylor, P.C., James, S.J., Pogribny, I.P., Miller, B.J., Henning, S.M., and Swendseid, M.E. (1998). Moderate folate depletion increases plasma homocysteine and decreases lymphocyte DNA methylation in postmenopausal women. *J Nutr* 128, 1204–1212.

101. Rampersaud, G.C., Kauwell, G.P., Hutson, A.D., Cerda, J.J., and Bailey, L.B. (2000). Genomic DNA methylation decreases in response to moderate folate depletion in elderly women. *Am J Clin Nutr* 72, 998–1003.

102. Pufulete, M., Al-Ghnaniem, R., Rennie, J.A., Appleby, P., Harris, N., Gout, S., Emery, P.W., and Sanders, T.A. (2005). Influence of folate status on genomic DNA methylation in colonic mucosa of subjects without colorectal adenoma or cancer. *Br J Cancer* 92, 838–842.

103. Fang, M.Z., Chen, D., Sun, Y., Jin, Z., Christman, J.K., and Yang, C.S. (2005). Reversal of hypermethylation and reactivation of p16INK4a, RARbeta, and MGMT genes by genistein and other isoflavones from soy. *Clin Cancer Res* 11, 7033–7041.

104. Wang, L.G., Beklemisheva, A., Liu, X.M., Ferrari, A.C., Feng, J., and Chiao, J.W. (2007). Dual action on promoter demethylation and chromatin by an isothiocyanate restored GSTP1 silenced in prostate cancer. *Mol Carcinog* 46, 24–31.

105. Shi, S.T., Wang, Z.Y., Smith, T.J., Hong, J.Y., Chen, W.F., Ho, C.T., and Yang, C.S. (1994). Effects of green tea and black tea on 4-(methylnitrosamino)-1-(3-pyridyl)-1-butanone bioactivation, DNA methylation, and lung tumorigenesis in A/J mice. *Cancer Res* 54, 4641–4647.

106. Day, J.K., Bauer, A.M., DesBordes, C., Zhuang, Y., Kim, B.E., Newton, L.G., Nehra, V., Forsee, K.M., MacDonald, R.S., Besch-Williford, C., Huang, T.H., and Lubahn, D.B. (2002). Genistein alters methylation patterns in mice. *J Nutr* 132, 2419S–2423S.
107. Olthof, M.R., Hollman, P.C., Zock, P.L., and Katan, M.B. (2001). Consumption of high doses of chlorogenic acid, present in coffee, or of black tea increases plasma total homocysteine concentrations in humans. *Am J Clin Nutr* 73, 532–538.
108. Beach, R.S., Gershwin, M.E., and Hurley, L.S. (1982). Gestational zinc deprivation in mice: Persistence of immunodeficiency for three generations. *Science* 218, 469–471.
109. Wallwork, J.C., and Duerre, J.A. (1985). Effect of zinc deficiency on methionine metabolism, methylation reactions and protein synthesis in isolated perfused rat liver. *J Nutr* 115, 252–262.
110. Davis, C.D., Uthus, E.O., and Finley, J.W. (2000). Dietary selenium and arsenic affect DNA methylation in vitro in Caco-2 cells and in vivo in rat liver and colon. *J Nutr* 130, 2903–2909.
111. Davis, C.D., and Uthus, E.O. (2003). Dietary folate and selenium affect dimethylhydrazine-induced aberrant crypt formation, global DNA methylation and one-carbon metabolism in rats. *J Nutr* 133, 2907–2914.
112. Di Croce, L., Raker, V.A., Corsaro, M., Fazi, F., Fanelli, M., Faretta, M., Fuks, F., Lo Coco, F., Kouzarides, T., Nervi, C., Minucci, S., and Pelicci, P.G. (2002). Methyltransferase recruitment and DNA hypermethylation of target promoters by an oncogenic transcription factor. *Science* 295, 1079–1082.
113. Sirchia, S.M., Ren, M., Pili, R., Sironi, E., Somenzi, G., Ghidoni, R., Toma, S., Nicolo, G., and Sacchi, N. (2002). Endogenous reactivation of the RARbeta2 tumor suppressor gene epigenetically silenced in breast cancer. *Cancer Res* 62, 2455–2461.
114. Rowling, M.J., McMullen, M.H., and Schalinske, K.L. (2002). Vitamin A and its derivatives induce hepatic glycine N-methyltransferase and hypomethylation of DNA in rats. *J Nutr* 132, 365–369.
115. Moreno, F.S., S.-Wu, T., Naves, M.M., Silveira, E.R., Oloris, S.C., da Costa, M.A., Dagli, M.L., and Ong, T.P. (2002). Inhibitory effects of beta-carotene and vitamin A during the progression phase of hepatocarcinogenesis involve inhibition of cell proliferation but not alterations in DNA methylation. *Nutr Cancer* 44, 80–88.
116. Benbrahim-Tallaa, L., Waterland, R.A., Styblo, M., Achanzar, W.E., Webber, M.M., and Waalkes, M.P. (2005). Molecular events associated with arsenic-induced malignant transformation of human prostatic epithelial cells: Aberrant genomic DNA methylation and K-ras oncogene activation. *Toxicol Appl Pharmacol* 206, 288–298.
117. Chen, H., Li, S., Liu, J., Diwan, B.A., Barrett, J.C., and Waalkes, M.P. (2004). Chronic inorganic arsenic exposure induces hepatic global and individual gene hypomethylation: Implications for arsenic hepatocarcinogenesis. *Carcinogenesis* 25, 1779–1786.
118. Uthus, E.O., and Davis, C. (2005). Dietary arsenic affects dimethylhydrazine-induced aberrant crypt formation and hepatic global DNA methylation and DNA methyltransferase activity in rats. *Biol Trace Elem Res* 103, 133–145.
119. Choi, S.W., Stickel, F., Baik, H.W., Kim, Y.I., Seitz, H.K., and Mason, J.B. (1999). Chronic alcohol consumption induces genomic but not p53-specific DNA hypomethylation in rat colon. *J Nutr* 129, 1945–1950.

120. Lu, S.C., Huang, Z.Z., Yang, H., Mato, J.M., Avila, M.A., and Tsukamoto, H. (2000). Changes in methionine adenosyltransferase and S-adenosylmethionine homeostasis in alcoholic rat liver. *Am J Physiol Gastrointest Liver Physiol* 279, G178–G185.

121. Marutha Ravindran, C.R., and Ticku, M.K. (2004). Changes in methylation pattern of NMDA receptor NR2B gene in cortical neurons after chronic ethanol treatment in mice. *Brain Res Mol Brain Res* 121, 19–27.

122. Bonsch, D., Lenz, B., Reulbach, U., Kornhuber, J., and Bleich, S. (2004). Homocysteine associated genomic DNA hypermethylation in patients with chronic alcoholism. *J Neural Transm* 111, 1611–1616.

123. Ishida, E., Nakamura, M., Ikuta, M., Shimada, K., Matsuyoshi, S., Kirita, T., and Konishi, N. (2005). Promotor hypermethylation of p14ARF is a key alteration for progression of oral squamous cell carcinoma. *Oral Oncol* 41, 614–622.

124. Chang, H.W., Ling, G.S., Wei, W.I., and Yuen, A.P. (2004). Smoking and drinking can induce p15 methylation in the upper aerodigestive tract of healthy individuals and patients with head and neck squamous cell carcinoma. *Cancer* 101, 125–132.

125. Hass, B.S., Hart, R.W., Lu, M.H., and Lyn-Cook, B.D. (1993). Effects of caloric restriction in animals on cellular function, oncogene expression, and DNA methylation in vitro. *Mutat Res* 295, 281–289.

126. Miyamura, Y., Tawa, R., Koizumi, A., Uehara, Y., Kurishita, A., Sakurai, H., Kamiyama, S., and Ono, T. (1993). Effects of energy restriction on age-associated changes of DNA methylation in mouse liver. *Mutat Res* 295, 63–69.

127. Lillycrop, K.A., Phillips, E.S., Jackson, A.A., Hanson, M.A., and Burdge, G.C. (2005). Dietary protein restriction of pregnant rats induces and folic acid supplementation prevents epigenetic modification of hepatic gene expression in the offspring. *J Nutr* 135, 1382–1386.

128. Burdge, G.C., Slater-Jefferies, J., Torrens, C., Phillips, E.S., Hanson, M.A., and Lillycrop, K.A. (2007). Dietary protein restriction of pregnant rats in the F0 generation induces altered methylation of hepatic gene promoters in the adult male offspring in the F1 and F2 generations. *Br J Nutr* 97, 435–439.

129. Lillycrop, K.A., Slater-Jefferies, J.L., Hanson, M.A., Godfrey, K.M., Jackson, A.A., and Burdge, G.C. (2007). Induction of altered epigenetic regulation of the hepatic glucocorticoid receptor in the offspring of rats fed a protein-restricted diet during pregnancy suggests that reduced DNA methyltransferase-1 expression is involved in impaired DNA methylation and changes in histone modifications. *Br J Nutr* 97, 1064–1073.

130. Demary, K., Wong, L., and Spanjaard, R.A. (2001). Effects of retinoic acid and sodium butyrate on gene expression, histone acetylation and inhibition of proliferation of melanoma cells. *Cancer Lett* 163, 103–107.

131. Rada-Iglesias, A., Enroth, S., Ameur, A., Koch, C.M., Clelland, G.K., Respuela-Alonso, P., Wilcox, S., Dovey, O.M., Ellis, P.D., Langford, C.F., Dunham, I., Komorowski, J., and Wadelius, C. (2007). Butyrate mediates decrease of histone acetylation centered on transcription start sites and down-regulation of associated genes. *Genome Res* 17, 708–719.

132. Kida, Y., Shimizu, T., and Kuwano, K. (2006). Sodium butyrate up-regulates cathelicidin gene expression via activator protein-1 and histone acetylation at the promoter region in a human lung epithelial cell line, EBC-1. *Mol Immunol* 43, 1972–1981.

133. Druesne, N., Pagniez, A., Mayeur, C., Thomas, M., Cherbuy, C., Duee, P.H., Martel, P., and Chaumontet, C. (2004). Diallyl disulfide (DADS) increases histone acetylation and p21(waf1/cip1) expression in human colon tumor cell lines. *Carcinogenesis* 25, 1227–1236.
134. Pogribny, I.P., Tryndyak, V.P., Muskhelishvili, L., Rusyn, I., and Ross, S.A. (2007). Methyl deficiency, alterations in global histone modifications, and carcinogenesis. *J Nutr* 137, 216S–222S.
135. Park, P.H., Miller, R., and Shukla, S.D. (2003). Acetylation of histone H3 at lysine 9 by ethanol in rat hepatocytes. *Biochem Biophys Res Commun* 306, 501–504.
136. Shukla, S.D., and Aroor, A.R. (2006). Epigenetic effects of ethanol on liver and gastrointestinal injury. *World J Gastroenterol* 12, 5265–5271.
137. Mahadev, K., and Vemuri, M.C. (1998). Ethanol-induced changes in hepatic chromatin and nonhistone nuclear protein composition in the rat. *Alcohol* 15, 207–211.
138. Kim, J.S., and Shukla, S.D. (2006). Acute in vivo effect of ethanol (binge drinking) on histone H3 modifications in rat tissues. *Alcohol Alcohol* 41, 126–132.
139. Sharma, R., Nakamura, A., Takahashi, R., Nakamoto, H., and Goto, S. (2006). Carbonyl modification in rat liver histones: Decrease with age and increase by dietary restriction. *Free Radic Biol Med* 40, 1179–1184.
140. Uthus, E.O., Ross, S.A., and Davis, C.D. (2006). Differential effects of dietary selenium (se) and folate on methyl metabolism in liver and colon of rats. *Biol Trace Elem Res* 109, 201–214.
141. Detich, N., Theberge, J., and Szyf, M. (2002). Promoter-specific activation and demethylation by MBD2/demethylase. *J Biol Chem* 277, 35791–35794.
142. Ghoshal, K., Li, X., Datta, J., Bai, S., Pogribny, I., Pogribny, M., Huang, Y., Young, D., and Jacob, S.T. (2006). A folate- and methyl-deficient diet alters the expression of DNA methyltransferases and methyl CpG binding proteins involved in epigenetic gene silencing in livers of F344 rats. *J Nutr* 136, 1522–1527.
143. Aviram, A., Zimrah, Y., Shaklai, M., Nudelman, A., and Rephaeli, A. (1994). Comparison between the effect of butyric acid and its prodrug pivaloyloxymethylbutyrate on histones hyperacetylation in an HL-60 leukemic cell line. *Int J Cancer* 56, 906–909.

chapter nine

Nutrition, epigenetics, and cancer

Sharon A. Ross

Contents

Compelling evidence suggests that diet and dietary factors are important in cancer etiology by inhibiting or enhancing the cancer process. Because diet may contribute significantly to the causation of many human cancers, it is important to uncover the molecular mechanisms of action of dietary bioactive factors in cancer prevention, as well as those stimulating neoplastic cell transformations. The role of epigenetic mechanisms in the etiology of disease, including cancer development and progression, has been increasingly recognized in recent years. The importance of epigenetic mechanisms is highlighted by their influence on gene expression and chromatin stability, which thereby impact the regulation of cell cycle control, DNA damage, apoptosis, differentiation, and other cancer-related processes. Evidence suggests that environmental factors, such as diet, may be significant regulators of epigenetic events, including DNA methylation and histone posttranslational modulation. For example, it has long been known that folate participates in the generation of S-adenosylmethionine, which acts as a methyl donor in the methylation of cytosines in DNA and participates in posttranslational methylation of histones. A classic example for the role of diet in epigenetics and cancer is the finding that dietary methyl deficiency (folate, choline, and methionine) in a rat model has been shown to alter hepatic DNA methylation patterns and induce hepatocarcinogenesis in the absence of a carcinogen. Several other bioactive food components (BFCs), including genistein, epigallocatechin gallate, diallyl disulfide, and sulforaphane have been suggested to impact epigenetic mechanisms. Many of these examples will be presented, as well as the next steps in diet, epigenetic events, and cancer prevention research.

9.1   Introduction

Several epidemiological and preclinical studies have suggested that the increased intake of selected BFCs, including folate, zinc, genistein, epigallocatechin gallate, diallyl disulfide, and sulforaphane may modulate cancer risk. However, the specific molecular mechanisms for these BFCs and the quantities needed (as well as issues of frequency, duration, and timing of exposure in the life span) to bring about the antitumorigenic effects remain largely unresolved. Diet and BFCs may alter the cellular milieu by modulating several cellular processes, including DNA repair, hormonal regulation, differentiation, inflammation, apoptosis, cell cycle control/proliferation, carcinogen metabolism, and angiogenesis, among others. Cancer has been hypothesized to develop from a clone of cells that have escaped normal regulation of such processes, as well as an interruption of normal intercellular relationships. These abnormalities of function are believed to derive from disordered expression of key genes, resulting in altered cellular phenotype.[1] Such anomalous gene expression may result from genetic mutation or from epigenetic modulation that may silence genes that should be active or switch on genes that should be silent. Diet and BFCs may directly influence both processes.

Many studies provide intriguing evidence that part of the anticancer properties attributed to several BFCs may relate to modulation of epigenetic processes, including DNA methylation and histone posttranslational modification. We have previously delineated[2] at least four ways in which nutrients may be interrelated with DNA methylation. The first is that nutrients may influence the supply of methyl groups for the formation of *S*-adenosylmethionine. The second mechanism is that nutrients may modify utilization of methyl groups by processes including altered DNA methyltransferase activity. A third possible mechanism may relate to DNA demethylation activity. Finally, the DNA methylation patterns may influence the response to a nutrient. Intriguingly, such interactions may apply similarly to the way in which diet impacts histone methylation marks and processes. The interrelationship between nutrients, epigenetics, and cancer will be further explored in this review by providing additional examples and highlighting areas for further research.

9.2 Epigenetics and cancer

Epigenetic marks and processes—such as DNA methylation of the cytosine phosphate guanine dinucleotide (CpG) islands in promoters and other regions of the genome, chromatin remodeling and higher-order chromatin structural alterations, posttranslational ATP-dependent modifications, which include methylation, acetylation, ubiquitination, and phosphorylation of histone tail domains, as well as gene regulation through noncoding RNAs—impart control on gene activity and chromatin structure. The most widely studied epigenetic modification in humans is the cytosine methylation of DNA within the dinucleotide CpG.[3] Regions rich in CpG dinucleotides, known as CpG islands, span the 5′ end region (promoter, untranslated region and exon 1) of many genes and are usually unmethylated in normal cells.[4] This unmethylated status is associated with the ability of CpG-island-containing genes to be transcribed in the presence of the necessary transcriptional activators. Conversely, the covalent modification of cytosine to 5-methylcytosine contributes to the transcriptional regulation of specific genes and participates in regional chromatin conformation by affecting the binding properties of methylation-sensitive DNA-binding proteins, thereby blocking transcription.[5] In cancer cells, the transcriptional silencing of tumor-suppressor genes by CpG-island-promoter hypermethylation is thought to be an early response in the tumorigenic process.[6] In addition to region-specific hypermethylation, widespread global DNA hypomethylation[7] and increased DNA methyltransferase[8] activity are common characteristics of tumor cells. Importantly, DNA methylation changes are thought to be inherited mitotically in somatic cells, providing a potential mechanism by which environmental effects on the epigenome can have long-term effects on gene expression.[9]

Histone modifications of nucleosomes distinguish euchromatic (open) from heterochromatic (closed) chromatin states. In particular, acetylation of specific residues in histones H3 and H4 has been associated with an open chromatin configuration and a permissive gene transcription state.[10] Histone acetylation is regulated by several enzymatic activities with the capacity either to transfer acetyl groups or to induce histone deacetylation, which is associated with gene silencing. Recent findings have suggested a link between histone posttranslational modifications and cancer. For example, the loss of monoacetylation and trimethylation of histone H4 is a common hallmark of human tumor cells.[11] Additionally, an imbalance of histone acetyltransferase (HAT) and histone deacetylase (HDAC) activities has also been observed in cancer cells.[12] Moreover, aberrant targeting of HDACs has been found to be associated with transcriptional silencing of tumor-suppressor genes, including *p21*, which is a cyclin-dependent kinase inhibitor that blocks cell cycle progression from G_1 into S phase.[13] The expression of *p21* has been found to be defective in many different tumors, allowing uncontrolled cell division. Interestingly, HDAC inhibitors have been shown to reactivate *p21* expression and thereby prevent tumor cell proliferation.[13] In fact, the HDAC inhibitor-induced expression of *p21* has been found to correlate with an increase in the acetylation of histones associated with the *p21* promoter region. Such early discoveries have led to the development of HDAC inhibitors for cancer chemotherapy, which is a promising current clinical research emphasis.[12]

The role of small noncoding RNA molecules in the regulation of gene expression has only recently begun to be understood. Noncoding RNAs have been shown to modulate posttranscriptional silencing (i.e., the targeted degradation of mRNAs) and there is much interest in studying deregulation of these small RNAs in various diseases, including cancer.[14] Moreover, epigenetic modifications have recently been found to be induced and directed by small RNA molecules in human cells.[15] In fact, small RNA-mediated transcriptional gene silencing was shown to be correlated with changes in chromatin structure at the targeted promoter. Specifically, silencing was correlated with decreases in certain active-state histone modifications, increases in certain silencing histone methylation marks, and in some instances, increases in DNA methylation at the targeted promoter. The impact of this epigenetic mechanism in cancer development is currently being explored.

Additional epigenetic regulators, such as the Polycomb group (PcG) proteins, which function as transcriptional repressors that silence specific sets of genes through chromatin modification, may also contribute to the pathogenesis of cancer.[16] The PcG actually comprise two distinct complexes, PcG complex 1 and 2. Initially, PcG complex 2 silences chromatin and encodes a histone mark by methylating histone H3 at lysine 27 (K27me3); next PcG complex 1 is recruited through recognition of this histone mark, and thereby ubiquitinates histone H2A and/or inhibits chromatin remodeling to maintain the silenced states of the locus.[17] PcG-deficient mice have provided biological evidence that PcGs are essential for sustaining stem cell activity. In addition to being correlated with cancer progression and prognosis, PcGs are also associated with cancer stem cell activity. The SWItch/Sucrose NonFermentable (SWI/SNF) complex is a chromatin-remodeling complex that uses the energy of ATP hydrolysis to modify chromatin structure in order to regulate gene expression and recent observations link an aberrant SWI/SNF complex to cancer.[18] How and in what context these and other epigenetic mechanisms and regulatory factors may interact to regulate chromatin structure, dynamics and gene expression in cancer development and prevention is an active area of research.

9.3 Dietary exposure in utero: Agouti model

Increasing evidence from animal studies indicates that prenatal and early postnatal environmental factors; including nutritional supplementation,[19–24] xenobiotic chemical exposure,[25–27] behavioral cues,[28,29] reproductive factors,[30,31] and low-dose radiation[32] alters epigenetic marks and processes and subsequent changes in the risk of developing disease. Intriguingly, evidence also suggests that epigenetic alterations might also be inherited transgenerationally, thus potentially affecting the health of future generations.[27,33–37] The results of these studies support the fetal basis or developmental origins of the adult-onset disease hypothesis. This intriguing idea implies that an organism can adapt to environmental signals during early life, but that these adaptations can also increase the risk of developing chronic diseases, including cancer, later in life when there is a mismatch between the perceived environment and that which is encountered in adulthood.

Evidence using the viable yellow agouti (A^{vy}) model suggests that dietary supplementation to dams in utero can lead to changes in DNA methylation as well as profound effects on phenotype of the offspring.[19–22,38] In the viable yellow agouti (A^{vy}) mice an endogenous retrovirus-like transposon sequence is inserted close to the gene coding for the Agouti protein.[39] Normally, a cryptic promoter within the retrotransposon is silenced by methylation allowing normal tissue-specific and regulated *agouti* expression. However, if this site is undermethylated the promoter is active and drives constitutive ectopic expression of the *agouti* gene, leading to yellow coat color and obesity (and increased susceptibility to other chronic diseases, including cancer). Dietary supplementation of maternal diets with folic acid, vitamin B12, choline, betaine, and zinc was associated with a change in coat color from a yellow to an agouti coat in the offspring. This phenotype change is typically associated with a lower risk of cancer, diabetes, and obesity and prolonged life in this model.[19,38] Furthermore, these investigators examined DNA methylation in representative phenotypes and found that the representative yellow mice displayed more hypomethylated long terminal repeats 5′ of the *agouti* gene and that the representative agouti or brown coat mice were found to have a greater degree of hypermethylation in the long terminal repeat 5′ of the *agouti* gene.

Another group of investigators has also examined the effect of methyl donor supplementation (folic acid, vitamin B12, choline, and betaine without zinc) to the maternal diet in the agouti model and found similar effects on the phenotypic expression of the offspring.[20] These researchers characterized a shift in the distribution of coat color and CpG methylation of the *agouti* locus in methyl-supplemented compared to nonsupplemented animals. They found that changes in pigmentation of mouse pup hair coat, ranging from yellow to brown, were significantly associated with supplementation of the pregnant mother's diet. Furthermore, these coat color changes were directly linked to alterations in DNA methylation with a distribution shift toward increased CpG methylation at the A^{vy} locus with methyl supplementation. Moreover, by a comparison of tail DNA at 21 days and liver DNA at 100 days these investigators found that the coat color phenotype and A^{vy} methylation relationship persisted into adulthood. This study clearly demonstrates that maternal methyl donor supplementation during gestation can alter offspring phenotype by methylating the epigenome. It is not yet clear, however, which of the dietary components are necessary for the DNA methylation and phenotypic change.

In a more recent study by Dolinoy et al.,[22] similar alterations in coat color were induced in offspring through maternal ingestion of genistein, the major phytoestrogen in soy, at doses comparable to those a human might receive through a high soy diet (250 mg/kg diet). Most interestingly, the methylation changes at the A^{vy} locus with genistein supplementation appeared to protect the mouse offspring against obesity in adulthood, demonstrating that maternal dietary supplementation is associated with not only altered fetal methylation patterns but also methylation-dependent susceptibility to disease. The mechanism of how genistein affects methylation and epigenetic pathways has yet to be determined. These investigators did not find an association between genistein supplementation and S-adenosylmethionine or S-adenosylhomocysteine concentrations, suggesting the change in methylation was independent of the one-carbon pathway. Changes in specific nuclear transcription factors or their regulation are a logical site of action of genistein, but additional research is needed to identify the specific site of action of genistein.

The A^{vy} mouse has also been used further as an environmental biosensor to evaluate the effects on the fetal epigenome of maternal dietary exposure to a xenobiotic chemical.[40] In utero or neonatal exposure to bisphenol A (BPA), a high-production volume chemical used in the manufacture of polycarbonate plastic, is associated with higher body weight, increased breast and prostate cancer, and altered reproductive function. Maternal exposure to this endocrine active compound (50 mg of BPA/kg) shifted the coat color distribution of A^{vy} mouse offspring toward yellow by decreasing CpG methylation in an IAP retrotransposon upstream of the *agouti* gene. Moreover, maternal nutritional supplementation of the BPA diet with either methyl donors or the phytoestrogen genistein resulted in a control coat color distribution and negated the DNA hypomethylating effect of BPA. These studies present compelling evidence that early developmental exposure to a xenobiotic chemical such as BPA can change offspring phenotype by stably altering the epigenome, an effect that can be counteracted by maternal dietary supplements.

It is important to clarify how observations in the agouti model may relate to human disease. Although the A^{vy} locus—a retrovirus-like transposon sequence—is not found in the human genome, there is the possibility that metastable epialleles ("metastable" refers to the labile nature of the epigenetic state of these alleles; "epiallele" defines their potential to maintain epigenetic marks transgenerationally[41]) associated with other transposable elements could similarly be influenced by methylation via in utero exposure to dietary factors. Whitelaw and Martin have proposed that transposable elements in the mammalian genome cause considerable phenotypic variability, making each individual mammal a "compound epigenetic mosaic."[42] Whether such an epigenetic mosaic can be modulated by early diet and how such phenotypes alter susceptibility to chronic disease, including cancer, in adulthood requires further study. Other regions of the genome that may be vulnerable to epigenetic variation need to be identified and characterized in human tissues. There is also a need to further our understanding of the interaction between diet, epigenetics, and crucial times of exposure during development and throughout the entire life span.

9.4 Methyl-deficient diet induced hepatocarcinogenesis

The methyl-deficient model of endogenous hepatocarcinogenesis in rodents is unique in that dietary omission rather than the addition of chemical carcinogens can lead to tumor formation.[43] Specifically, deficiency of the major dietary sources of methyl groups—methionine, choline, folic acid, and vitamin B12—is sufficient to induce liver tumor formation in male rats and certain mouse strains.[44–47] The methyl deficiency induced in these rodent animals has been associated with several defects, including increased genome-wide and gene-specific hypomethylation.[47–50] Importantly, the aberrant epigenetic alterations imposed by this diet have been hypothesized to be the primary mechanism responsible for malignant transformation of rat liver cells.[47,48,50–52] The effects of feeding a methyl-deficient diet followed by a methyl-adequate diet on liver DNA methylation and on the formation and evolution of altered hepatic foci have been investigated.[51] These investigators fed a methyl-deficient diet for 9, 18, 24, and 36 weeks to male F344 rats, followed by refeeding a methyl-adequate diet for a total of 54 weeks. Three major effects were observed: (1) a rapid decrease in hepatic *S*-adenosylmethionine levels, which was completely reversible upon refeeding the methyl-adequate diet; (2) refeeding the complete diet restored DNA methylation to normal levels only in the group that had been fed the methyl-deficient diet for 9 weeks; and (3) the formation of persistent altered hepatic foci, as measured by placental isoform of glutathione-*S*-transferase (GSTpi)-positive lesions, at all investigated time points. The results suggest that biological and biochemical changes associated with the early stages of hepatocarcinogenesis occurred between 9 and 18 weeks of methyl deprivation. The persistence of altered hepatic foci in liver after withdrawal of methyl-deficient diet suggests the carcinogenic potential of a methyl-deficient diet. Furthermore, the association between DNA hypomethylation and expansion of foci suggests that stable DNA hypomethylation is a promoting factor for clonal expansion of initiated cells. These results provide experimental evidence and a mechanistic basis by which epigenetic alterations may contribute to the initiation and promotion steps of carcinogenesis and also point to the importance of timing of an environmental impact in carcinogenesis. In other recent studies examining the early stages of hepatocarcinogenesis induced by methyl deficiency in rats, substantial alterations in other aspects of the epigenetic machinery have been observed, including aberrant expression of DNA methyltransferases and methyl CpG binding proteins,[53] defects in histone methyltransferase protein expression and histone posttranslational modifications,[52] and changes in the expression of microRNAs.[54] Evidence has suggested that early dysregulation of microRNAs in the process of hepatocarcinogenesis could be reversed by restoring methyl donors. The epigenetic changes observed in the methyl-deficiency induced hepatocarcinogenesis model are thought to be important contributing factors in the formation of epigenetically reprogrammed cells that become neoplastic. How these epigenetic mechanisms are interrelated and which mechanism is the earliest trigger toward fixing the neoplastic state requires further study. It is interesting to note that the sequence of pathological and molecular events in the methyl-deficient model of liver carcinogenesis is remarkably similar to the development of human hepatocellular carcinoma associated with viral hepatitis B and C infections, alcohol exposure, and metabolic liver diseases.[55] The biochemical and molecular events predisposing to cancer in the methyl-deficient induced hepatocarcinogenesis are the result of chronic metabolic stress and the model provides an ideal system to study progressive epigenetic alterations that might occur during human carcinogenesis.

9.5   Dietary polyphenols reactivate silenced genes via epigenetic mechanisms

The aberrant patterns of DNA methylation and histone posttranslational modifications in a neoplastic cell may influence the response to BFCs. Interestingly, the ability of dietary factors to reduce proliferation in normal cells has been observed to be less than that in neoplastic cells. It may be that such differences in sensitivity to dietary factors are related to variation in epigenetic marks and processes in different cell types. Furthermore, prevention or reversal of hypermethylation-induced inactivation of key tumor suppression genes or receptor genes in cancer cells could be an effective approach for cancer prevention. In this regard, epigallocatechin 3-gallate (EGCG) (5 to 50 μM) from green tea and genistein (2 to 20 μmol/L) from soybean have been found to restore methylation patterns and gene expression of tumor suppressor genes in neoplastic cells in culture.[56–58] Experimental evidence from this laboratory suggests that both dietary factors inhibit DNA methyltransferases (DNMT) in vitro. This inhibitory activity was associated with demethylation of CpG islands in the gene promoters and the reactivation of methylation-silenced genes such as *p16INK4a*, retinoic acid receptor beta, O6-methylguanine methyltransferase, human mutL homolog 1, and glutathione *S*-transferase-pi.[56–58] These activities have been observed in human esophageal, colon, prostate, and mammary cancer cell lines and were also associated with inhibited cell growth in these systems.

Other investigators have observed epigenetic modulation by EGCG in cancer cells. In MCF-7 breast cancer cells, EGCG treatment (100 μM) induced apoptosis through decreased transcription of *hTERT*, which is the catalytic subunit essential for the proper function of telomerase.[59] The decreased *hTERT* transcription observed in this study was correlated with epigenetic modulations, including reduction of DNA methylation at the *hTERT* promoter and H3 lys9 acetylation. The atypical correlation between demethylation and decreased transcription found in this study was hypothesized to be due to decreased capacity of DNMT1 to maintain methylation, leading to demethylation of the key E2F-1 sites, thereby allowing the repressor to bind and block transcription.[59] Another suggested possibility was that EGCG-induced demethylation facilitated the loss of methylation at CTCF (a multifunctional transcription factor) binding regions, within the first exon, allowing for repression of *hTERT*. Interestingly, at least one laboratory has replicated the finding that EGCG inhibits DNA methyltransferase activity in vitro with IC_{50} values ranging from 0.21 to 0.47 μM,[60] while another has not (using a mean IC_{20} concentration of 10 μM).[61] In vivo research is needed to clarify the importance of inhibition of DNA methyltransferase activity by EGCG.

As for genistein, a recent report suggested that this dietary factor (at both 10 and 25 μmol/L) induced the expression of the tumor suppressor genes *p21* and *p16* (*INK4a*) with a concomitant decrease in cyclins in prostate cancer cells, but that DNA methylation analysis revealed the absence of *p21* promoter methylation prior to genistein exposure.[62] These investigators, however, found that genistein increased acetylation of histones H3, H4, and H3/K4 at the *p21* and *p16* transcription start sites with concomitant increased expression of histone acetyltransferases. Furthermore, these same investigators found that genistein (50 μM) activated expression of several aberrantly silenced tumor suppressor genes that have unmethylated promoters such as *PTEN*, *CYLD*, *p53*, and *FOXO3a* in prostate cancer cells.[63] Instead of activating tumor suppressor genes through promoter demethylation, these investigators found that genistein influenced remodeling of the heterochromatic domains at promoters by modulating histone H3-Lysine 9 (H3-K9) methylation and deacetylation. These findings strengthen the understanding of how genistein may be protective against cancers with different epigenetic profiles. Furthermore, the relationship between histone modifications and DNA methylation in gene reactivation, which may be gene specific, is not entirely clear and requires additional study.

Because of the relatively low bioavailability of most polyphenolic compounds, the exact effect dietary polyphenols would have on DNA methylation or histone modifications in humans is not clear.[56] The effect of normal dietary consumption of a single polyphenolic compound is not likely to affect individuals. However, the combinational and additive effects of polyphenols with various epigenetic activities may, in theory, produce biological consequences. On the other hand, the consumption of excessive amounts of polyphenols from dietary supplements would seem to be more likely to affect DNA methylation and/or histone methylation/ acetylation status. All these possibilities remain to be examined. Although genistein and EGCG are thought to selectively induce apoptosis or reduce proliferation in cancer cells but not in normal cells, additional research is also warranted to determine beneficial versus deleterious responses to these BFCs during vulnerable periods of the life span.

9.6 Histone deacetylase (HDAC) inhibition by dietary factors

Several dietary factors, including butyrate (formed in the colon from the fermentation of dietary fiber), diallyl disulfide (present in garlic and other *Allium* vegetables), and sulforaphane (found in cruciferous vegetables) have the ability to inhibit type I and II HDAC enzymes.[64,65] These dietary compounds have been associated with cancer prevention in various preclinical and clinical studies. Moreover, evidence suggests that inhibition of HDAC activity may be associated with the cancer protective effects of these dietary components. Butyrate, diallyl disulfide, and sulforaphane have all been shown to inhibit cell proliferation and stimulate apoptosis in a manner analogous to other nondietary HDAC inhibitors.

HDAC inhibition and increased acetylation of histones has been reported in a number of cell lines treated with butyrate.[65] These butyrate-induced alterations in histone marks have been associated with several processes, including cellular differentiation, cell cycle arrest, apoptosis and inhibition of invasion and metastasis. Furthermore, butyrate has been found to alter transcriptional regulation in a manner analogous to other HDAC inhibitors, such as trichostatin A.[66] Similar to trichostatin A, butyrate caused downregulation of c-myc mRNA expression, which may account for its effect on inhibiting cell proliferation.[67] Furthermore, in chromatin immunoprecipitation (ChIP) experiments, an increase in histone H3 and H4 acetylation within the *CDKN1A* promoter, which regulates the p21 protein, was induced by either trichostatin A or butyrate in Colo-320 and SW116 cells.[68] Because only 2% of genes are thought to be regulated by butyrate, specificity of HDAC inhibition and consequent transcription/gene regulation may be conferred by genes with butyrate response elements in their promoter region.[69] Genome-wide epigenetic analysis should assist in uncovering such specificity.

Diallyl disulfide (DADS) has been shown to induce cell cycle arrest in the G_2/M phase in both HT-29 and Caco-2 human colon cancer cell lines. These antiproliferative effects were associated with increased CDKN1A mRNA and p21 protein levels, as well as increased H4 and/or H3 acetylation within the *CDKN1A* promoter.[70,71] The results suggest that histone hyperacetylation of the promoter region may account for the cell cycle arrest induced by DADS. DADS (200 mg/kg body weight) has also been shown to modify histone acetylation in rat liver and transplanted Morris hepatoma 7777 cells, demonstrating that altered acetylated histone status is achievable in vivo.[72] In a nontumorigenic animal model, DADS (200 mg/kg) treatment increased histone H4 and H3 acetylation in isolated colonocytes.[73] Additional studies are necessary, comparing the effects of garlic constituents on normal and cancer cells, in order to decipher the biological effects. Another organosulfur compound from garlic, *S*-allyl-mercaptocysteine (at low micromolar range) has also been reported to induce growth arrest in various cell lines and increase the levels of acetylated histones H3 and H4 at physiologic concentrations.[74] Much of the work described utilized a very large dose of garlic constituent (i.e., 200 μM) so there is a need to perform dose response experiments to delineate the physiological versus pharmacological effects that may provide indications for either prevention or therapy.

Sulforaphane (SFN) (3 to 15 μM) has been shown to inhibit HDAC activity and concomitantly increase acetylated histones in human embryonic kidney 293 cells, HCT116 human colorectal cancer cells, and various prostate epithelial cells lines (BPH-1, LnCaP, and PC-3).[65] The increased histone acetylation induced by sulforaphane was associated with increased apoptosis and more cells in G_2/M cell cycle arrest than control treated cells.[65] Moreover these effects were associated with increased acetylated histone H4 in the *p21* promoter and increased p21 protein expression.[75] Furthermore, in a ChIP assay, sulforaphane dose-dependently increased the amount of acetylated histone H4 associated with the *p21* promoter.[76] Sulforaphane (443 mg/kg diet) was also found to suppress tumor development in *Apc*[min] mice, and there was an increase in acetylated histones in gastrointestinal polyps, including acetylated histones specifically associated with the promoter region of the *p21* and *bax* genes.[77] Most interesting is the finding that in healthy human subjects ($N = 3$), a single ingestion of 68 g (1 cup) of broccoli sprouts inhibited HDAC activity in circulating peripheral blood mononuclear cells 3 to 6 h after consumption, with concomitant induction of histone H3 and H4 acetylation.[78] The biological consequences of reduced HDAC activity and enhanced histone acetylation in normal as well as in cancer cells require further study. Although SFN has been shown to selectively induce apoptosis in cancer cells but not in normal cells, additional research is warranted to determine beneficial versus deleterious responses to BFCs during vulnerable periods. More recently, another isothiocyanate present in cruciferous vegetables, namely phenethyl isothiocyanate (1 μM), was found to inhibit the level and activity of HDACs in prostate cancer cells and induce selective histone acetylation and methylation for chromatin unfolding.[79] These results demonstrate that isothiocyanates can inhibit HDAC activity in vitro and suggest that this inhibition might contribute to the cancer protective effects of cruciferous vegetables.

With regard to dietary induced histone posttranslational modifications, the majority of the research has examined the effects of dietary HDAC inhibitors as described above. Additional histone posttranslational modifications and their enzymatic partners have been shown to be influenced by dietary factors that have also been implicated in cancer prevention. These include interactions between curcumin and histone acetyltransferases (HATs),[80] methyl-deficient diet and histone methylation,[52] and the nutrient biotin and histone biotinylation.[81] These reports provide evidence for the impact of dietary factors on histone modification and in determining whether the chromatin is in the open (active) or closed (inactive) state. Research efforts should support the continued identification and characterization of triggers of histone modifications and associated effects such as gene silencing or activation. There is also the need to examine specificity of bioactive food factors for particular HDACs and HATs as well as to utilize epigenome approaches to map the numerous histone posttranslational marks in normal and cancer cells following dietary exposure.

9.7   Dietary modulation of polycomb repressive complexes

Histone modifications via Polycomb repressive complex signaling are thought to be important during embryonic stem (ES) cell differentiation.

During differentiation, PcG complex 2 binding, which mediates trimethylation of lysine 27 on histone H3 (K27me3), is lost on developmental genes that are transcriptionally induced. The active vitamin A constituent retinoic acid (RA) is known to be involved in differentiation of ES cells as well as differentiation of various cancer cells in culture. Interestingly, a global decrease in K27me3 was recently observed in as little as 3 days after differentiation of mouse ES cells induced by RA (1 μM) treatment.[82] Global levels of the enzyme that mediates the K27me3 mark (histone K27 methyltransferase EZH2) also decreased with RA treatment. A loss of EZH2 binding and K27me3 was observed locally on PcG complex 2 target genes induced after 3 days of RA, including the gene nestin. In contrast, direct RA-responsive genes that are rapidly induced, such as *Hoxa1*, showed a loss of EZH2 binding and K27me3 after only a few hours of RA treatment. These results suggest that there are likely temporal stages of derepression of Polycomb complex target genes during early differentiation and also emphasize the complexity of the histone code in regulating gene transcription as increased histone acetylation was found to override the K27me3 repressive mark to induce gene transcription in some genes.

After the PcG complex 2 binds and increases the K27me3 mark in a specific region, the second Polycomb repressive complex 1 (PcG complex 1), which contains the protein Bmi-1, binds to the K27me3 in histone H3 and catalyzes the ubiquitinylation of histone H2A. This cooperation between the two PcG complexes leads to silencing of gene expression. PcG complex 1, including *Bmi-1*, appears to remain anchored to the chromatin after these events are completed. *Bmi-1* is overexpressed in some human cancers, including colorectal cancer,[83] and human non-small cell lung cancer.[84] Bmi-1 levels have also been found to be markedly elevated in epidermal squamous cell carcinoma cells.[85]

The impact of EGCG on this chromatin remodeling factor in cultured squamous cell carcinoma cells was recently examined.[86] These investigations were initiated to determine whether Bmi-1 mediates or antagonizes the ability of EGCG to reduce skin cancer cell survival. EGCG (40 μM) was found to suppress Bmi-1 levels and reduce Bmi-1 phosphorylation, resulting in displacement of the Bmi-1 Polycomb protein complex from chromatin and reducing survival of transformed cells. Such studies suggest that dietary agents may reduce cancer cell survival by altering epigenetic control of gene expression. The importance of the Polycomb repressive complexes in the development of cancer is currently an active research endeavor. An important area for future research will be to clarify the role of dietary regulation of PcGs (primarily focusing on cancer stem cells) during cancer prevention as well as cancer progression and during other periods of vulnerability.

9.8   Epigenome mapping to identify targets of dietary exposure

It has become increasingly clear that individual epigenetic modifications may not be critical targets or markers of a process. The genomes of higher eukaryotes are known to contain numerous epigenetic modifications and thus a more detailed look on a large scale may provide clues about which modifications are critical for a particular process. An epigenome can be described as the epigenomic profile of a specific cell or tissue type which reflects its biological condition or state (e.g., normal or diseased, perturbed in response to environmental exposure) and defines its transcriptional potential. Thus, characterizing an epigenome could provide clues about how epigenetic processes may regulate cellular function. The epigenome does not exist in the same way as the genome of a species or an individual may exist. Rather, many epigenomes or epigenomic profiles exist and can be cell or tissue specific. Each epigenomic profile directs a specific gene expression profile, thereby influencing the phenotype of a cell or tissue. Such profiles are highly dynamic as the cell responds to its environment and biological condition. There are several efforts under way to characterize epigenomic profiles, including the Human Epigenome Project.[87] One research group, in order to understand the dynamics of methylation reprogramming during development on a large scale, has taken a comprehensive genomewide analysis of promoter methylation in the mouse genome, comparing pluripotent and multipotent cell types (ES, embryonic germ, and trophoblast stem cells) with germ cells (sperm), and differentiated cells (primary embryonic fibroblasts).[88] This genomewide methylation study showed for the first time that epigenetic reprogramming is crucial for maintaining the pluripotency of germ and embryonic stem cells.

To further encourage epigenomic research, the National Institutes of Health (NIH) has recently developed an NIH Roadmap Epigenomics Program (http://nihroadmap.nih.gov/epigenomics/index.asp) consisting of several areas of research support. The NIH interest in epigenomics is based on the hypothesis that the origins of health and susceptibility to disease are, in part, the result of epigenetic regulation of the genetic blueprint. For example, epigenetic mechanisms that control stem cell differentiation and organogenesis contribute to the biological response to endogenous and exogenous forms of *stimuli* that result in disease. Furthermore, the time is likely ripe to identify the chemical changes and relationships between chromatin constituents that provide functional control to the genetic code because the technology is at hand to begin defining human epigenomes (genewide epigenetic marks) at high resolution.[89] The NIH Roadmap Epigenomics Program includes the following initiative topics: centers to map reference epigenomes as well as to coordinate the data for public use, technology development for epigenetics research, discovery of novel epigenetic marks in mammalian cells, and characterization of epigenomic maps in human health and disease. The goals of the reference epigenome mapping centers are to develop reference epigenomes of government-approved human embryonic stem cells, differentiating cells, and selected differentiated cell lines and human primary cells that are relevant to complex human disease. The ultimate objective is to utilize the reference epigenomes as a resource for the scientific community to identify potential therapeutic targets, pursue therapeutic opportunities in stem cell-based and tissue regeneration strategies, enhance understanding of disease mechanisms, provide additional insights to genetic susceptibility of disease, gather new information regarding environmental interactions, including diet, with disease, and collect information about normal differentiation, development, and aging/senescence. Among the topics that might be supported by the epigenomic maps in human health and disease initiative is an epigenomewide analysis in primary cancer cells/tissues before and after a dietary exposure that contributes to increased cancer risk or cancer prevention. Thus, the reference epigenomes and other epigenomic research endeavors will provide new opportunities in the near future for nutrition science. The ability to characterize reference epigenomes (be it profiles of DNA methylation or histone modifications) will greatly impact the ability to determine, on a global level, how diet impacts differential epigenetic effects on normal versus diseased tissue, elucidate epigenetic changes resulting from dietary exposures during critical periods of prenatal and postnatal development, adolescence, and senescence, as well as investigate the potential impact of diet on transgenerational transmission of epigenetic changes.

9.9   Conclusions

Diet and bioactive food factors may alter the cellular milieu by modulating several cellular processes that participate in cancer risk and prevention, including DNA repair, hormonal regulation, differentiation, inflammation, apoptosis, cell cycle control/proliferation, carcinogen metabolism, and angiogenesis, among others. Additionally, the genes involved in these processes may be regulated and influenced by epigenetic processes. Recent evidence suggests that dietary components—as diverse as folate, retinoids, and sulforaphane—exert cancer protective effects through modulation of epigenetic mechanisms, such as DNA methylation, histone posttranslational modifications, microRNA, and Polycomb repressive complexes.

   In the near future, epigenomic approaches are likely to assist in characterizing genomewide epigenetic marks that are targets for dietary regulation. Emerging research also suggests that the relationship between genetics and epigenetics may provide additional insights about transcriptional regulation in cancer risk and prevention. Just how dietary factors impact these interactions will likely need to be unraveled. Moreover, the identification and characterization of novel epigenetic marks and mechanisms with the capacity to influence gene expression and function are likely to surface over the next few years. Understanding how diet and dietary factors influence these mechanisms will provide additional research opportunities.

Although the cancer epigenetic field has grown exponentially in the last decade, much remains to be discovered, especially with respect to potential modification by bioactive dietary components. Issues remain about the quantity of dietary components needed to bring about a biological effect, the timing of exposure, and other variables that can influence the response. Importantly, for the future of nutrigenomics and personalized nutrition, epigenetic marks and features may be useful as biomarkers of cancer prevention, early disease, or nutritional status, as well as serve as potential molecular targets that are modulated by dietary interventions.

References

1. Wiseman, M. (2008). The Second World Cancer Research Fund/American Institute for Cancer Research Expert Report. Food, nutrition, physical activity, and the prevention of cancer: A global perspective. *Proc Nutr Soc* 67, 253–256.
2. Ross, S.A. (2003). Diet and DNA methylation interactions in cancer prevention. *Ann NY Acad Sci* 983,197–207.
3. Esteller, M. (2005). Aberrant DNA methylation as a cancer-inducing mechanism. *Annu Rev Pharmacol Toxicol* 45, 629–656.
4. Esteller, M. (2007). Cancer epigenomics: DNA methylomes and histone-modification maps. *Nat Rev Genet* 8, 286–298.
5. Li, E. (2002). Chromatin modification and epigenetic reprogramming in mammalian development. *Nat Rev Gene* **3**, 662–673.
6. Belinsky, S.A. (2005). Silencing of genes by promoter hypermethylation: Key event in rodent and human lung cancer. *Carcinogenesis* 26, 1481–1487.
7. Ehrlich, M. (2002). DNA methylation in cancer: too much, but also too little. *Oncogene* 21, 5400–5413.
8. Kautiainen, T.L., and Jones, P.A. (1986). DNA methyltransferase levels in tumorigenic and nontumorigenic cells in culture. *J Biol Chem* 261, 1594–1598.
9. Wolffe, A.P. (1994). Inheritance of chromatin states. *Dev Genet* 15: 463–470.
10. Garcia-Manero, G., and Issa, J.P. (2005). Histone deacetylase inhibitors: A review of their clinical status as antineoplastic agents. *Cancer Invest* 23, 635–642.
11. Fraga, M.F., Ballestar, E., Villar-Garea, A., Boix-Chornet M., Espada, J., Schotta, G., et al. (2005). Loss of acetylation at Lys16 and trimethylation at Lys20 of histone H4 is a common hallmark of human cancer. *Nat Genet* 37, 391–400.
12. Rosato, R.R., and Grant, S. (2003). Histone deacetylase inhibitors in cancer therapy. *Cancer Biol Ther* 2, 30–37.
13. Gibbons, R.J. (2005). Histone modifying and chromatin remodeling enzymes in cancer and dysplastic syndromes. *Hum Mol Genet* 14, R85–R92.

14. Fabbri, M., Croce, C.M., and Calin, G.A . (2008). MicroRNAs. *Cancer J* 14, 1–6.
15. Hawkins, P.G., and Morris, K.V. (2008). RNA and transcriptional modulation of gene expression. *Cell Cycle* 7, 602–607.
16. Sparmann, A., and van Lohuizen, M. (2006). Polycomb silencers control cell fate, development and cancer. *Nature Reviews Cancer* 6, 846–856.
17. Takihara, Y. (2008). Role of Polycomb-group genes in sustaining activities of normal and malignant stem cells. *Int J Hematol* 87, 25–34.
18. Medina, P.P., and Cespedes, M.S. (2008). Involvement of the chromatin-remodeling factor BRG1/SMARCA4 in human cancer. *Epigenetics* 3, 64–68.
19. Wolff, G.L., Kodell, R.L., Moore, S.R., and Cooney, C.A. (1998). Maternal epigenetics and methyl supplements affect agouti gene expression in Avy/a mice. *FASEB J* 12, 949–957.
20. Waterland, R.A., and Jirtle, R.L. (2003). Transposable elements: Targets for early nutritional effects on epigenetic gene regulation. *Mol Cell Biol* 23, 5293–5300.
21. Cropley, J.E., Suter, C.M., Beckman, K.B., and Martin, D.I. (2006). Germ-line epigenetic modification of the murine A vy allele by nutritional supplementation. *Proc Natl Acad Sci USA* 103, 17308–17312.
22. Dolinoy, D.C., Weidman, J.R., Waterland, R.A., and Jirtle, R.L. (2006). Maternal genistein alters coat color and protects A^{vy} mouse offspring from obesity by modifying the fetal epigenome. *Environ Health Perspect* 114, 567–572.
23. Waterland, R.A., Dolinoy, D.C., Lin, J.R., Smith, C.A., Shi, X., and Tahiliani, K.G. (2006). Maternal methyl supplements increase offspring DNA methylation at *Axin fuse*. *Genesis* 44, 401–406.
24. Waterland, R.A., Lin, J.R., Smith, C.A, and Jirtle, R.L. (2006). Post-weaning diet affects genomic imprinting at the insulin-like growth factor 2 (*IGF2*) locus. *Hum Mol Genet* 15, 705–716.
25. Li, S., Hansman, R., Newbold, R., Davis, B., McLachlan, J.A., and Barrett, J.C. (2003). Neonatal diethylstilbestrol exposure induces persistent elevation of *c-fos* expression and hypomethylation in its exon-4 in mouse uterus. *Mol Carcinog* 38, 78–84.
26. Ho, S.M., Tang, W.Y., Belmonte de Frausto, J., and Prins, G.S. (2006). Developmental exposure to estradiol and bisphenol A increases susceptibility to prostate carcinogenesis and epigenetically regulates phosphodiesterase type 4 variant 4. *Cancer Res* 66, 5624–5632.
27. Anway, M.D., and Skinner, M.K. (2006). Epigenetic transgenerational actions of endocrine disruptors. *Endocrinology* 147, S43–S49.
28. Weaver, I.C., Cervoni, N., Champagne, F.A., D'Alessio, A.C., Sharma, S., Seckl, J.R., Dymove, S., Szyf, M., and Meaney, M.J. (2004). Epigenetic programming by maternal behavior. *Nature Neurosci* 7, 847–854.
29. Weaver, I.C., Champagne, F.A., Brown, S.E., Dymov, S., Sharma, S., Meaney, M.J., and Szyf, M. (2005). Reversal of maternal programming of stress responses in adult offspring through methyl supplementation: Altering epigenetic marking later in life. *J Neurosci* 25, 11045–11054.
30. Niemitz, E.L., and Feinberg, A.P. (2004). Epigenetics and assisted reproductive technology: A call for investigation. *Am J Hum Genet* 74, 599–609.
31. Rossignol, S., Steunou, V., Chalas, C., Kerjean, A., Rigolet, M., Viegas-Pequignot, E., Jouannet, P., Le Bouc, Y., and Gicquel, C. (2006). The epigenetic imprinting defect of patients with Beckwith–Wiedemann syndrome born after assisted reproductive technology is not restricted to the 11p15 region. *J Med Genet* 43, 902–907.

32. Koturbash, I., Baker, M., Loree, J., Kutanzi, K., Hudson, D., Pogribny, I., Sedelnikova, O., Bonner, W., and Kovalchuk, O. (2006). Epigenetic dysregulation underlies radiation-induced transgenerational genome instability in vivo. *Int J Radiat Oncol Biol Phys* 66, 327–330.

33. Morgan, H.D., Sutherland, H.G., Martin, D.I., and Whitelaw, E. (1999). Epigenetic inheritance at the agouti locus in the mouse. *Nature Genet* 23, 314–318.

34. Lane, N., Dean, W., Erhardt, S., Hajkova, P., Surani, A., Walter, J., and Reik, W. (2003). Resistance of IAPs to methylation reprogramming may provide a mechanism for epigenetic inheritance in the mouse. *Genesis* 35, 88–93.

35. Rakyan, V.K., Chong, S., Champ, M.E., Cuthbert, P.C., Morgan, H.D., Luu, K.V., and Whitelaw, E. (2003). Transgenerational inheritance of epigenetic states at the murine *Axin(Fu)* allele occurs after maternal and paternal transmission. *Proc Natl Acad Sci USA* 100, 2538–2543.

36. Anway, M.D., Cupp, A.S., Uzumcu, M., and Skinner, M.K. (2005). Epigenetic transgenerational actions of endocrine disruptors and male fertility. *Science* 308, 1466–1469.

37. Pembrey, M.E., Bygren, L.O., Kaati, G., Edvinsson, S., Northstone, K., Sjöström, M., and ALSPAC Study Team. (2006). Sex-specific, male-line transgenerational responses in humans. *Eur J Hum Genet* 14, 159–166.

38. Cooney, C.A., Dave, A.A., and Wolff, G.L. (2002). Maternal methyl supplements in mice affect epigenetic variation and DNA methylation of offspring. *J Nutr* 132, 2393S–2400S.

39. Duhl, D.M., Vrieling, H., Miller, K.A., Wolff, G.L., and Barsh, G.S. (1994). Neomorphic agouti mutations in obese yellow mice. *Nat Genet* 8, 59–65.

40. Dolinoy, D.C., Huang, D., and Jirtle, R.L. (2007). Maternal nutrient supplementation counteracts bisphenol A-induced DNA hypomethylation in early development. *Proc Natl Acad Sci USA* 104, 13056–13061.

41. Rakyan, V.K., Blewitt, M.E., Druker, R., Preis, J.I., and Whitelaw, E. (2002). Metastable epialleles in mammals. *Trends Genet* 18, 348–351.

42. Whitelaw, E., and Martin, D.I. (2001). Retrotransposons as epigenetic mediators of phenotypic variation in mammals. *Nat Genet* 27, 361–365.

43. Pogribny, I.P., Tryndyak, V.P., Muskhelishvili, L., Rusyn, I., and Ross, S.A. (2007). Methyl deficiency, alterations in global histone modifications, and carcinogenesis. *J Nutr* 137, 216S–222S.

44. Newberne, P.M. (1986). Lipotropic factors and oncogenesis. *Adv Exp Med Biol* 206, 223–251.

45. Poirier, L.A. (1994). Methyl group deficiency in hepatocarcinogenesis. *Drug Metab Rev* 26, 185–199.

46. Denda, A., Kitayama, W., Kishida, H., Murata, N., Tsutsumi, M., Tsujiuchi, T., Nakae, D., and Konishi, Y. (2002). Development of hepatocellular adenomas and carcinomas associated with fibrosis in C57BL/6J male mice given a choline-deficient, L-amino acid-defined diet. *Jpn J Cancer Res* 93, 125–132.

47. Christman, J.K. (2003). Diet, DNA methylation and cancer. In *Molecular Nutrition*, ed. H. Daniel, and J. Zempleni, 237–265. Oxon, UK: CABI Publishing.

48. Wainfan, E., and Poirier, L.A. (1992). Methyl groups in carcinogenesis: Effects on DNA methylation and gene expression. *Cancer Res* 52, 2071S–2077S.

49. Christman, J.K., Sheikhnejad, G., Dizik, M., Abileah, S., and Wainfan, E. (1993). Reversibility of changes in nucleic acid methylation and gene expression in rat liver by severe dietary methyl deficiency. *Carcinogenesis* 14, 551–557.

50. Pogribny, I.P., James, S.J., Jernigan, S., and Pogribna, M. (2004). Genomic hypomethylation is specific for preneoplastic liver in folate/methyl deficient rats and does not occur in non-target tissues. *Mutat. Res* 548, 53–59.

51. Pogribny, I.P., Ross, S.A., Wise, C., Pogribna, M., Jones, E.A., Tryndyak, V.P., James, S.J., Dragan, Y.P., and Poirier, L.A. (2006). Irreversible global DNA hypomethylation as a key step in hepatocarcinogenesis induced by dietary methyl deficiency. *Mutat Res* 593, 80–87.

52. Pogribny, I.P., Ross, S.A., Tryndyak, V.P., Pogribna, M., Poirier, L.A, and Karpinets, T.V. (2006). Histone H3 lysine 9 and H4 lysine 20 trimethylation and the expression of Suv-20h2 and Suv-39h1 histone methyltransferases in hepatocarcinogenesis induced by methyl deficiency in rats. *Carcinogenesis* 27, 1180–1186.

53. Ghoshal, K., Li, X., Datta, J., Bai, S., Pogribny, I., Pogribny, M., Huang, Y., Young, D., and Jacob, S.T. (2006). A folate- and methyl-deficient diet alters the expression of DNA methyltransferases and methyl CpG binding proteins involved in epigenetic gene silencing in livers of F344 rats. *J Nutr* 136, 1522–1527.

54. Kutay, H., Bai, S., Datta, J., Motiwala, T., Pogribny, I., Frankel, W., Jacob, S.T., and Ghoshal, K. (2006). Downregulation of miR-122 in the rodent and human hepatocellular carcinomas. *J Cell Biochem* 99, 671–678.

55. Powell, C.L., Kosyk, O., Bradford, B.U., Parker, J.S., Lobenhofer, E.K., Denda, A., Uematsu, F., Nakae, D., and Rusyn, I. (2005). Temporal correlation of pathology and DNA damage with gene expression in a choline-deficient model of rat liver injury. *Hepatology* 42, 1137–1147.

56. Fang, M., Chen, D., and Yang, C.S. (2007). Dietary polyphenols may affect DNA methylation. *J Nutr* 137, 223S–228S.

57. Fang, M.Z., Wang, Y., Ai, N., Hou, Z., Sun, Y., Lu, H., Welsh, W., and Yang, C.S. (2003). Tea polyphenol (-)-epigallocatechin-3-gallate inhibits DNA methyltransferase and reactivates methylation-silenced genes in cancer cell lines. *Cancer Res* 63, 7563–7570.

58. Fang, M.Z., Chen, D., Sun, Y., Jin, Z., Christman, J.K., and Yang, C.S. (2005). Reversal of hypermethylation and reactivation of p16INK4a, RARbeta, and MGMT genes by genistein and other isoflavones from soy. *Clin Cancer Res* 11, 7033–7041.

59. Berletch, J.B., Liu, C., Love, W.K., Andrews, L.G., Katiyar, S.K., and Tollefsbol, T.O. (2008). Epigenetic and genetic mechanisms contribute to telomerase inhibition by EGCG. *J Cell Biochem* 103, 509–519.

60. Lee, W.J., Shim, J.Y., and Zhu, B.T. (2005). Mechanisms for the inhibition of DNA methyltransferases by tea catechins and bioflavonoids. *Mol Pharmacol* 68, 1018–1030.

61. Stresemann, C., Brueckner, B., Musch, T., Stopper, H., and Lyko, F. (2006). Functional diversity of DNA methyltransferase inhibitors in human cancer cell lines. *Cancer Res* 66, 2794–2800.

62. Majid, S., Kikuno, N., Nelles, J., Noonan, E., Tanaka, Y., Kawamoto, K., Hirata, H., Li, L.C., Zhao, H., Okino, S.T., Place, R.F., Pookot, D., and Dahiya, R. (2008). Genistein induces the p21WAF1/CIP1 and p16INK4a tumor suppressor genes in prostate cancer cells by epigenetic mechanisms involving active chromatin modification. *Cancer Res* 68, 2736–2744.

63. Kikuno, N., Shiina, H., Urakami, S., Kawamoto, K., Hirata, H., Tanaka, Y., Majid, S., Igawa, M., and Dahiya, R. (2008). Genistein mediated histone acetylation and demethylation activates tumor suppressor genes in prostate cancer cells. *Int J Cancer* 123, 552–560.

64. Garfinkel, M.D., and Ruden, D.M. (2004). Chromatin effects in nutrition, cancer and obesity. *Nutrition* 20, 56–62.

65. Myzak, M.C., and Dashwood, R.H. (2006). Histone deacetylases as targets for dietary cancer preventive agents: Lessons learned with butyrate, diallyl disulfide and sulforaphane. *Current Drug Targets* 7, 443–452.

66. Mariadason, J.M., Corner, G.A., and Augenlicht, L.H. (2000). Genetic reprogramming in pathways of colonic cell maturation induced by short chain fatty acids: Comparison with trichostatin A, sulindac, and curcumin and implications for chemoprevention of colon cancer. *Cancer Res* 60, 4561–4572.

67. Bernhard, D., Ausserlechner, M.J., Tonko, M., Löffler, M., Hartmann, B.L., Csordas, A., and Kofler, R. (1999). Apoptosis induced by the histone deacetylase inhibitor sodium butyrate in human leukemic lymphoblasts. *FASEB J* 13, 1991–2001.

68. Fang, Y.J., Chen, Y.X., Lu, J., Lu, R., Yang, L., Zhu, H.Y., Gu, W.Q., and Lu, L.G. (2004). Epigenetic modification regulates both expression of tumor-associated genes and cell cycle progressing in human colon cancer cell lines: Colo-320 and SW1116. *Cell Res* 14, 217–226.

69. Davie, J.R. (2003). Inhibition of histone deacetylase activity by butyrate. *J Nutr* 133, 2485S–2493S.

70. Druesne, N., Pagniez, A., Mayeur, C., Thomas, M., Cherbuy, C., Dhée, P.H., Martel, P., and Chaumontet, C. (2004). Diallyl disulfide (DADS) increases histone acetylation and p21$^{waf1/cip1}$ expression in human colon tumor cell lines. *Carcinogenesis* 25, 1227–1236.

71. Druesne-Pecollo, N., Pagniez, A., Thomas, A., Cherbuy, C., Dhée, P.H., Martel, P., and Chaumontet, C. (2006). Diallyl disulfide increases CDKN1A promoter-associated histone acetylation in human colon tumor cell lines. *J Agric Food Chem* 54, 7503–7507.

72. Lea, M.A., and Randolph, V.M. (2001). Induction of histone acetylation in rat liver and hepatoma by organosulfur compounds including diallyl disulfide. *Anticancer Res* 21, 2841–2846.

73. Druesne-Pecollo, N., Chaumontet, C., Pagniez, A., Vaugelade, P., Bruneau, A., Thomas, M., Cherbuy, C., Dhée, P.H., and Martel, P. (2007). In vivo treatment by diallyl disulfide increases histone acetylation in rat colonocytes. *Biochem Biophys Res Commun* 354, 140–147.

74. Lea, M.A., Rasheed, M., Randolph, V.M., Khan, F., Shareef, A., and desBordes, C. (2002). Induction of histone acetylation and inhibition of growth of mouse erythroleukemia cells by S-allylmercaptocysteine. *Nutr Cancer* 43, 90–102.

75. Myzak, M.C., Karplus, A., Chung, F.-L., and Dashwood, R.H. (2004). A novel mechanism of chemoprotection by sulforaphane: Inhibition of histone deacetylase. *Cancer Res* 64, 5767–5774.

76. Myzak, M.C., Hardin, K., Wang, R., Dashwood, R.H., and Ho, E. (2006). Sulforaphane inhibits histone deacetylase activity in BPH-1, LnCaP and PC-3 prostate epithelial cells. *Carcinogenesis* 27, 811–819.

77. Myzak, M.C., Dashwood, W.M., Orner, G.A., Ho, E., and Dashwood, R.H. (2006). Sulforaphane inhibits histone deacetylase in vivo and suppresses tumorigenesis in *APC*^min mice. *FASEB J* 20, 506–508.

78. Myzak, M.C., Tong, P., Dashwood, W.M., Dashwood, R.H., and Ho, E. (2007). Sulforaphane retards the growth of human PC-3 xenografts and inhibits HDAC activity in human subjects. *Exp Biol Med (Maywood)* 232, 227–234.

79. Wang, L.G., Belkemisheva, A., Liu, X.M., Ferrari, A.C., Feng, J., and Chiao, J.W. (2007). Dual action on promoter demethylation and chromatin by an isothiocyanate restored GSTP1 silenced in prostate cancer. *Molecular Carcinogenesis* 46, 24–31.

80. Kang, J., Chen, J., Shi, Y., Jia, J., and Zhang, Y. (2005). Curcumin-induced histone hypoacetylation: The role of reactive oxygen species. *Biochem Pharmacol* 69, 1205–1213.

81. Hassan, Y.I., and Zempleni, J. (2006). Epigenetic regulation of chromatin structure and gene function by biotin. *J Nutr* 136, 1763–1765.

82. Lee, E.R., Murdoch, F.E., and Fritsch, M.K. (2007). High histone acetylation and decreased polycomb repressive complex 2 member levels regulate gene specific transcriptional changes during early embryonic stem cell differentiation induced by retinoic acid. *Stem Cells* 25, 2191–2199.

83. Kim, J.H., Yoon, S.Y., Kim, C.N., Joo, J.H., Moon, S.K., Choe, I.S., Choe, Y.K., and Kim, J.W. (2004). The Bmi-1 oncoprotein is overexpressed in human colorectal cancer and correlates with the reduced p16INK4a/p14ARF proteins. *Cancer Lett* 203, 217–224.

84. Vonlanthen, S., Heighway, J., Altermatt, H.J., Gugger, M., Kappeler, A., Borner, M.M., van Lohuizen, M., and Betticher, D.C. (2001). The bmi-1 oncoprotein is differentially expressed in non-small cell lung cancer and correlates with INK4A-ARF locus expression. *Br J Cancer* 84, 1372–1376.

85. Lee, K., Adhikary, G., Balasubramanian, S., Gopalakrishna, R., McCormick, T., Dimri, G.P., Eckert, R.L., and Rorke, E.A. (2008). Expression of Bmi-1 in epidermis enhances cell survival by altering cell cycle regulatory protein expression and inhibiting apoptosis. *J Invest Dermatol* 128, 9–17.

86. Balasubramanian, S., Lee, K., Adhikary, G., Gopalakrishnan, R., Rorke, E.A., and Eckert, R.L. (2008). The Bmi-1 Polycomb group gene in skin cancer: Regulation of function by (-)-epigallocatechin-3-gallate (EGCG). *Nutrition Rev* 66 (Suppl 1), S65–S68.

87. Brena, R.M., Huang, T.H., and Plass, C. (2006). Toward a human epigenome. *Nat Genet* 38, 1359–1360.

88. Farthing, C.R., Ficz, G., Ng, R.K., Chan, C.F., Andrews, S., Dean, W., Hemberger, M., and Reik, W. (2008). Global mapping of DNA methylation in mouse promoters reveals epigenetic reprogramming of pluripotency genes. *PLoS Genet* 4, e1000116.

89. Jones, P.A., and Martienssen, R. (2005). A Blueprint for a Human Epigenome Project: The AACR Human Epigenome Workshop. *Cancer Research* 65, 11241–11246.

chapter ten

Conclusions and future perspectives

Sang-Woon Choi and Simonetta Friso

Although we have a generic understanding of the role of genetics, there is still much to investigate in the post-genomic project era: a series of modifications in DNA and DNA associated structures, which currently falls under the umbrella of epigenetics. These epigenetic modifications are heritable from one generation to the next, like genetic inheritance. However, these modifications affect the genome very differently from genetic inheritance.

The human epigenome projects, global maps of DNA methylation and histone modifications, started to identify and interpret epigenetic patterns of all human genes. It is now emerging that epigenetic patterns are as important as genetic sequences for gene function and subsequently for physiologic and pathologic processes. In fact, epigenetic phenomena are modifiable genomic parameters that can change gene function under exogenous influence, thereby constituting a link between genetics and environment; a concept that is widely thought to play a critical role in the etiology of most human pathologies (refer to Chapter 9). Diet is one of the most important environmental factors to which we are exposed during our lifetime. It is well known that nutrients and bioactive food components found in a typical daily diet can modulate the epigenetic phenomena in our cells, thereby affecting critical gene expression. This is one mechanism by which lifestyle factors affect physiologic and pathologic processes in our body. Thus, we can speculate that a certain nutrient deficiency may induce an abnormality in the epigenetic condition, and a proper nutritional intervention program may reverse disordered epigenetic patterns.

As discussed in this book, epigenetic phenomena are DNA methylation, a chemical modification of the DNA itself, and modifications of histones: proteins closely associated with DNA. Histones are modified posttranslationally by various enzymatic reactions at their flexible N-terminals. These modifications play an important role in modulating chromatin structure. In fact, chromatin is much more than a structure for packaging and condensing genomic DNA with histones. The regulation of chromatin structures through epigenetic mechanisms is critical for the proper control of DNA accessibility that controls transcription, replication, recombination and repair. The effect of chromatin modification by itself is so variable; it could be local or far-reaching, and short lived or life-long lasting. Chromatin remodeling enzymes and histone modifications are also essential for proper DNA methylation patterns and the connections among these epigenetic phenomena are important for the control of chromosome structure and gene expression (refer to Chapters 2, 3 and 4).

It is known that nutrients can affect embryonic development, aging, and aging-associated chronic diseases through epigenetic mechanisms. During the embryonic development, when most of the initial cell differentiation occurs, differentiation patterns of each cell are established by epigenetic mechanisms to define the patterns of gene expression. Maternal diets have a strong effect on their offsprings' embryonic development and the epigenetic patterns influenced by diet can persist during the embryonic development period. Nevertheless, these established epigenetic patterns are not always immutable; aging can change the epigenetic pattern by interacting with life style factors. This age-dependent epigenetic change may result in the reduced function of genes. However, age-associated aberrant methylation does not occur in all cells and the epigenetic pattern is cell specific as well as organ specific. Currently, the links between nutrition, epigenetics and aging are largely unknown and must be regarded as a very intriguing topic for future research (refer to Chapters 7 and 8).

Epigenetic phenomena are highly associated with carcinogenesis. Epigenetic silencing of critical genes precedes genetic changes such as mutation and loss of heterozygosity, and can push cells to the dysplastic condition. Current understanding is that epigenetic phenomena not only initiate carcinogenesis but are also involved in the progression of cancer; mutation, invasion, metastasis and even relapse. Since epigenetic phenomena are reversible, it appears that nutrients or bioactive food components, which can modify epigenetic phenomena, might be useful to limit the carcinogenetic process (refer to Chapters 5 and 9).

Nutrients can modulate epigenetic phenomena by inhibiting enzymes such as DNA methyltransferases and histone deacetylases or by affecting one-carbon metabolism, a biochemical pathway that regulates biological methylation by altering the supply of S-adenosylmethionone, which is the unique methyl donor for epigenetic methylation, or by accumulation of S-adenosylhomocysteine, a known methyltransferase inhibitor. Current evidence is not yet strong enough to consider a clinical therapeutic use of those nutrients but several pharmacologic inhibitors of methyltransferases or histone deacetylases are already approved by the U.S. Food and Drug Administration and many other epigenetic drugs are now under evaluation at various stages of clinical trials. This suggests that, in the future, nutritional agents that have proven effects on epigenetic phenomena

similar to those of known drugs can be comfortably used in clinical prac-
tice, since nutrients are a more physiologic approach and have fewer side
effects compared to potent drugs that directly inhibit epigenetic phenomena. Thus, nutrients may be used in the future to prevent cancer, to delay
the onset of cancer or as an ancillary modality for the use of pharmacologic agents (refer to Chapters 5, 6 and 9).

In the diet there are many different types of nutrients. Whether we
need them by the gram (macronutrients) or by the microgram (micronutrients) order of measurement, all these nutrients are certainly essential
for maintaining our life. In our food there are, however, also many other
different types of bioactive components. They are not considered essential
components, yet they are required to maintain health. It is known that both
nutrients and bioactive food components can modulate epigenetic phenomena but so far the function of only a few have been tested. Since such food
elements interact with genes and other lifestyle factors, it is very difficult
to determine the precise effects of nutrients or bioactive food components
on each epigenetic phenomenon, as well as their possible effect on physiologic and pathologic processes in our body. It is therefore strongly recom-
mended that researchers continue to pursue this fascinating field to unveil
more nutrients or functional components that may be potentially useful.
A deeper understanding in this field will serve to protect our health with
nutritional modulation that is certainly more physiologic than the use of
pharmacological agents (refer to Chapters 6, 8 and 9).

In conclusion, during our life, nutrients can modify our physiologic
and pathologic processes through epigenetic phenomena. Modulation of
those processes through diet or specific nutrients may maintain biological
homeostasis and health. There is a growing list of nutrients and bioactive food components that have shown effects on epigenetic phenomena
(refer to Chapters 5 and 6). Exploring this area of research may open up
a greater understanding of the role of diet in altering epigenetic patterns
and guide research to develop new strategies for disease prevention.

Index

T - #0407 - 071024 - C8 - 234/156/12 - PB - 9780367385644 - Gloss Lamination